More on Mediterranean Diets

World Review of Nutrition and Dietetics

Vol. 97

Series Editor

Artemis P. Simopoulos
The Center for Genetics, Nutrition and Health, Washington, D.C., USA

Advisory Board

Regina C. Casper USA
Cuiqing Chang China
Claudio Galli Italy
Uri Goldbourt Israel
C. Gopalan India
Tomohito Hamazaki Japan
Michel de Lorgeril France

Leonard Storlien Sweden
Ricardo Uauy-Dagach Chile
Antonio Velázquez Mexico
Mark L. Wahlqvist Australia
Paul Walter Switzerland
Bruce A. Watkins USA

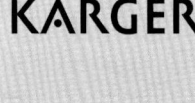

More on Mediterranean Diets

Volume Editors

Artemis P. Simopoulos
The Center for Genetics, Nutrition and Health, Washington, D.C., USA

Francesco Visioli
Institute of Pharmacological Sciences, University of Milan, Milan, Italy

36 figures, and 27 tables, 2007

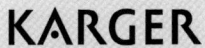

Basel · Freiburg · Paris · London · New York ·
Bangalore · Bangkok · Singapore · Tokyo · Sydney

Artemis P. Simopoulos
The Center for Genetics,
Nutrition and Health
Washington, D.C. (USA)

Francesco Visioli
Institute of Pharmacological Sciences
University of Milan
Milan (Italy)

Library of Congress Cataloging-in-Publication Data

More on Mediterranean diets / volume editors, Artemis P. Simopoulos, Francesco Visioli.
    p. ; cm. – (World review of nutrition and dietetics, ISSN 0084-2230 ; v. 97)
  Includes bibliographical references and index.
  ISBN-13: 978-3-8055-8219-3 (hard cover : alk. paper)
  ISBN-10: 3-8055-8219-6 (hard cover : alk. paper)
  1. Nutrition. 2. Diet–Mediterranean Region. I. Simopoulos, Artemis P., 1933- II. Visioli, F. (Francesco) III. Series.
  [DNLM: 1. Diet, Mediterranean–Mediterranean Region. 2. Diet Therapy–Mediterranean Region. W1 WO898 v.97 2007 / QT 235 M835 2007]
  QP141.M77 2007
  613.209182'2–dc22

                                                                    2006036381

Bibliographic Indices. This publication is listed in bibliographic services, including Current Contents® and Index Medicus.

Disclaimer. The statements, options and data contained in this publication are solely those of the individual authors and contributors and not of the publisher and the editor(s). The appearance of advertisements in the book is not a warranty, endorsement, or approval of the products or services advertised or of their effectiveness, quality or safety. The publisher and the editor(s) disclaim responsibility for any injury to persons or property resulting from any ideas, methods, instructions or products referred to in the content or advertisements.

Drug Dosage. The authors and the publisher have exerted every effort to ensure that drug selection and dosage set forth in this text are in accord with current recommendations and practice at the time of publication. However, in view of ongoing research, changes in government regulations, and the constant flow of information relating to drug therapy and drug reactions, the reader is urged to check the package insert for each drug for any change in indications and dosage and for added warnings and precautions. This is particularly important when the recommended agent is a new and/or infrequently employed drug.

All rights reserved. No part of this publication may be translated into other languages, reproduced or utilized in any form or by any means electronic or mechanical, including photocopying, recording, microcopying, or by any information storage and retrieval system, without permission in writing from the publisher.

© Copyright 2007 by S. Karger AG, P.O. Box, CH–4009 Basel (Switzerland)
www.karger.com
Printed in Switzerland on acid-free paper by Reinhardt Druck, Basel
ISSN 0084–2230
ISBN-10: 3–8055–8219–6
ISBN-13: 978–3–8055–8219–3

Contents

XI Preface

1 Modified Cretan Mediterranean Diet in the Prevention of Coronary Heart Disease and Cancer: An Update
de Lorgeril, M.; Salen, P. (Grenoble)

2 Recent Epidemiological Studies about Mediterranean Diets and Coronary Heart Disease
3 Summary of the Lyon Diet Heart Study Results
4 The Experimental Diet Tested in the Lyon Trial
8 Coronary Heart Disease Is an Inflammatory Disease
9 Role of Inflammation and Oxidation in Plaque Rupture and Progression of Coronary Heart Disease
10 Lipids and Inflammation in Coronary Heart Disease
11 Fatty Acids and the Experimental Modified Cretan Diet
12 Omega-3 Fatty Acids in the Med Diets and in Coronary Heart Disease
15 Folate, Homocysteine, Nitric Oxide Pathway, Coronary Heart Disease and the Med Diets
16 Selenium and the Protective Effect of the Med Diets against Cancers
18 Metabolic Syndromes and Mediterranean Diets
19 Polyphenols in Med Diets
23 Conclusions
24 References

33 Endothelial Nitric Oxide Synthase as a Mediator of the Positive Health Effects of Mediterranean Diets and Wine against Metabolic Syndrome
Leighton, F.; Urquiaga, I. (Santiago)

33 Plasma Lipid Metabolism
35 Hemostatic Mechanisms
37 Endothelial Function
38 Antioxidant Defense Mechanisms
39 Metabolic Syndrome and Its Relationship with Mediterranean Diets and Alcohol Consumption
41 Pathogenesis of the Metabolic Syndrome: A Central Role for Endothelial Nitric Oxide Synthase
42 Potential Role of Mediterranean Diets, Omega-3 Fatty Acids, Antioxidants and Red Wine, as Endothelial Nitric Oxide Synthase Enhancers, in the Control of the Metabolic Syndrome
44 Acknowledgements
44 References

52 Effects of an Omega-3-Enriched Mediterranean Diet (Modified Diet of Crete) versus a Swedish Diet
Friberg, P.; Johansson, M. (Göteborg)

52 Components of a Mediterranean Diet
53 Epidemiology and Mediterranean Diets
54 Type of Diet and Unsaturated Fatty Acids and Blood Components/Inflammation
58 Mediterranean Diet and Blood Vessels
60 Mediterranean Diet and Unsaturated Fatty Acids and Their Importance for Metabolic and Blood Pressure Control
61 Mediterranean Diet, Unsaturated Fatty Acids and Overweight/Obesity
62 Mediterranean Diet and Heart Rate
63 Conclusions
63 Acknowledgements
63 References

67 Dietary Fat Intake of European Countries in the Mediterranean Area: An Update
Marangoni, F.; Martiello, A.; Galli, C. (Milan)

69 Fats in the Mediterranean Diet
70 Vegetable Fats
70   Visible
72 Food Consumption as Sources of Invisible Fats
72   Consumption of Plant Foods
73   Consumption of Animal Foods
74   Composition of Selected Foods (Fatty Acid Profile and Content): Animal and Vegetable

78	Relevant Fatty Acids in the Mediterranean Diets (Content and Health Properties): Oleic Acid and Omega-3
79	New Findings about Omega-9 MUFA
81	ALA Content in Mediterranean Foods
82	Menus for Optimal Intakes of ALA
82	Conclusions
83	References

85 The Mediterranean Diet in Italy: An Update
Rubba, P. (Naples); Mancini, F.P. (Naples/Benevento); Gentile, M.; Mancini, M. (Naples)

88	Dietary Scores
90	Macronutrients and Coronary Heart Disease
94	Nutrition, Hypertension and Stroke in Italy
95	Vitamins
97	Mediterranean Diet and Obesity
98	Mediterranean Diet and Cancer in Italy
104	Mediterranean Diet in the Elderly
106	Conclusions
107	Acknowledgement
107	References

114 A Mediterranean Diet Is Not Enough for Health: Physical Fitness Is an Important Additional Contributor to Health for the Adults of Tomorrow
Castillo-Garzón, M.J.; Ruiz, J.R.; Ortega, F.B.; Gutierrez-Sainz, A. (Granada)

114	Is It Only Diet?
115	The Spanish-Mediterranean Life-Style (and Diet)
116	Diet and Physical Activity Interaction
118	Physical Activity, Physical Exercise and Physical Fitness
119	Physical Fitness as a Health Determinant
120	Physical Fitness and Cardiovascular Risk Factors in Mediterranean Adolescents
120	Cardiorespiratory Fitness and Traditional Cardiovascular Risk Factors
121	Cardiorespiratory Fitness and Emerging Cardiovascular Risk Factors
127	Muscle Strength and Cardiovascular Risk Factors
129	Body Composition and Cardiovascular Risk Factors in Mediterranean Adolescence
129	Physical Activity, Fitness and Total Body Fat
129	Total Body Fat in Young Populations
130	Associations of Total Body Fat with Physical Activity and Fitness
130	Physical Activity, Fitness and Body Fat Distribution
130	Body Fat Distribution in Young Populations
132	Associations of Body Fat Distribution with Physical Activity and Fitness
134	Conclusion
134	Acknowledgements
134	References

139 Mediterranean Diet in the Maghreb: An Update
Zeghichi-Hamri, S. (La Tronche); Kallithraka, S. (Athens)

- 140 Recent Dietary Trends in Algeria, Libya, Morocco and Tunisia
- 144 Time Trends
- 146 Fruits and Vegetables
- 147   Nutritional Aspects
- 149 Animal Products
- 151 Animal Fats and Vegetable Oils
- 153   Nutritional Aspects
- 155 The Maghreb Diet and Cancer
- 158 Conclusion
- 158 References

162 Antioxidants in the Mediterranean Diets: An Update
Bogani, P.; Visioli, F. (Milan)

- 162 Oxidation Processes and Human Pathology
- 163 Cancer
- 164 Mediterranean Antioxidants: Selected Examples
- 165 Is Lycopene the 'Active Ingredient' of Tomato?
- 166 Olive Oil and Red Wine: Do We Have Solid Human Evidence?
- 166   Olive oil
- 169   Wine
- 170 Phenolic Antioxidants: Wild Plants and Endothelial Function
- 170 Conclusions
- 171 Acknowledgements
- 171 References

180 Olive Oil
Boskou, D. (Thessaloniki)

- 181 Olive Oil Composition
- 181   Fatty Acids and Triacylglycerols
- 182   Partial Glycerides
- 182   Free Fatty Acids
- 182   Minor Constituents
- 182   Hydrocarbons
- 183   Sterols
- 185   Fatty Alcohol, Waxes and Diterpene Alcohols
- 186   Diterpene Alcohols
- 186   Tocopherols
- 187   Volatile and Aroma Compounds
- 187   Other Minor Constituents
- 187   Triterpene Acids
- 187   Phospholipids
- 189   Proteins

189	Polar Phenolic Compounds
190	Polyphenols and Keepability (Shelf Life)
191	Polyphenols and Sensory Properties
192	Antioxidant Properties
196	Quality and Genuineness
196	Definitions
197	Characteristics of Extra Virgin Olive Oil (EVOO) and Virgin Olive Oil (VOO)
197	Organoleptic Assessment
197	Metals
198	Moisture and Volatile Matter
198	Trans Unsaturated Fatty Acids
198	Saturated Fatty Acids at 2-Position
198	Delta CN 42 Values
199	Erythrodiol and Uvaol
199	Waxes
199	Stigmastadiene
199	Other Properties Used to Evaluate Quality not Included in International Standards
199	Olive Oil Extraction
200	Olive Oil Production and Consumption. Traditional and Modern Use
200	Olive Oil Production
201	Consumption Trends
201	Traditional and Modern Use
202	New Applications
204	Cloudy and Unfiltered Oil
204	Conclusions
205	References

211 Melatonin in Edible Plants (Phytomelatonin): Identification, Concentrations, Bioavailability and Proposed Functions
Reiter, R.J.; Tan, D.; Manchester, L.C. (San Antonio, Tex.);
Simopoulos, A.P. (Washington, D.C.); Maldonado, M.D.; Flores, L.J.;
Terron, M.P. (San Antonio, Tex.)

212	Preparation of Plant Tissues for Melatonin Measurement
215	Melatonin Levels and Proposed Functions in Plant Tissues
222	Evidence of Melatonin Synthesis in Plants
224	Bioavailability of Melatonin from Consumed Plant Material
225	Unresolved Issues
226	Concluding Remarks and Perspectives
227	References

231 Author Index

232 Subject Index

Preface

This is the second volume on Mediterranean diets in the series of *World Review of Nutrition and Dietetics*. The first volume, *Mediterranean Diets*, was published in the year 2000 (vol. 87). Since then, many studies have been published on the beneficial effects of the diets in the Mediterranean region. In addition, studies in which the traditional diet of the country was modified to resemble the traditional diet of Crete (Greece), by increasing the intake of fruits, vegetables, fish, and flax oil, have led to decreases in the omega-6:omega-3 ratio in the plasma and inflammatory biomarkers, indicating that the traditional diet of Greece has anti-inflammatory properties. Investigators have carried out epidemiological and cross-sectional studies using a diet 'score' to define adherence to the Mediterranean diet and its relationship to various chronic diseases. Such studies have shown decreased mortality from cardiovascular disease and cancer, while others have related the Mediterranen diet score to levels of adiponectin. But, the Mediterranean diet score is a crude measurement that does not provide any information on the nutritional composition or nutritional quality of the diet, particularly on fatty acids, types of antioxidants, or other nutrients with antithrombotic, anti-inflammatory and anticarcinogenic properties. Furthermore, it is well known that foods in different climates have different nutritional composition and properties on health. When a dietary score is used, two major requirements have to be achieved in order to obtain an accurate and valid nutritional methodology, namely a precise definition of the composition of the Mediterranean diet, and the validation of the dietary score by means of biomarkers. Therefore, in this volume specific nutrients and their mechanisms of action are discussed and their relationship to health and disease are presented. Because many of the beneficial effects of Mediterranean diets are synergistic with the health effects of physical fitness, a special paper is included on this subject.

In the previous volume, the papers included dietary patterns of different Mediterranean countries and precise descriptions of olive oil and wine, two major constituents of the Mediterranean diets, and for the first time, the concept that there is no such thing as one Mediterranean diet was extensively discussed. In the current volume the emphasis is on the contribution of foods and nutrients in clinical intervention studies and updated information on olive oil as well as new discoveries of nutrients, such as melatonin, which is high in purslane (*Portulaca oleracea*), nuts, cherries, and other foods that are commonly eaten in some of the Mediterranean countries. Melatonin is a potent antioxidant and anticarcinogenic agent.

The volume begins with the paper 'Modified Cretan Mediterranean Diet in the Prevention of Coronary Heart Disease and Cancer: An Update' by Michel de Lorgeril and Patricia Salen. The authors clearly show that a modified diet of Crete, just like the one used in the Lyon Heart Study, i.e. a dietary pattern that combines high intake of natural antioxidants, low intake of saturated fat, but high intake of oleic acid, with low intake of omega-6 fatty acids, and high intake of omega-3 fatty acids, has a high cardioprotective effect. The Lyon Heart Study (which was a randomized single-blind clinical trial) was the first clinical trial to pay particular attention to the omega-6:omega-3 ratio, with the experimental group having a ratio of 4:1 of omega-6:omega-3. The traditional diet of Crete (Greece) has an omega-6:omega-3 ratio of 2:1 to 1:1, similar to the Paleolithic diet. In addition to the importance of omega-3 fatty acids in the secondary prevention of coronary heart disease, the authors discuss the role of folate, homocysteine, and the nitric oxide pathway. The role of selenium in cancer protection is reviewed along with an extensive discussion of polyphenols that are the most abundant dietary antioxidant.

A number of studies have shown a decreased prevalence of the metabolic syndrome in patients following a Mediterranean diet. Drs. Leighton and Urquiaga in their paper 'Endothelial Nitric Oxide Synthase as a Mediator of the Positive Health Effects of Mediterranean Diets and Wine against Metabolic Syndrome' present a critique and focus on the influence of omega-3 fatty acids, antioxidants, and red wine as the important enhancers of endothelial nitric oxide synthase (eNOS) in the prevention of the metabolic syndrome. The authors provide data from their laboratory as well as other laboratories to support their hypothesis that metabolic improvements following consumption of Mediterranean diets, including red wine, are mediated by eNOS. Although many genes are involved, the participation of eNOS is a constant feature. The recent findings that the eNOS knockout mice present a cluster of cardiovascular risk factors comparable to those of the metabolic syndrome, suggest that defects in eNOS function may cause human metabolic syndrome. These mice are hypertensive, insulin resistant, and dyslipidemic. Further support for a pathogenic role of eNOS comes from the finding in humans, that eNOS polymorphisms are associated with insulin resistance and diabetes, hypertension, inflammatory and oxidative stress markers and with albuminuria. The data support the hypothesis that eNOS enhancement should reduce the incidence of metabolic syndrome and its consequences. The authors conclude that the hypothesis is supported by epidemiological and observational studies but needs experimental validation with human intervention studies.

Drs. Friberg and Johansson in their paper 'Effects of an Omega-3 Enriched Mediterranean Diet (Modified Diet of Crete) versus a Swedish Diet' comment on the various components and their function of a modified diet of Crete and describe their own study in normal Swedish volunteers. The purpose of the study was to change from the standard Swedish diet to a Mediterranean-inspired diet rich in fish and flaxseed oil, similar to the modified diet of Crete used in the Lyon Heart Study, and to measure anti-inflammatory biomarkers, and changes of the omega-6:omega-3 ratio in the plasma. This is a very important study because it shows that (1) changing the diet was not a problem; (2) the omega-6:omega-3 plasma ratio decreased, and (3) the inflammatory biomarkers decreased.

The next paper by Drs. Marangoni, Martiello and Galli on 'Dietary Fat Intake of European Countries in the Mediterranean Area: An Update' focuses on the contribution of various components of the diets in European Mediterranean countries to the overall fat consumption versus Northern European countries. The authors discuss the protective effects of oleic acid, omega-3 fatty acids, and especially the land-based omega-3 fatty acid alpha-linolenic acid (ALA), and their interactions, and provide practical recommendations on how to formulate menus, including specific amounts of health-promoting fatty acids.

Although changes have occurred in the diet of both Greece and Italy in comparison to the diets prior to 1960 at the time of the beginning of the Seven Countries Study, and despite the effects of globalization, Greeks continue to eat more fish, fruits and vegetables along with increasing intake of meat and dairy products. Rubba's group provides a review and critique of epidemiologic studies, and diet and health, in various parts of Italy, and the consequences of dietary changes on health. It appears that for the past 10 years there is a return to a much healthier and traditional dietary pattern. The authors discuss micronutrients and coronary heart disease, hypertension and stroke, vitamins, Mediterranean diet and obesity, and Mediterranean diet and cancer in Italy. The authors are puzzled that obesity is so prevalent in the European area where diet is still of the Mediterranean type and ask, 'Could the high consumption of bread, pasta, pizza, olive oil and wine facilitate adiposity?' But, the high fiber content of green vegetables and fresh fruit typical of Mediterranean diets reinforces satiety, a strong anti-obesity effect. Diet alone is not enough to prevent obesity. Physical activity is a very important aspect of health and the prevention of obesity. Epidemiological studies show an increase in sedentary life styles in the Mediterranean region as in other parts of the world, particularly in Western countries.

This point is reinforced in the next paper 'A Mediterranean Diet Is Not Enough for Health: Physical Fitness Is an Important Additional Contributor to Health for the Adults of Tomorrow' by Dr. Castillo-Garzón and co-workers. In addition to diet, a sedentary life-style is another major risk factor for non-communicable diseases. Diet and physical activity interact in the development (or prevention) of coronary heart disease and several other health conditions. Regular physical activity stimulates the functional adaptation of all tissues and organs in the body (e.g. improves fitness and decreases fatness), thereby also making them less vulnerable to lifestyle-related degenerative and chronic diseases. The authors explain that it is not only physical activity. Results obtained from Spanish adolescents and other European and American peers have shown that physical fitness (especially cardiorespiratory fitness and muscle strength) is strongly associated with cardiovascular risk factors. Cardiorespiratory fitness has been shown to be associated with traditional risk factors such as triglycerides, total cholesterol, high and low density lipoprotein cholesterol, glucose, waist circumference, total body fat, but also with emerging risk factors such as C-reactive protein, C3, and homocysteine. Muscle strength has been suggested to be inversely associated with all-cause mortality in adults; however, less is known about the association between muscle strength and risk factors in adolescents. For public health strategies and preventive purposes it is of interest to understand the associations of diet, physical activity and fitness on cardiovascular risk factors from an early age.

A book on the Mediterrranean diets would not be complete without an update on the dietary and health aspects of the North African region called the 'Maghreb'. Drs. Sabrina Zeghichi-Hamri and Stamatina Kallithraka in their paper 'Mediterranean Diet in the Maghreb: An Update' present data on recent dietary trends in Algeria, Libya, Morocco and Tunisia. These four countries do not have a uniform dietary pattern but relatively specific diets. For example, Moroccans have the highest intake of cereals and sweeteners, and the lowest milk, fats and oils among the four Maghreb countries whereas Tunisians consume the highest amount of fish and other seafood and fruit. In general, the diet of the Maghreb is relatively low in total fat and animal products but high in cereals and vegetables. Alcohol and wine – an important aspect of a healthy diet in Greece, Italy, France and Spain – is very low due to religious restrictions. The authors illustrate the differences among the Maghreb countries by calculating the contribution of the various food groups to total energy supply for the period 2000–2003. Their paper clearly illustrates that the 'Mediterranean diet' is not a homogenous nutritional model because there are several Mediterranean dietary patterns as a result of different cultures, traditions, religions and income, resulting in a wide variety of the dietary patterns within the Mediterranean region.

In epidemiological studies, high amounts of fruits and vegetables in the diet are associated with lower levels of coronary heart disease and cancer. Because fruits and vegetables are high in antioxidant vitamins and minerals, polyphenols, etc., intervention studies with vitamin E, vitamin C, and carotenoids were carried out but failed to support the hypothesis. In fact, the opposite was shown. Studies examining total antioxidant capacity revealed a higher level of total antioxidant capacity than those based on the sum of the antioxidant vitamins and minerals. This finding has led to studies looking at the antioxidant effect of other constituents in fruits, vegetables, wine, olive oil, and wild plants. In their paper on 'Antioxidants in the Mediterranean Diets: An Update', Drs. Bogani and Visioli define antioxidants and their relationship to cancer. The authors report on Mediterranean antioxidants and give selective examples, specifically, lycopene and its properties, olive oil and wine, and conclude with a section on phenolic antioxidants, wild plants and endothelial function. In their studies, edible wild plants increase the production of nitric oxide. The authors conclude, '... the answer to the debate on the efficacy of antioxidant supplements is likely to be found in the adoption of a Mediterranean-style diet, in which the abundance of bioactive compounds provided by fruits, vegetables, wine, and olive oil grants a higher protection toward ROS (reactive oxygen species)-induced diseases'.

Dr. Dimitrios Boskou's paper on 'Olive Oil' presents the latest information on olive oil composition, fatty acids and triglycerides, partial glycerides, free fatty acids, and minor constituents, which are divided into two categories (1) fatty acid derivatives, and (2) components with different chemical structures. Special focus is given to squalene sterols, fatty alcohol, waxes, diterpene alcohols, tocopherols, volatile and aroma compounds, and other minor constituents. Triterpene acids and various phospholipids, such as phosphatidlycholine, phosphatidylinositol and phosphatidylserine. A major section is devoted to polar phenolic compounds in terms of shelf life, sensory properties, antioxidant properties, isoprostane formation, and scavenging of radicals and other reactive species. There is a section on olive oil quality. The quest for quality is based on the applications of clearly defined rules during the growing and processing of olives, and retail packing of the oil. Dr. Boskou provides definitions of the various types of olive oil, the characteristics of extra virgin olive oil and virgin olive oil, organoleptic assessment, metals, moisture, and volatile matter. There is a special section on olive oil extraction and the changes that have taken place over the past 30–40 years, the culinary aspects and new applications. The phenolic compounds in olive oil diminish during heating. Therefore, the antioxidant activity of the oil, determined by the ABTS radical decolorization assay or the DPPH radical test, diminishes. It is therefore important to further study the nature of the monoglyceride components of olive oil and to improve methods to quantify and preserve functional ingredients.

Edible wild plants have been one of our areas of investigation in attempting to precisely define the traditional diet of Greece prior to 1960. In the past, we focused our studies on the contribution of omega-3 fatty acids from both animal and plant sources. More recently, we studied the antioxidant content of edible wild plants in terms of vitamins, minerals, glutathione and melatonin. Melatonin is a broad-spectrum direct radical scavenger and indirect antioxidant.

Melatonin, n-acetyl-5-methoxtryptamine, was long thought to be an endogenously generated molecule found exclusively in vertebrates (pineal gland, retina) that synchronizes circadian and circannual rhythms. Lately, melatonin has been found in insects, unicellular organisms, bacteria, and most recently in plants. Because physiologic concentrations of melatonin in the blood are known to correlate with the total antioxidant capacity of the serum, consuming food stuffs containing melatonin may be helpful in lowering oxidative stress.

Melatonin directly detoxifies the hydroxyl radical (*OH), hydrogen peroxide, nitric oxide, peroxynitrite anion, peroxynitrous acid, and hypochlorous acid. The products from each of these reactions have been identified in pure chemical systems, and in at least one case in vivo: The interaction product of melatonin with the *OH, i.e. cyclic 3-hydroxymelatonin is found in the urine of humans and rats. Melatonin increases the efficiency of mitochondrial oxidative phosphorylation and reduces electron leakage (thereby lowering free radical formation). Melatonin reduces the initiation of cancer by limiting oxidative damage to DNA. It also curtails the growth of tumors once they are established by inhibiting the uptake of growth factors, such as omega-6 fatty acids, by cancer cells. Melatonin's effects on cancer inhibition are achieved at physiological concentrations, and phytomelatonin such as that found in purslane has been proven as a potential means of limiting the growth on established tumors.

In the paper by Reiter, Simopoulos and co-workers on 'Melatonin in Edible Plants (Phytomelatonin): Identification, Concentrations, Bioavailability and Proposed Function', the authors indicate that except for the potato tuber, all other plants that have been investigated contain various amounts of melatonin ranging from nanograms to picograms per gram of tissue. The paper contains information on the melatonin levels of some edible plant foods, indicating a wide variation in the concentration of melatonin. Purslane (*Portulaca oleracea*), a commonly eaten wild plant in Greece and other parts of the world, has been shown to have the highest amount of the omega-3 fatty acid ALA. It is not surprising that purslane also has one of the highest amounts of melatonin.

Melatonin, being a potent antioxidant, is needed to stabilize the high amount of ALA found in the purslane. Purslane in the diet further contributes to the antioxidant and anticarcinogenic properties of the Greek diet. At the level of 19 ng/g, it has one of the highest amounts of melatonin among edible plant foods. Here, then is another dietary constituent that adds to the armamentarium of the beneficial constituents of the traditional diet of Greece contributing to health.

The new advances reported in this volume should serve as a strong incentive for the initiation of clinical intervention trials and studies that will test the effects of specific dietary patterns as well as specific nutrients in the prevention and management of chronic diseases.

This volume should be of interest to physicians, cardiologists, cancer specialists, nutritionists, dietitians, agriculturists, food scientists and policy makers in government, private industry and international organizations, as well as the informed public.

Artemis P. Simopoulos, MD

Modified Cretan Mediterranean Diet in the Prevention of Coronary Heart Disease and Cancer: An Update

Michel de Lorgeril, Patricia Salen

Laboratoire Nutrition, Vieillissement et Maladies Cardiovasculaires (NVMCV), Faculté de Médecine, Université Joseph Fourier, Grenoble, France

Prospective studies of the epidemiology of coronary heart disease (CHD) and cancer have shown that mortality from these diseases differs greatly among populations and that at least some of the differences are associated with differences in dietary habits [1, 2]. Mediterranean populations, for instance, are protected from CHD and certain cancers, and the particular composition of the Mediterranean (Med) diet has been put forth to explain this [3–5]. However, epidemiological studies only provide associations between the risk factors and clinical endpoints, not causal relationships. Several confounding factors may play a part in the associations. The economic situation and the presence or absence of extended social support systems have been proposed to explain the low prevalence of CHD in some Mediterranean countries. Although an effect of these factors cannot be totally excluded, data from Albania, where a low CHD rate was associated until recently with economic misery and modest health services, do not agree with this possibility [6, 7].

Randomized trials are the only way to make sure that a given dietary pattern results in a significant cardioprotective and/or anticancer effect.

Some dietary trials in primary or secondary prevention of CHD have reported an impressive reduction of CHD risk, especially in terms of mortality [8–10]. In contrast, other dietary trials specifically aimed at reducing blood cholesterol failed to significantly improve the prognosis of the dieters [11]. The successful trials tested dietary patterns characterized by a low intake of total, saturated and omega-6 polyunsaturated fats [8, 9] and an increased intake of omega-3 fatty acids [8–10, 12]. Their aim, with the exception of one assay [8], was not to primarily reduce blood cholesterol. Two of these trials [8, 9] also included a high intake of fresh fruits and vegetables, legumes and cereals containing large amounts of fiber, antioxidants, minerals, vegetable proteins and vitamins of the B group. The credibility of these trials was considerably reinforced by a number of studies showing major cardioprotective effects of most of these foods and nutrients [13–21], with a particular emphasis on omega-3 fatty acids [10–12, 16, 17] and on folates for their role in hyperhomocysteinemia and in the arginine-nitric oxide-BH4 pathway [17–21].

The Lyon Diet Heart Study was a randomized single-blind secondary prevention trial aimed at testing whether an experimental modified Cretan diet (Exp) may reduce the risk of recurrence after a first myocardial infarction (MI). A significant reduction of the rates of cardiovascular complications was reported [9, 22, 23], and no major bias was detected in the trial [23, 24]. In addition, the trial suggested that patients following the cardioprotective Exp diet may also be protected from cancer [25]. Although further trials are warranted to confirm the cancer data, those obtained from the Lyon trial are in line with several studies [26], in particular prospective studies with heavy emphasis on the role of selenium (of which the various typical Med diets contain large amounts) in the reduction of the incidence of, and mortality from, carcinomas at several sites [27]. Olive oil (both oleic acid and phenolic compounds) and the vegetable components of the Med diet also might be important [28–30], whereas the effects of omega-3 fatty acids from either plant or marine sources are still controversial [31–36].

Recent Epidemiological Studies about Mediterranean Diets and Coronary Heart Disease

Since the publication of Volume 87 of *World Review in Nutrition and Dietetics* about Med Diets in 2000 [37], prospective cohort and case-control studies about Med diets and CHD have been reported. One randomized trial, the 'Indo-Mediterranean diet trial', also reported protective effects but raised concerns about some ethical and scientific aspects [38]. For that reason, and even though the article was not withdrawn by the publisher and the data not retracted by the authors, we prefer to wait some time before further discussing this potentially important report.

Regarding the epidemiological studies, and whatever the country where the studies were conducted and the general context of each study (international comparison or monocentric analysis, primary or secondary prevention), the data are impressive [39–45]. None of these studies suggests that the Med diet is not highly protective against CHD and not associated with longer survival. One problem with these studies, however, is the way to define, and then to quantify, the traditional Med diet. In general, the technique used by the investigators was to calculate a Med score from individual data obtained through an extensive, validated food-frequency questionnaire. It is clear that this technique does not fully reflect the complexity of a dietary pattern such as the traditional Med diet. However, the combination of Med foods in a given person or patient can actually be summed up as a score, which can provide some information if there is a statistically significant correlation with clinical endpoints. Another weakness of these studies was the lack of biomarkers, for instance blood antioxidants and vitamin B, or plasma or red cell fatty acids. This, in fact, raises the major question of whether one should define a diet in terms of foods or in terms of nutrients. We think, as shown in our own studies [22–25] and discussed below, that the preferred technique is probably to use both foods and nutrients to define the kind of Med diet that we are exploring, and then to quantify the dietary habits of individuals or populations. In spite of these technical limitations and differences in the way of evaluating Med scores, investigators report that adherence to a Med diet style is associated with a reduction in total mortality. The effect on mortality was seen in both primary and secondary prevention of CHD and also was attributable to a reduced risk of cancer death [40, 41, 43–45]. This emphasized the importance of dietary habits in the prevention of CHD and cancer, and confirmed beyond any doubt both the results of the Lyon Diet Heart Study and the relevance of the Med diet.

Summary of the Lyon Diet Heart Study Results

The design and methods of the trial have been reported [9, 22–24]. Briefly, statistical analyses were done on the intention-to-treat principle. Event-free survival for MI, cardiovascular death (CD) and three composite outcomes (CO) were estimated using the Kaplan-Meier method. The Cox proportional hazard model was used to calculate the risk ratios and to quantify the associations between each traditional risk factor and the different COs, namely MI plus CD (CO 1) or MI plus CD plus major secondary events (CO 2) or the precedents plus minor events requiring hospital admission (CO 3). In the Exp group, CO 1 was reduced (14 events against 44, $p > 0.0001$), as were CO 2 (27 events against 90, $p > 0.0001$) and CO 3 (95 events against 180, $p > 0.0002$). Adjusted risk ratios ranged from 0.28 to 0.53 [23].

In CHD patients, adopting a slightly modified Cretan diet resulted in a 50–70% decrease in the risk of recurrence.

Among the traditional risk factors, total blood cholesterol (1 mmol/l being associated with an increase in risk by 18–28%), systolic blood pressure (1 mm Hg being associated with an increase in risk by 1–2%), leukocyte count (adjusted risk ratios ranging from 1.64 to 2.86 at counts >9 giga/l), female gender (adjusted risk ratios: 0.27–0.46) and aspirin use (adjusted risk ratios: 0.59–0.82) were each significantly and independently associated with recurrence. The data indicate that the Exp diet did not alter, at least qualitatively, the usual relationships between major risk factors of CHD (e.g. elevated cholesterol and blood pressure) and recurrence. This is a very important point for the physicians in charge of the patients, since it means that pharmacological treatment (with aspirin, blood pressure- and cholesterol-lowering drugs) and dietary prevention are not mutually exclusive but have additional and independent beneficial effects, although further trials combining the two approaches are warranted.

Finally, the fact that the two groups of the Lyon trial were similar in terms of traditional risk factors during the study [9, 23] should not be interpreted as meaning that the Exp diet did not have any effect on blood lipids or blood pressure in patients with established CHD. In fact, the vast majority of the patients of both groups were taking blood pressure-lowering drugs (prescribed by their attending physicians) as part of a systematic secondary prevention treatment, which resulted in low blood pressure levels in both groups and probably masked any blood pressure-lowering effect of the Exp diet. It has been shown that a diet including high intakes of vegetables and reduced intakes of meat and high-fat dairy products (a diet quite similar to the traditional Med diets) could indeed reduce blood pressure [46], and data from investigators in Italy found that such diets, also in the Med context, actually lower blood pressure [47]. Thus, the cardioprotective effect of the Med diet may be also due to an unidentified effect on factors regulating blood pressure and presumably involved in the pathogenesis of CHD.

The same reasoning applies for blood lipids. One third of each group of patients in the Lyon trial was taking cholesterol-lowering drugs, with a trend towards more patients being treated in the Western group during the trial [24]. Thus, a small effect of the Exp diet on blood cholesterol may have been masked by the drug therapy. In fact, any lipid-lowering effect of a Med diet should be evaluated by comparing patients following a Med diet with patients following a typical Western diet, including high intakes of saturated fats and dietary cholesterol. Thus, the evaluation of the true effect of any type of Med diet on cholesterol level in CHD patients with various dyslipidemias warrants further investigations and trials specifically designed for that purpose.

The Experimental Diet Tested in the Lyon Trial

The theoretical principles of the Exp Med diet (a modified Cretan diet) tested in the trial have been described [9, 11, 22–24]. The Seven Countries

Study showed that mortality from CHD is lower in Crete than in the other Southern Mediterranean countries [1] where the amount of fat in the diet (about 30% of total energy) is considerably lower than in Crete (about 40%). In these other Mediterranean countries (Italy and Spain for instance), people do not eat as many wild plants, walnuts and legumes as the people in Crete and their intake of alpha-linolenic acid (ALA) is lower. What is so special about the Cretan diet is the much higher ALA content and lower linoleic acid content, with higher amounts of fruits and less meat, along with the otherwise traditional components of the Med diet.

Briefly, in terms of lipids, the Exp diet would supply about 30% of energy from fats and less than 10% of energy from saturated fats. Regarding the essential fatty acids, the intake of $18:2\omega6$ (linoleic acid, LA) should be restricted to 4% of energy and the intake of $18:3\omega3$ (ALA) should compose more than 0.6% of energy. In practical terms, the dietary instructions were detailed and customized to each patient [9] and could be summarized as: more bread, more cereals, more legumes and beans, more fresh vegetables and fruits, more fish, less meat (beef, lamb, pork) and delicatessen food, which are to be replaced by poultry; no more butter and cream, to be replaced by an experimental, canola oil-based margarine. This margarine was chemically comparable with olive oil but slightly enriched in $18:2\omega6$ and mostly in $18:3\omega3$, the two essential fatty acids. The concentrations of trans fatty acids were around 5% in the first part of the trial (first two years) and about 0% thereafter. Finally, the oils recommended for salad and food preparation were exclusively olive and canola (erucid acid-free rapeseed oil) oils. What the patients of the Exp and Western diet groups actually ate during the trial has been reported [9, 23]. Patients of the Western group followed a prudent diet, with about 34% of energy as total fats, 12% saturated fats and a mean of 312 mg/day of dietary cholesterol. These patients were assuredly not following a typical Western diet, rather a prudent diet not too different from the US National Cholesterol Education Program (NCEP) step I. In contrast, patients of the Exp group were close to step II of the NCEP recommended for survivors of a previous infarct (except for the omega-3 and omega-6 fatty acids), with 30% as total fats, 7–8% saturated fats and 200 mg/day of cholesterol. Intake of the main food groups has been reported [9, 23] and is summarized in table 1. The main points concerned the consumption of bread, fresh fruits and vegetables, meat and delicatessen food, oils, and butter (and cream) versus the canola oil-based margarine. The exclusive use of olive and canola oils and of canola-oil based margarine to prepare meals and salad is a major issue in that study since it resulted in major differences in the fatty acid composition of both circulating plasma lipids (essentially lipoproteins) and membrane cell phospholipids (tables 2–4), which in turn were probably associated with critical effects on the major mechanisms involved in the occurrence of the cardiovascular complications, as discussed below.

Table 1. Summary of the intake of the main food groups recorded at the last visit of the patients in the Lyon trial: results in g/day, mean ± SD

	Western	Exp	p
Bread	140 (58)	171 (86)	0.004
Other cereals	69.7 (116)	97.0 (132)	0.11
Vegetables (without potatoes)	340 (203)	427 (222)	0.004
Fruits	214 (201)	271 (218)	0.05
Potatoes	82.2 (123)	66.6 (129)	0.38
Delicatessen foods	21 (42)	3.0 (14)	0.0001
Meat	53.4 (70)	35.1 (62)	0.04
Poultry and lean meat	57.1 (75)	48.1 (62)	0.30
Fish	32.8 (68)	47.9 (72)	0.12
Whole milk	19.8 (83)	3.10 (37)	0.09
Skimmed milk and light milk	147 (202)	118 (178)	0.30
Cheese	36.3 (30)	29.7 (30)	0.12
Butter and cream	12.4 (13)	2.60 (7)	0.0001
Margarine	7.9 (10)	17.4 (15)	0.0001
Oil	15.5 (13)	18.9 (12)	0.05

Table 2. Plasma fatty acid differences (Diff) in patients following either an experimental modified diet of Crete (Exp) or a prudent Western (West) type of diet

Ratio	After 2 months			After 1 year		
	Exp (n = 236)	West (n = 247)	Diff %	Exp (n = 141)	West (n = 139)	Diff %
18:1/18:2	0.809	0.658	+23	0.799	0.668	+20
18:2/18:3	42	76	−45	44	79	−44
20:4/20:5	6.8	9.1	−25	6.2	9.1	−32

All differences are statistically significant (p < 0.05).
18:1 is oleic acid (18:1 omega-9); 18:2 is linoleic acid (18:2 omega-6); 18:3 is alpha-linolenic acid (18:3 omega-3); 20:4 is arachidonic acid (20:4 omega-6); 20:5 is eicosapentaenoic acid (20:5 omega-3).

Finally, it must be mentioned that the main antioxidant vitamins, alpha-tocopherol and ascorbic acid, were significantly higher in the plasma in the Exp group than in the Western group [9], which stresses the potent antioxidant effect of the Exp diet. This is not surprising because beyond the obvious effects of the Exp diet on the fatty acid composition of lipids (which is by itself an antioxidant

Table 3. Platelet phospholipids fatty acids

	Exp	West	p
Saturated fatty acids			
14:0	0.28 ± 0.01	0.31 ± 0.01	<0.05
16:0	14.70 ± 0.25	14.39 ± 0.17	NS
18:0	15.81 ± 0.17	16.35 ± 0.14	0.01
Sum	30.79 ± 0.28	31.05 ± 0.21	NS
Unsaturated fatty acids			
Omega-9 family			
18:1ω9	12.56 ± 0.32	11.64 ± 0.14	0.01
20:1ω9	0.88 ± 0.04	0.74 ± 0.03	0.01
20:3ω9	0.16 ± 0.01	0.15 ± 0.01	NS
Sum	13.50 ± 0.35	12.43 ± 0.15	0.01
Omega-6 family			
18:2ω6	5.09 ± 0.16	5.46 ± 0.17	NS
20:3ω6	1.22 ± 0.03	1.31 ± 0.05	NS
20:4ω6	25.89 ± 0.33	26.45 ± 0.28	NS
22:4ω6	2.72 ± 0.09	3.02 ± 0.10	<0.05
Sum	34.93 ± 0.42	36.26 ± 0.29	0.01
Omega-3 family			
20:5ω3	0.57 ± 0.04	0.48 ± 0.04	NS
22:5ω3	2.11 ± 0.08	1.94 ± 0.06	NS
22:6ω3	2.59 ± 0.10	2.38 ± 0.10	NS
Sum	5.27 ± 0.17	4.81 ± 0.16	0.05

Results are mean ± SEM.
NS = Nonsignificant.

Table 4. Comparisons of the different families of platelet phospholipids fatty acids

Ratios	Exp	West	p
Omega-6/omega-9	2.70 ± 0.12	2.95 ± 0.05	0.05
Omega-6/omega-3	6.92 ± 0.27	7.88 ± 0.29	≤0.05
Omega-6/omega-9 + omega-3	1.90 ± 0.06	2.13 ± 0.04	≤0.005
Saturated/omega-6	0.88 ± 0.01	0.86 ± 0.01	0.13
Saturated/omega-9 + omega-3	1.68 ± 0.05	1.82 ± 0.03	0.01
Saturated/unsaturated	0.57 ± 0.01	0.58 ± 0.01	0.90

intervention as it modifies the main substrate of oxidation), this diet actually provided large amounts of various antioxidant compounds including vitamins, trace elements and polyphenols, including flavonoids [48]. The Exp diet is a non-strict vegetarian diet, low in saturated and polyunsaturated fat and high in oleic acid, omega-3 fatty acids, fiber, vitamins of the B group and various antioxidants.

Coronary Heart Disease Is an Inflammatory Disease

Most investigators now agree that atherosclerosis and CHD are chronic inflammatory diseases [49]. Proinflammatory factors (free radicals caused by cigarette smoking, hyperhomocysteinemia, diabetes, peroxidized lipids, hypertension, elevated and modified blood lipids) contribute to injuries of the vascular endothelium resulting in alterations of its antiatherosclerotic and antithrombotic properties. This is thought to be a major step in the initiation and formation of arterial fibrostenotic lesions [49]. From a clinical point of view, however, an essential distinction should be made between unstable, lipid-rich and leukocyte-rich lesions and stable, lipid-poor and acellular fibrotic lesions, because the propensity of these two types of lesion to rupture into the lumen of the artery, whatever the degree of stenosis and lumen obstruction, is totally different. We hypothesized the role of inflammation and leukocytes in the onset of acute CHD events many years ago [50], and this was confirmed later [51–54]. One of the main mechanisms underlying the sudden onset of acute syndromes, including unstable angina MI and sudden death, is the erosion or rupture of an atherosclerotic lesion [51, 52], triggering thrombotic complications and considerably increasing the risk of ventricular arrhythmias [53, 54]. Leukocytes have been also implicated in the occurrence of ventricular arrhythmias in the clinical and experimental settings [55, 56], and they contribute to myocardial damage during both ischemia and reperfusion [55].

Clinical and pathological evidence showed the importance of inflammatory cells and immune mediators in the occurrence of acute CHD events [49, 57, 58] and prospective epidemiological studies showed a strong and consistent association between acute CHD and systemic markers of inflammation [59, 60].

Any theory to explain the efficiency of the Cretan diet to reduce the rate of CHD should take into account the importance of inflammation in CHD.

The next question is whether the Med diet might be associated with a lower prevalence of inflammatory syndromes. At least three studies testing some forms of traditional Med diet, including 2 randomized trials, recently showed that the adoption of a Med diet reduces inflammatory markers such as serum

C-reactive protein, interleukins, TNF-α, P-selectin, fibrinogen or white blood cell counts [61–64]. Interestingly, two of them were also associated with an improvement of endothelial function, a marker of the risk of CHD complications such as plaque erosion or rupture [61, 63] as discussed below.

Role of Inflammation and Oxidation in Plaque Rupture and Progression of Coronary Heart Disease

Another critical question is why macrophages and activated lymphocytes [49] are present in atherosclerotic lesions, and how they get there, with the associated issues of local inflammation, plaque rupture and attendant acute CHD complications. In 1989, Steinberg et al. [65] hypothesized that lipoprotein oxidation causes accelerated atherogenesis. Elevated plasma levels of low-density lipoproteins (LDL) are a risk factor of CHD, and the reduction of blood LDL levels resulted in less CHD in many trials, although the effect on mortality was either small or non-significant in most recent statin trials conducted in patients with optimal drug treatment [66–70]. However, the mechanism(s) behind the effect of high LDL levels is not fully understood. The notion that LDL oxidation is a key characteristic of unstable lesions is supported by many reports [49]. Two processes have been proposed. First, when LDL particles become trapped in the arterial wall, they are progressively oxidized and internalized by macrophages, which results in the formation of the typical atherosclerotic foam cells. Oxidized LDL is chemotactic for other immune and inflammatory cells and up-regulates the expression of monocyte and endothelial cell genes involved in the inflammatory reaction [49, 65, 71, 72]. The inflammatory response itself can have a profound effect on LDL [48], thus creating a vicious circle of LDL oxidation, inflammation and further LDL oxidation.

Second, oxidized LDL circulates in the plasma for a period sufficiently long to enter and accumulate in the arterial intima, suggesting that the entry of oxidized lipoproteins within the intima may be another mechanism of lesion inflammation, in particular in patients without hyperlipidemia [73–75]. Elevated plasma levels of oxidized LDL are associated with CHD, and the plasma level of malondialdehyde-modified LDL is higher in patients with unstable CHD syndromes (usually associated with plaque rupture) than in patients with clinically stable CHD [76]. In the accelerated form of CHD typical of post-transplantation patients, higher levels of lipid peroxidation [77–79] and of oxidized LDL [80] were found compared with the stable form of CHD in non-transplanted patients. Reactive oxygen metabolites and oxidants influence thrombus formation [81], and platelet reactivity is significantly higher in transplanted patients than in non-transplanted CHD patients [82]. However, platelet phospholipid fatty acids (which partly determine platelet function) are different from those of non-transplanted CHD patients [82], which may explain, at least partly, the high platelet reactivity of transplanted patients. Since the effects of reactive oxygen metabolites on platelet function are quite complex [83], further studies are warranted to conclusively answer the question of the relations between lipid peroxidation and platelet function in CHD.

Another question is whether antioxidant intervention might alter the risk of CHD. There are different types of antioxidant treatment, including either a global dietary approach (aimed both at reducing oxidant stress and at increasing antioxidant defenses, with the Med diet as a good example) or a pharmacological approach using capsules of various antioxidants. The second approach has been extremely disappointing.

With respect to antioxidant vitamins and CHD, randomized trials have failed to fulfill the promises of observational epidemiological studies, which were also supported by a body of evidence from basic research suggesting plausible biological mechanisms [84].

This does not mean that oxidized lipids do not have a role in CHD complications. However, there is clearly a missing link in the current theory, and further research is needed before we can recommend systematic antioxidant supplementation for the prevention of CHD.

Lipids and Inflammation in Coronary Heart Disease

The oxidized LDL theory is not inconsistent with the well-established lipid-lowering treatment of CHD, as there is a positive correlation between plasma LDL levels and lipid peroxidation markers [78, 85]. Low LDL levels actually result in reduced amounts of LDL available for oxidative modification. The lowering of LDL can be achieved by drugs or by reducing saturated fats in the diet. Reduction of the oxidative susceptibility of LDL was reported when dietary fat was replaced with carbohydrates [86]. This is rather in line with the first approach (global dietary approach) described above and different from the pharmacological antioxidant approach.

Pharmacological/quantitative (lowering of cholesterol) and nutritional/qualitative (increased antioxidant defenses, reduction of oxidative stress) approaches of the prevention of CHD are not mutually exclusive but additive and complementary.

An alternative way to reduce LDL concentrations is to replace saturated fats with polyunsaturated fats. However, diets high in polyunsaturated fatty acids increase the polyunsaturated fatty acid content of LDL particles render them more susceptible to oxidation [87] and increase oxidative stress, which would argue against the use of such diets. As a matter of fact, in the secondary prevention of CHD, such diets failed to improve the prognosis of the patients [11]. In this context, the Exp diet tested in the Lyon trial, which included both low saturated and polyunsaturated fat intakes, appears to be the best choice. However, diets rich in oleic acid increase the resistance of LDL to oxidation independently of the antioxidant content [88, 89] and result in leukocyte inhibition [90, 91]. Thus, oleic acid-rich diets decrease the proinflammatory properties of oxidized LDL. Constituents of olive oil other than oleic acid may also inhibit LDL oxidation [92]. Various components of the Med diets may also affect LDL oxidation. For instance, alpha-tocopherol or vitamin C or a diet combining reduced fat, low-fat dairy products and high intakes of fruits and vegetables were shown to favorably affect LDL oxidation itself and/or the cellular consequences of LDL oxidation [93–96]. Finally, a significant correlation was found between certain dietary fatty acids and the fatty acid composition of human atherosclerotic plaques [97, 98], suggesting that dietary fatty acids are rapidly incorporated into the plaques. This implies a direct influence of dietary fatty acids on plaque formation and the process of plaque rupture. It is conceivable that fatty acids that stimulate LDL oxidation (omega-6 fatty acids) induce plaque rupture, while those which inhibit LDL oxidation (oleic acid) or leukocyte function (omega-3 fatty acids) [99] help stabilize the dangerous lesions.

Thus, any dietary pattern combining high intakes of natural antioxidants, low intakes of saturated fatty acids, high intakes of oleic acid, low intakes of omega-6 fatty acids and high intakes of omega-3 fatty acids would logically result in a highly cardioprotective effect. Such a dietary pattern has now been tested in a randomized trial [22–25], and the results of the 'Lyon Diet Heart Study' were confirmed by several epidemiological studies [39–45].

Thus, the concept of Med diet with its multiple approaches (including the notion that the main targets of oxidative stress within the LDL are the polyunsaturated fatty acids, while monounsaturated fatty acids are resistant to oxidation) leads to reconcile a body of inconsistent data. Large doses of non-natural antioxidant vitamins (as they were tested in randomized trials) in the absence of consideration for the target of oxidation might be pro-oxidant in certain patients or certain conditions, and this may explain the failure to prevent CHD complications in these trials. We believe that any antioxidant intervention must be included in a more global dietary approach such as the Med diet.

Fatty Acids and the Experimental Modified Cretan Diet

Tables 1–4 summarize dietary, plasma and cell fatty acid data from the patients of the Lyon trial. They provide a scientific rationale to explain, at least partly, the clinical results of the trial. In table 2, for instance, the differences between groups in the plasma 18:1/18:2 ratio could be considered an indicator of lipid oxidizability as fatty acids are transported by the lipoproteins and are the main determinants of LDL oxidizability. However, while circulating blood lipids are crucial in the development of CHD, cell membrane lipids are also important because they are also affected by oxidant stress. The cell membrane consists of a bilayer primarily composed of phospholipids and cholesterol. Embedded in this essential matrix are also a variety of proteins, such as receptors, transporters and enzymes, performing important cellular functions. The requirement for a dynamic state of lipids in the bilayer is one of the fundamental features of the fluid-mosaic model of membrane structure [100]. Any factors modifying cell membrane fatty acid or the nature and/or content of the proteins must also influence the physical state of the bilayer and, as a consequence, alter cellular function [101]. Any consistent variation in the dietary intake of fats will be reflected in the composition of structural lipids within cell membrane, as shown in tables 3 and 4 of this study. Significant differences were observed for individual saturated fatty acids and for the 3 main families of unsaturated fatty acids (table 3). The exact physiological and pathophysiological significance of these differences is not yet clearly identified. However, the data suggest that cell membrane lipids in the Exp group were less oxidizable than those in the Western group (table 4). Further studies are warranted to examine the molecular and cellular consequences of these variations in the fatty acid composition on cellular function in the various types of cells involved in CHD (platelets, endothelial cells, leukocytes and smooth muscle cells). However, this reasoning includes only theoretical explanations based on the quantitative or qualitative (oxidized LDL theory) aspects of the lipoprotein and lipid paradigm. In fact, the dramatic cardioprotective effect resulting from the adoption of the Exp Med diet may be explained through the modification of other metabolic pathways that we will briefly discuss in the next sections.

Omega-3 Fatty Acids in the Med Diets and in Coronary Heart Disease

Sandker et al. [102] reported high concentrations of omega-3 fatty acids, in particular ALA, in the plasma of the Greek population, and Simopoulos and coworkers [103, 104] confirmed that ALA is a major component of the Cretan diet. There is now a large body of evidence indicating that dietary ALA is a major protective factor against CHD, including fatal complications of CHD [105–109]. Thus, there is no doubt that a high intake of ALA is a major feature of the Cretan Med diet, as also confirmed in the Lyon Diet Heart Study [22–25]. On the other hand, consumption of fish once or twice a week is clearly associated with a significant reduction in CHD mortality [110–115]. This effect has been attributed to the cardioprotective effect of long-chain omega-3 fatty acids. In particular, experimental and clinical studies provided convincing evidence that long-chain omega-3 fatty acids prevent ventricular arrhythmia, the main cause of sudden cardiac death [114, 115]. In contrast, the prudent NCEP diet, either step I or II, was not reported to have any effect on sudden cardiac death. While some people may still debate whether a high intake of fish or fish oils is actually protective against CHD, this is no longer an issue. However, it is not clear whether other components of fish (protein types, certain trace elements such as zinc and selenium) may also have a role to play in the cardioprotective effect of fish. In the Lyon trial, the intake of fish was slightly higher in the Exp group than in the Western group [9, 22]. The differences in the concentrations in the long-chain omega-3 fatty acids in plasma and cell phospholipids in the Exp group were related to both the higher intake of fish and the higher intake of ALA through the consumption of canola oil-based margarine. Table 2 shows the large differences (from 25 to 45%) between groups in the omega-6/omega-3 ratios for both the 18- and 20-carbon fatty acids in plasma. The differences between groups were less drastic for platelet phospholipids (because of tight endogenous regulations), but statistically significant (tables 3, 4). It should be noted that platelets have a particular regulation of fatty acid metabolism and do not reflect the actual concentrations in omega-3 fatty acids in the heart or in leucocytes.

Changes in plasma and cell membrane omega-6/omega-3 fatty acid ratios are among the main biological effects of the Cretan diet as tested in the Lyon trial.

Another important aspect of how the various families of fatty acids are involved in CHD is their role in the metabolism of eicosanoids. Although it is probably a major point to understand the cardioprotective effects of the Exp diet, this complex issue is beyond the scope of the present review. Plasma and cell concentrations of omega-6 and omega-3 fatty acids and their ratios illustrate their interference with different pathways involved in CHD. First, there is competition between linoleic acid (the main 18-carbon omega-6 fatty acid, which represents about 30% of total plasma fatty acids) and ALA (the main 18-carbon omega-3 fatty acid, which represents only 0.30% of total plasma fatty acids) for desaturation and elongation to synthesize either arachidonic acid (the main 20-carbon omega-6 fatty acid) or eicosapentanoic acid (the main 20-carbon omega-3 fatty acid) which are the main substrates for the metabolism of eicosanoids [116]. Despite a huge difference in the plasma concentrations of linoleic acid and ALA (a ratio of 100 to 1), there is evidence that elongases and desaturases prefer omega-3 to omega-6 fatty acids [116]. Small increases in the intake of ALA result in significant changes in the omega-6/omega-3 ratios in both plasma and cell membranes, as shown in tables 2 and 4.

The second competition point between omega-6 and omega-3 fatty acid families is at the level of eicosanoid metabolism. Arachidonic acid (AA) and eicosapentanoic acid (EPA) are the precursors to a broad array of structurally diverse and potent bioactive lipids that include prostaglandins, thromboxanes, leukotrienes, lipoxins as well as other oxygenated fatty acids. Collectively, these molecules are termed eicosanoids [117, 118]. In human tissues, eicosanoid biosynthesis is initiated by cyclooxygenases (present in two forms, a constitutive one and an inducible one) that can give rise to prostaglandins, thromboxanes and prostacyclins, as well as three major lipoxygenases [118]. These various compounds are doubtlessly involved in the inflammatory process that characterizes both early and advanced stages of CHD (even in patients on aspirin) as well as myocardial diseases and the chronic heart failure syndrome [119–122]. The discovery that prostaglandins, thromboxanes and leukotrienes derived from EPA have different biological properties from those derived from AA stimulated research on the nutritional aspect of eicosanoid metabolism. When the omega-6/omega-3 ratios decrease, as a result of dietary changes, EPA competes with AA for eicosanoid metabolism at the cyclooxygenase and lipoxygenase levels in platelets and leukocytes. As a result, the balance between metabolites stimulating platelets and leukocytes (and also with vasoconstrictive properties) and metabolites with opposing properties shifts towards those with antithrombotic, anti-inflammatory and vasodilative properties. Thus, the ability to modify membrane fatty acid composition in vivo by diet, even when essential fatty acids are adequately provided, demonstrates the importance of dietary fatty acids in CHD beyond their role in the resistance of LDL to oxidation.

Diet-induced modification of the fatty acid composition of cell membranes affects the generation of products (eicosanoids) directly derived from their fatty acid precursors, indicating that dietary fats potentially affect key processes in cell function.

Decreasing the concentration of AA may have other advantages as prostaglandin-like compounds could be formed from nonenzymatic free radical catalyzed peroxidation of AA. Morrow and co-workers have demonstrated that prostaglandin-like isomers, termed F2 isoprostanes, were formed as the result of oxidant attack of cell membrane phospholipids or LDL [123, 124]. Increased formation of F2 isoprostanes is associated with hypercholesterolemia [125] and chronic heart failure [126] and these compounds are present in human atherosclerotic lesions [127]. In the apoE-deficient mouse model, vitamin E supplementation suppresses isoprostane generation in vivo and reduces atherosclerosis without altering cholesterol levels [128]. These data are important because, given the ubiquitous distribution of AA, isoprostane generation can occur in virtually all of the cellular players of CHD as well as in LDL.

Finally, in a recent report, Pitsavos et al. [129] studied the effect of the Med diet (evaluated through a Med score) on total antioxidant capacity (TAC), an integrated measurement of antioxidant defenses in the body, and oxidized LDL in more than 3,000 Greek adults who had no clinical evidence of CHD. They found a positive association between the Med score and the TAC and an inverse association with oxidized LDL. The TAC was positively correlated with the consumption of olive oil and of fruit and vegetables, again indicating that the benefits of the Med diet cannot be confined to the effects of a few fatty foods or nutrients but result from a combination of multiple factors, including some not related to fat. Interestingly, similar results (a decrease in circulating oxidized LDL particles) were obtained in a non-Med population in a nutritional intervention promoting a Med food pattern [130].

Folate, Homocysteine, Nitric Oxide Pathway, Coronary Heart Disease and the Med Diets

High intakes of cereals (in particular wheat flour), legumes, vegetables and fruits (including nuts) are major characteristics of the Med diets and of the Exp diet tested in the Lyon trial. These foods are important sources of folates [5] known to lower plasma homocysteine levels [131]. On the other hand, out of over 40 well-conducted studies, all but a few have shown that moderate hyperhomocysteinemia is an independent risk factor for CHD. The risk appears to be graded across the whole distribution of plasma homocysteine levels and there are a number of plausible biological mechanisms to account for the toxic nature of homocysteine on arteries and veins [131–133]. Finally, several studies have now linked elevated homocysteine levels with decreased plasma levels of folates and vitamins B_6 and B_{12}. Of these, low folate level is the most significant and intervention studies have demonstrated that elevated plasma homocysteine levels can be normalized by moderate doses of folate alone or in combination with vitamins B_6 and B_{12} [134, 135]. Further, a prospective study found low plasma folate to be directly associated with an increased risk of CHD [136].

Finally, folic acid is also involved in the nitric oxide pathway, as 5-methyltetrahydrofolate, the active form of folic acid, was shown to restore endothelial function in hypercholesterolemic patients [20]. Nitric oxide formation is indeed critically dependent on the presence of the cofactor tetrahydrobiopterin (BH4), which stimulates conversion of arginine to citrulline and nitric oxide by nitric oxide synthase, and it has been demonstrated that administration of BH4 can restore impaired nitric oxide activity in hypercholesterolemia. In fact, BH4 itself is active only in its reduced form, and folates have been suggested to stimulate endogenous regeneration of BH4 from its oxidized form [137]. Although further studies on the role of folates on the nitric oxide pathway are required, these data suggest that folates may be important not only for the prevention of hyperhomocysteinemia but also in other conditions (dyslipidemia, hypertension, diabetes) where the nitric oxide pathway is altered. Although specific studies are needed to confirm the point, it is likely that a significant part of the cardioprotective effect of the Med diets, including the Exp diet tested in the Lyon trial, is related to folates.

However, randomized trials testing the effects of vitamins B on clinical endpoints have provided conflicting data [138–142], in some way reproducing the antioxidant story with impressive data from epidemiological studies and negative results from randomized trials. Studies on the interaction between adherence to a Med diet and genetic polymorphism (for instance the methylenetetrahydrofolate reductase 677C-T mutation) may help to understand this kind of discrepancy. Dedoussis and colleagues have reported that a Med score was not associated with homocysteine concentrations in a Greek healthy adult population [143]. However, after control for potential confounders, they found that adherence to a Med diet was associated with reduced homocysteine in persons with certain genotypes but not with other genotypes. This suggests that certain subjects with a specific genotype require higher folate intakes than subjects with other genotypes to achieve similar homocysteine concentrations, which points to complex interactions between genes and nutrition.

Selenium and the Protective Effect of the Med Diets against Cancers

Although it was not specifically designed to study cancer rate, the Lyon trial did suggest that the Exp diet favorably influences clinical manifestations of cancer. Fewer cancers of the urinary and digestive tracts and of the throat were actually diagnosed in the Exp than in the Western group [25]. When excluding the cases diagnosed within the first 24 months following entry into the trial, the arithmetic difference between the 2 groups (12 vs. 2) was still greater [25]. These results are not surprising, for several reasons. First, the Exp diet included several nutrients (fiber, natural antioxidants, a low omega-6/omega-3 fatty acid ratio, for instance) that have been shown, when taken separately, to potentially prevent cancer initiation or spread [144–148]. Second, mortality statistics from the WHO have clearly documented the low incidence of most neoplasms and the long survival of people in the Mediterranean regions, despite a high prevalence of smoking [149]. As migrant studies (from Mediterranean regions to the USA or Australia, for instance) were not in favor of a familial, hereditary (genetic) protection, this means that it is probably the Med diets that are protective. In fact, since the publication of the cancer data of the Lyon trial in 1998, several groups of epidemiologists have reported an inverse association between adherence to a Med diet and either mortality from cancer or cancer prevalence [41, 43, 45]. The Lyon trial is the first controlled dietary trial to show that such a protection may be achieved in a non-Med population through a well-designed dietary intervention. However, although the study has the strength of a prospective randomized trial with complete follow-up, which minimizes confounding and bias, this does not completely compensate for the relatively small sample size, and further studies are warranted to confirm these data. Another question is the plausibility that the Med diets can be protective against various tumor types. Most tumors eventually take a common final pathway to grow, spread and metastasize. This requires an adequate local (e.g. angiogenic and inflammatory factors) and systemic (immunological factors) environment. We know (as discussed above) that this environment can be influenced by dietary changes modifying cell membrane fatty acid composition and cell function, as also clearly shown on animal models [148]. Thus, certain angiogenic and inflammatory factors (prostaglandin and leukotrienes) involved in the final common pathway of most cancers can be modified by the fatty acid profile characteristic of Med diets, in particular the Exp diet tested in the Lyon trial. Finally, Med diets are also characterized by large amounts of fresh vegetables and fruits providing high amounts of various natural antioxidants, which may prevent carcinogenesis [144, 150, 151]. Large epidemiological studies have actually shown that people consuming more beta-carotene and carotenoids have a lower risk of various cancers [145]. Unfortunately, clinical trials (using, however, nonnatural antioxidant supplements) were disappointing [152–155]. In the Lyon trial, patients of the Exp group consumed more vitamin C, more fiber and probably more trace elements (including selenium) and polyphenols than patients of the Western group. A recent randomized trial in the USA has provided evidence that selenium supplementation (200 µg daily) decreases the incidence of prostate, lung and colorectal cancers over a mean follow-up of 4.5 years [27]. Another study has revealed an inverse association between advanced prostate cancer and toenail selenium concentrations, a surrogate of long-term selenium intake [156]. These data are in line with those of the Lyon trial since the Med diets, rich in grains and marine products (100 g of cooked octopus, the Greek national dish, provides about 90 µg of selenium), are selenium-rich diets. Also, in both the Lyon and the US selenium trials, the benefits became apparent within 3–4 years. Finally, as selenium was shown to interfere with carcinogens in animal models through several possible mechanisms [157], the anticancer selenium hypothesis appears to be realistic. Supplementation with omega-3 fatty acid results in higher concentrations of long-chain omega-3 fatty acids, known to interfere with eicosanoid metabolism and inflammation as well as leukocyte and platelet function, as discussed above. Although the link between cancer and inflammation is by no means a simple one [158], it is possible that the anticancer effect shown in the Lyon trial partly resulted from a local anti-inflammatory effect of omega-3 fatty acids. This agrees with findings from animal models showing that diets high in omega-3 fatty acids result in diminished tumor development and a longer tumor latency period [148]. In contrast, diets rich in omega-6 fatty acids (these fatty acids were significantly reduced in both the diet and plasma of the patients of the Exp group) enhance tumor development [147]. Also, dietary omega-3 fatty acids have been shown in vivo in humans to down-regulate gene expression of potent carcinogenetic growth factors [159]. EPA, the omega-3 fatty acid which competes with AA in the cyclooxygenase pathway, was lower in the Western than the Exp group and blockade of the cyclooxygenase pathway has indeed been proposed as prophylaxis against colorectal cancer [160].

Although these data do not conclusively prove an anticancer effect of the Med diets, they should be a strong incentive to initiate dietary intervention trials testing the effect of specific dietary patterns.

Both adherence to and compliance with the Exp diet were excellent in the Lyon trial [9, 23], suggesting that such a diet should not be so difficult for high-risk patients to follow, and allowing a long-term test of anticancer hypotheses. Further basic studies are also needed to examine how the local lipid environment of cancer cells may influence tumor growth, since certain fatty acids or, more precisely, certain fatty acid profiles seem to be able to delay the clinical manifestation of certain cancers. Unfortunately, it may take a long time before a dietary trial actually provides a clear demonstration of the anticancer effect of the Exp diet tested in the Lyon trial. The information obtained by current epidemiological data about Med populations and the results of the Lyon trial should nonetheless lead high-risk persons to adopt the Exp diet. No harmful side effects are to be expected and, in view of the frequency and severity of most cancers, there is no convincing argument against such a prudent attitude.

Metabolic Syndromes and Mediterranean Diets

The metabolic syndromes consist of a constellation of factors that increase the risk of CHD and type II diabetes. Estimates suggest that metabolic syndromes, whatever their definitions, are highly prevalent in most Western countries, up to 25% of the population being affected in certain countries such as the USA. Their clinical identification is based on measures of elevated blood pressure, glucose intolerance, abdominal obesity, and dyslipidemia.

Studies also suggest that a pro-inflammatory state is one component of metabolic syndromes. Thus, a Med diet might be effective in reducing the prevalence of metabolic syndromes, as suggested in a recent randomized trial [63], but not confirmed by another study [161]. Other studies suggest that the Med diet and/or olive oil consumption are associated with a reduced incidence of hypertension [162] or inversely associated with blood pressure [163]. Furthermore, in a Spanish population, adherence to the traditional Med diet was inversely associated with body mass index and obesity [164]. These findings were not confirmed by another study conducted in a Greek population [165]. Finally, in an obese Med population, central obesity was positively associated with omega-6 fatty acids and inversely associated with monounsaturated fatty acids and omega-3 fatty acids in adipose tissue [166], suggesting that some key lipid characteristics of the Med diet seem to be protective against central obesity, a major component of the metabolic syndromes. However, further studies are needed to confirm the importance of the Med diet model in preventing the development of metabolic syndromes and of dangerous forms of obesity.

Polyphenols in Med Diets

Polyphenols are the most abundant antioxidants in our diets, and epidemiological studies have suggested associations between the consumption of polyphenol-rich foods (fruit and vegetables) or beverages (wine and tea) and the prevention of major chronic diseases such as cancers and CHD. No trial results have been published to date. Med diets are extremely rich in polyphenols from various foods and beverages, and there is no doubt that the protection they provide against various diseases is partly related to polyphenols.

Polyphenols are characterized by a considerable diversity of structures, and several thousands of natural polyphenols have been identified in plants and plant foods. In order to understand their impact on human health, we need to know the nature of the main polyphenols ingested with our daily diet and their bioavailability [167]. Another issue is how (by which methods) the effects of exposure to dietary polyphenols should be assessed. Several studies have tried and identified the nature of the polyphenols to which circulating cells and tissues are exposed in vivo. Dietary polyphenols actually undergo extensive modifications during first-pass metabolism, so that the forms entering the blood and tissues are generally not the same as the dietary sources. Thus, great efforts are warranted to define the biological activities of polyphenols in humans, taking into account their specific bioavailability and metabolism [168].

The main classes of polyphenols are defined according to the nature of their carbon skeleton: simple phenols and phenolic acids (1), flavonoids (2), the

Table 5. Main polyphenols

Simple phenols and phenolic acids	Flavonoids	Stilbenes and lignans	Ill-defined phenolic polymers
Tea	See table 6	Red grapes	Wines
Coffee		Wine	Tea
Vanilla		Berries	
Cherry		Peanuts	
Blueberry			
Citrus fruit		Flaxseed	
Plum		Whole-grain foods	
Whole-grain foods		Prunes	
		Garlic	
		Asparagus	

Table 6. Main flavonoids according to Scalbert et al. [167]

Isoflavones	Proanthocyanidins (polymeric flavanols)	Anthocyanins	Flavonols	Flavones	Flavanols	Flavanones
Soy beans	Fruit (pears, apples, grapes, …)	Berries	Onion	Parsley	Apricot	Citrus fruit
Red clover leaf		Wine	Curly kale	Red pepper	Tea	
Barley	Wine	Grapes	Leek	Celery	Red wine	
Brown rice	Tea	Tea	Broccoli	Citrus fruit	Grapes	
Whole wheat			Blueberry	Onion	Chocolate	
Flaxseed			Red wine		Apple	
			Green tea			
			Tomatoes			

less common stilbenes and lignans (3) and other ill-defined phenolic polymers (4). See table 5 for a schematic description of polyphenols.

Phenolic acids are very abundant in foods. The most common one is caffeic acid, often found in the form of esters (chlorogenic acid) that are present in many fruits and in coffee.

Flavonoids are the most abundant polyphenols in our diet. They can be divided into several classes according to the degree of oxidation of oxygen heterocycles (table 6): flavones, flavonols, flavanols, isoflavones, flavanones, anthocyanins and proanthocyanidins. However, the occurrence of some of these flavonoids is restricted to a few foodstuffs. For instance, the main source of isoflavones is soy, which contains about 1 mg of genistein and daidzein per gram of dry bean and has received considerable attention due to its estrogenic properties. Citrus fruits are the main sources of flavanones, the most commonly consumed form being hesperidin from oranges. Other flavonoids are common to various foods. The main flavonol in our diet is quercetin, which is present in many fruits, vegetables and beverages (wine). It is particularly abundant in onions and tea. Flavones are less common and were identified in red pepper and celery. The main flavanols are catechins, which are very abundant in tea. An infusion of green tea contains about 1 g/l catechins, whereas their content in black tea is reduced by about 50% due to fermentation. Other major sources of catechins are red wine and chocolate. Proanthocyanidins are polymeric flavanols present in plants as complex polymer blends. They are responsible for the astringency of foods. They are present in many fruits, including pears, apples and grapes, and in beverages such as wine and tea. Anthocyanins are pigments in red fruits such as berries, cherries, plums and grapes.

Stilbenes are not common in food plants. One of them, resveratrol, has recently received considerable attention for its potential anticarcinogenic properties and presence in very large amounts in wine. The dietary sources of lignans are essentially flaxseed (linseed) and flaxseed oil. These substances have been recognized as phytoestrogens.

Other dietary polyphenols are ill-defined chemical entities, usually resulting from food processing (fermentation, storage, cooking and other processes). These phenolic compounds are the main polyphenols in black tea and wine [167].

For a number of reasons, it is difficult to estimate the average daily intake of polyphenols. Most authors refer to data published more than 25 years ago and reporting a daily intake of 1 g of total phenols [169]. Plasma concentrations of the intact parent polyphenols are often low and do not account on their own for the increase in the antioxidant capacity of the plasma [167]. Metabolites also contribute to increase this antioxidant capacity. For instance, polyphenols can be methylated, and about 20% of the catechin present in the plasma 1 h only after the ingestion of red wine has been found to be methylated [170]. Microbial metabolites formed in the colon are also important, and equol may be 3–4 times more abundant in the plasma than the parent isoflavones [171]. The measurement of total plasma antioxidant capacity after consuming polyphenol-rich foods allows comparing the relative contribution of metabolites and parent polyphenols. Scalbert et al. [167] have calculated that after drinking 300 ml of red wine containing about 500 mg of polyphenols, the total polyphenol concentration is about 10 times higher than the calculated peak concentration of parent polyphenols, indicating that the metabolites formed in our tissues or by the microflora in the colon significantly contribute to the acquired antioxidant activity.

Tea, a popular drink in Northern Africa, the Mediterranean Middle East and Turkey, is a major source of flavonoids, and seems to reduce the risk of CHD.

Several studies in various populations have indeed suggested an inverse association between tea consumption and CHD, and a meta-analysis has confirmed this trend in spite of highly heterogeneous results between studies [174]. Geographic variations may explain this heterogeneity. Interestingly, the negative associations were found among drinkers of either black tea, as in Saudi Arabia [175], or green tea, as in Japan [176]. Finally, it is noteworthy that tea consumption was associated with beneficial effects on some major risk factors of CHD such as hypertension [177], obesity and body fat distribution [178], as well as on the risk of osteoporosis [179] and cancers [180]. All these data are in line with the healthy effect of the Med diets. However, no data from randomized trials are available.

Wine is another polyphenol-rich beverage whose moderate consumption has been associated with a reduced risk of CHD. Contrary to tea, in which there is practically no substance other than water and polyphenols to explain any health effect, wine also contains ethanol which is, by itself, a potent cardioprotective compound especially when taken in moderate amounts [181, 182]. One question is whether wine is more protective against CHD than other alcoholic beverages in relation with the presence of high amounts of polyphenols [183–186]. The presence of polyphenols in abundance in wine, but not in beer or spirits, should intuitively lead to think that wine drinking results in better protection. In fact, clinical and epidemiological data do not provide a concluding answer, because no study has been prospectively and specifically designed to compare the effect of the various alcoholic beverages. On the other hand, experimental data suggest that in addition to an effect on various parameters assumed to be associated with CHD, polyphenols may have a specific protective effect on the ischemic myocardium, a phenomenon called preconditioning [187]. Among polyphenols, resveratrol has been particularly studied in various experimental models, and data suggest that it may act through an effect on nitric oxide (NO) synthase activity and NO generation [188].

Whole-grain foods are emerging as dietary constituent that delivers significant health benefits. Several studies have provided strong support for a beneficial role of whole grain intake in reducing the risk of CHD [189]. Whole grains supply complex carbohydrates, resistant starch, dietary fiber, minerals, vitamins, and phytochemicals that can act as antioxidants. Whole-grain foods are indeed rich in phenolic acids as well as lignans that are formed of two phenylpropane units (a structure not very different from that of resveratrol). The main dietary source of lignans in the Western diet is linseed (flaxseed). Other cereals (wheat), grains, fruit (prunes), and certain vegetables (garlic, asparagus) also contain traces of lignans that are metabolized to enterodiol and enterolactone by the intestinal microflora and found in the blood and urine of animals and humans. However, the low amounts of lignans supplied by our normal diet do not account for the high concentrations of their metabolites measured in blood and urine. Other dietary sources of lignans, the precursors of enterodiol and enterolactone, have yet to be identified [190]. In a recently published prospective study, Finnish investigators found an inverse relation between high serum enterolactone levels (as a marker of a diet high in fiber and vegetables) and the risk of CHD death [191]. They also found an inverse association between F2-isoprostanes, a measure of lipid peroxidation, and serum enterolactone levels, suggesting that lignans may be protective through an antioxidant effect [192].

Vegetables and fruit are major sources of the different classes of polyphenols [193]. Their importance in the prevention of CHD has been the subject of many reviews, and a high consumption of vegetables and fruit is now one of the major lifestyle recommendations of the American Heart Association, the European Society of Cardiology and various Scientific and Research Councils [194].

Conclusions

Twelve years after the publication of the first trial testing the effects of a Med diet (a modified diet of Crete), and following hundreds of reports about its health effects, there is now a consensus to recommend this dietary pattern for the prevention of chronic diseases including CHD and cancer. The most important issue, in contrast with the pharmacological approach of the prevention of CHD, is that adherence to the Med diet results in a striking effect on survival, as also shown in several epidemiological studies. The main explanation is that the Med diet is protective not only against CHD but also against various chronic diseases, including cancers. Furthermore, contrary to drugs, no harmful side effects have been reported following the adoption of that dietary pattern.

The effectiveness of the Med diet to decrease overall and cause-specific mortality probably results mainly from the multiple biological and physiological changes induced by this diet [195]. Many energetic and nonenergetic micro- and macro-nutrients characteristic of the Med diet interact in synergy to induce states of resistance to these chronic diseases. New researches are needed to understand these complex interplays. There is obviously not a single 'Med diet' around the Mediterranean Sea. Dietary habits, agriculture, the types of food produced and the crops vary considerably from one area to another [196]. Finally, what the various experts and scientists involved in that research field consider the 'optimal diet' for the prevention of chronic diseases also varies greatly [197–199]. There is no doubt, however, that the concept of Med diet has been, and still is the basis of thinking and action to preserve health for the present as well as the future generations throughout the world.

References

1 Keys AB: Seven Countries: A Multivariate Analysis of Death and Coronary Heart Disease. A Commonwealth Fund Book. Cambridge, Harvard University Press, 1980, pp 1–381.
2 Sans S, Kesteloot H, Kromhout D: The burden of cardiovascular diseases mortality in Europe. Eur Heart J 1997;18:1231–1248.
3 Serra-Majem L, Ferro-Luzzi A, Bellizzi M, Salleras L: Nutrition policies in Mediterranean Europe. Nutr Rev 1997;55:S42–S57.
4 Willett WC, Sacks F, Trichopoulou A, et al: Mediterranean diet pyramid: a cultural model for healthy eating. Am J Clin Nutr 1995;61(suppl):1402S–1406S.
5 de Lorgeril M: Mediterranean diet in the prevention of coronary heart disease. Nutrition 1998;14:55–57.
6 Gjonca A, Bobak M: Albanian paradox, another example of protective effect of Mediterranean lifestyle? Lancet 1997;350:1815–1817.
7 de Lorgeril M, Salen P: Lessons from Albania. Lancet 1998;351:1440.
8 Hjermann I, Holme I, Leren P: Oslo Study Diet and Antismoking Trial. Results after 102 months. Am J Med 1986;80:7–11.
9 de Lorgeril M, Renaud S, Mamelle N, et al: Mediterranean alpha-linolenic acid-rich diet in secondary prevention of coronary heart disease. Lancet 1994;343:1454–1459.
10 Burr ML, Fehily AM, Gilbert JF, et al: Effects of changes in fat, fish, and fibre intakes on death and myocardial reinfarction: diet and reinfarction trial (DART). Lancet 1989;334:757–761.
11 de Lorgeril M, Salen P, Monjaud I, Delaye J: The diet heart hypothesis in secondary prevention of coronary heart disease. Eur Heart J 1997;18:14–18.
12 GISSI-Prevenzione Investigators: Dietary supplementation with n–3 polyunsaturated fatty acids and vitamin E after myocardial infarction: results of the GISSI-Prevenzione trial. Lancet 1999;354:447–455.
13 Gilman MW, Cupples LA, Gagnon D, et al: Protective effect of fruits and vegetables on development of stroke in men. JAMA 1995;273:1113–1117.
14 Rimm EB, Ascherio A, Giovannucci E, et al: Vegetable, fruit and cereal fiber intake and risk of coronary heart disease among men. JAMA 1996;275:447–451.
15 Key TJ, Thorogood M, Appleby PN, Burr ML: Dietary habits and mortality in 11,000 vegetarians and health conscious people: results of a 17-year follow-up. BMJ 1996;313:775–779.
16 Albert CM, Hennekens CH, O'Donnell CJ, et al: Fish consumption and risk of sudden death. JAMA 1998;279:23–28.
17 Daviglus ML, Stamler J, Orencia AJ, et al: Fish consumption and the 30-year risk of fatal myocardial infarction. N Engl J Med 1997;336:1046–1053.
18 Robinson K, Arheart K, Refsum H, et al: Low circulating folate and vitamin B6 concentrations: risk factors for stroke, peripheral vascular disease and coronary heart disease. Circulation 1998;97:437–443.
19 Stampfer MJ, Rimm EB: Folate and cardiovascular disease: why we need a trial now. JAMA 1996;275:1929–1930.
20 Verhaar MC, Wever RM, Kastelein JJ, et al: 5-Methyltetrahydrofolate, the active form of folic acid, restores endothelial function in familial hypercholesterolemia. Circulation 1998;97:237–241.
21 Wever RM, Lüscher TF, Cosentino F, Rabelink TJ: Atherosclerosis and the two faces of endothelial nitric oxide synthase. Circulation 1998;97:108–112.
22 de Lorgeril M, Salen P, Martin JL, et al: Effect of a Mediterranean-type of diet on the rate of cardiovascular complications in coronary patients: insights into the cardioprotective effect of certain nutriments. J Am Coll Cardiol 1996;28:1103–1108.
23 de Lorgeril M, Salen P, Martin JL, et al: Mediterranean diet, traditional risk factors and the rate of cardiovascular complications after myocardial infarction. Final report of the Lyon Diet Heart Study. Circulation 1999;99:779–785.
24 de Lorgeril M, Salen P, Caillat-Vallet E, et al: Control of bias in dietary trial to prevent coronary recurrences. The Lyon Diet Heart Study. Eur J Clin Nutr 1997;51:116–122.

25 de Lorgeril M, Salen P, Martin JL, et al: Mediterranean dietary pattern in a randomized trial: prolonged survival and possible reduced cancer rate. Arch Intern Med 1998;158:1181–1187.
26 Cummings JH, Bingham SA. Diet and the prevention of cancer. BMJ 1998;317:1636–1640.
27 Clark LC, Combs GF, Turnbull BW, et al: Effects of selenium supplementation for cancer prevention in patients with carcinoma of the skin: a randomized controlled trial. JAMA 1996;276:1957–1963.
28 Menendez JA, Papadimitropoulou A, Vellon L, et al: A genomic explanation connecting 'Mediterranean diet', olive oil and cancer: oleic acid, the main monounsaturated fatty acid of olive oil, induces formation of inhibitory 'PEA3 transcription factor-PEA3 DNA binding site' complexes at the Her-2/neu (erbB-2) oncogene promoter in breast, ovarian and stomach cancer cells. Eur J Cancer 2006;42:2425–2432.
29 Hashim YZ, Eng M, Gill CI, et al: Components of olive oil and chemoprevention of colorectal cancer. Nutr Rev 2005;63:374–386.
30 Fung TT, Hu FB, McCullough ML, et al: Diet quality is associated with the risk of estrogen-negative breast cancer in postmenopausal women. J Nutr 2006;136:466–472.
31 MacLean CH, Newberry SJ, Mojica WA, et al: Effects of omega-3 fatty acids on cancer risk: a systematic review. JAMA 2006;295:403–415.
32 Bougnoux P, Maillard V, Chajes V: Omega-6/omega-3 polyunsaturated fatty acids ratio and breast cancer. World Rev Nutr Diet. Basel, Karger, 2005, vol 94, pp 158–165.
33 Chan JM, Gann PH, Giovannucci EL: Role of diet in prostate cancer development and progression. J Clin Oncol 2005;32:8152–8160.
34 Larsson SC, Kumlin M, Ingelman-Sundberg M, Wolk A: Dietary long-chain n-3 fatty acids for the prevention of cancer: a review of potential mechanisms. Am J Clin Nutr 2004;79:935–945.
35 Norat T, Bingham S, Ferrari P, et al: Meat, fish and colorectal cancer risk: the European prospective investigation into cancer and nutrition. J Natl Cancer Inst 2005;97:906–916.
36 Whelan J, McEntee MF: Dietary n-6 PUFA and intestinal tumorigenesis. J Nutr 2004;134:3421S–3426S.
37 de Lorgeril M, Salen P: Modified Cretan Mediterranean diet in the prevention of coronary heart disease and cancer. World Rev Nutr Diet. Basel, Karger, 2000, vol 87, pp 1–23.
38 Singh RB, Dubnov G, Niaz MA, et al: Effect of an Indo-Mediterranean diet on progression of coronary artery disease in high risk patients (Indo-Mediterranean Diet Heart Study): a randomised single-blind trial. Lancet 2002;360:1455–1456.
39 Martinez-Gonzalez MA, Fernandez-Jarne E, Serrano-Martinez M, et al: Mediterranean diet and reduction in the risk of a first acute myocardial infarction: an operational healthy dietary score. Eur J Nutr 2002;41:153–160.
40 Barzi F, Woodward M, Marfisi RM, et al: Mediterranean diet and all-cause mortality after myocardial infarction: results from the GISSI-Prevenzione Trial. Eur J Clin Nutr 2003;57:604–611.
41 Trichopoulou A, Costacou T, Barnia C, Trichopoulos D: Adherence to a Mediterranean diet and survival in a Greek population. N Engl J Med 2003;348:2599–2608.
42 Panagiotakos DB, Pitsavos C, Polychronopoulos E, et al: Can a Mediterranean diet moderate the development and clinical progression of coronary heart disease? A systematic review. Med Sci Monit 2004;10:RA193–RA198.
43 Knoops KT, de Groot L, Kromhout D, et al: Mediterranean diet, lifestyle factors, and 10-year mortality in elderly European men and women. The HALE Project. JAMA 2004;292:1433–1439.
44 Trichopoulou A, Barnia C, Trichopoulos D: Mediterranean diet and survival among patients with coronary heart disease in Greece. Arch Intern Med 2005;165:929–935.
45 Trichopoulou A, Orfanos P, Norat T, et al: Modified Mediterranean diet and survival: EPIC-elderly prospective cohort study. BMJ 2005;330;991–998.
46 Appel LJ, Moore TJ, Obarzanek E, et al: The effect of dietary patterns of blood pressure: results from the dietary approach to stop hypertension trial (DASH). N Engl J Med 1997;336:1117–1124.
47 Strazzullo P, Ferro-Luzzi A, Siani A, et al: Changing the Mediterranean diet: effects on blood pressure. J Hypertens 1986;4:407–412.
48 Fraser G: Diet and coronary heart disease: beyond dietary fats and low-density lipoprotein cholesterol. Am J Clin Nutr 1994;59(suppl):1117S–1123S.
49 Ross R: Atherosclerosis: an inflammatory disease. N Engl J Med 1999;340:115–126.
50 de Lorgeril M, Latour JG: Leukocytes, thrombosis and unstable angina. N Engl J Med 1987;316:1161.

51 Moreno PR, Falk E, Palacios JF, et al: Macrophage infiltration in acute coronary syndromes. Implications for plaque rupture. Circulation 1994;90:775–778.
52 Van der Wal AC, Becker EC, Van der Los DS, Das PK: Site of intimal rupture or erosion of thrombosed coronary atherosclerotic plaques is characterized by an inflammatory process irrespective of the dominant plaque morphology. Circulation 1994;89:36–44.
53 Farb A, Burk AP, Tang AL, et al: Coronary plaque erosion without rupture into a lipid core: a frequent cause of coronary thrombosis in sudden coronary death. Circulation 1996;93:1354–1363.
54 Davies MJ, Thomas A: Thrombosis and acute coronary-artery lesions in sudden cardiac ischemic death. N Engl J Med 1984;310:1137–1140.
55 de Lorgeril M, Basmadjian A, Lavalleée M, et al: Influence of leukopenia on collateral flow, reperfusion flow, reflow ventricular fibrillation, and infarct size in dogs. Am Heart J 1989;117:523–532.
56 Kuzuya T, Hoshida S, Suzuki K, et al: Polymorphonuclear leukocyte activity and ventricular arrhythmia in acute myocardial infarction. Am J Cardiol 1988;62:868–872.
57 Liuzzo G, Biasucci LM, Gallimore JR, et al: The prognostic value of C-reactive protein and serum amyloid a protein in severe unstable angina. N Engl J Med 1994;331:417–424.
58 Kovanen PT, Kaartinen M, Paavonen T: Infiltrates of activated mast cells at the site of coronary atheromatous erosion or rupture in myocardial infarction. Circulation 1995;92:1084–1088.
59 Ernst E, Hammerschmidt DE, Bagge U, Matrai A, Dormandy JA: Leukocytes and the risk of ischemic heart diseases. JAMA 1987;257:2318–2324.
60 Kruskal JB, Commerford PJ, Franks JJ, Kirsch RE: Fibrin and fibrinogen-related antigens in patients with stable and unstable coronary artery disease. N Engl J Med 1987;317:1361–1365.
61 Fuentes F, Lopez-Miranda J, Sanchez E, et al: Mediterranean and low-fat diets improve endothelial function in hypercholesterolemic men. Arch Intern Med 2001;134:1115–1119.
62 Chrysohoou C, Panagiotakos DB, Pitsavos C, et al: Adherence to the Mediterranean diet attenuates inflammation and coagulation process in healthy adults. The ATTICA Study. J Am Coll Cardiol 2004;44:152–158.
63 Esposito K, Marfella R, Ciotola M, et al: Effect of a Mediterranean-style diet on endothelial dysfunction and markers of vascular inflammation in the metabolic syndrome: a randomized trial. JAMA 2004;292:1440–1446.
64 Serrano-Martinez M, Palacios M, Martinez-Losa E, et al: A Mediterranean dietary style influences TNF-alpha and VCAM-1 coronary blood levels in unstable angina patients. Eur J Nutr 2005;44:348–354.
65 Steinberg D, Parthasarathy S, Carew TE, Khoo JC, Witztum JL: Beyond cholesterol: modifications of low-density lipoproteins that increase its atherogenicity. N Engl J Med 1989;320:915–924.
66 Heart Protection Study Collaborative Group: MRC:BHF heart protection study of cholesterol lowering with simvastatin in 20,536 high-risk individuals: a randomised placebo-controlled trial. Lancet 2002;360:7–22.
67 Shepherd J, Blauw JG, Murphy MB, et al: Pravastatin in elderly individuals at risk of vascular disease (PROSPER): a randomised controlled trial. Lancet 2002;360:1623–1630.
68 The ALLHAT Officers and Coordinators for the ALLHAT Collaborative Research Group: Major outcomes in moderately hypercholesterolemic, hypertensive patients randomized to pravastatin vs. usual care: the Antihypertensive and Lipid-Lowering Treatment to prevent Heart Attack Trial (ALLHAT-LLT). JAMA 2002;288:2998–3007.
69 Sever PS, Dahlöf B, Poulter NR, et al: Prevention of coronary and stroke events with atorvastatin in hypertensive patients who have average or lower-than average cholesterol concentrations in the Anglo-Scandinavian Cardiac Outcomes Trial – Lipid Lowering Arm (ASCOT-LLA): a multicentre randomised controlled trial. Lancet 2003;361:1149–1158.
70 Koren MJ, Hunninghake DB, ALLIANCE Investigators: Clinical outcomes in managed-care patients with coronary heart disease treated aggressively in lipid-lowering diseases management clinics. The ALLIANCE Study. JACC 2004;44:1772–1779.
71 Griendling KK, Alexander RW: Oxidative stress and cardiovascular disease. Circulation 1997;96:3264–3265.
72 Liao F, Andalibi F, Qiao JH, et al: Genetic evidence for a common pathway mediating oxidative stress, inflammatory gene induction and aortic fatty streak formation in mice. J Clin Invest 1994;94:877–884.

73 Avogaro P, Bon GB, Cazzolato G: Presence of modified low density lipoproteins in humans. Arteriosclerosis 1988;8:79–87.
74 Hodis HN, Kramsch DM, Avogaro P, et al: Biochemical and cytotoxic characteristics of an in vivo circulating oxidized low density lipoprotein. J Lipid Res 1994;35:669–677.
75 Juul K, Nielsen LB, Munkholm K, Stender S, Nordestgaard BG: Oxidation of plasma low-density lipoprotein accelerates its accumulation in the arterial wall in vivo. Circulation 1996;94: 1698–1704.
76 Holvoet P, Vanhaecke J, Janssens S, Van de Werf F, Collen D: Oxidized LDL and malondialdehyde-modified LDL in patients with acute coronary syndromes and stable coronary artery disease. Circulation 1998;98:1487–1494.
77 Holvoet P, Stassen JM, Van Cleemput J, Collen D, Vanhaecke J: Correlation between oxidized low density lipoproteins and coronary artery disease in heart transplant patients. Arterioscler Thromb Vasc Biol 1998;18:100–107.
78 Chancerelle Y, de Lorgeril M, Viret R, et al: Increased lipid peroxidation in cyclosporin-treated heart transplant recipients. Am J Cardiol 1991;68:813–817.
79 de Lorgeril M, Richard MJ, Arnaud J, et al: Lipid peroxides and antioxidant defenses in accelerated transplantation-associated arteriosclerosis. Am Heart J 1992;125:974–980.
80 Holvoet P, Perez G, Zhao Z, et al: Malondialdehyde-modified low density lipoproteins in patients with atherosclerotic disease. J Clin Invest 1995;95:2611–2619.
81 Ambrosio G, Tritto I, Golino P: Reactive oxygen metabolites and arterial thrombosis. Cardiovasc Res 1997;34:445–452.
82 de Lorgeril M, Dureau G, Boissonnat P, et al: Platelet function and composition in heart transplant recipients compared with nontransplanted coronary patients. Arterioscler Thromb 1992;12:222–230.
83 Ambrosio G, Golino P, Pascucci I, et al: Modulation of platelet function by reactive oxygen metabolites. Am J Physiol 1994;267:H308–H318.
84 Hollar D, Hennekens CH: Antioxidant vitamins and cardiovascular disease: randomized trials fail to fulfil the promises of observational epidemiology; in Bourassa MG, Tardif JC (eds): Antioxidant and Cardiovascular Diseases, ed 2. New York, Springer, 2006, pp 305–325.
85 Zock PL, Katan MB: Diet, LDL oxidation and coronary artery disease. Am J Clin Nutr 1998;68: 759–760.
86 Parks EJ, German JB, Davis PA, et al: Reduced oxidative susceptibility of LDL from patients participating in an intensive atherosclerosis treatment program. Am J Clin Nutr 1998;68:778–785.
87 Louheranta AM, Porkkala-Sarataho EK, Nyyssönen MK, Salonen RM, Salonen JT: Linoleic acid intake and susceptibility of very-low-density and low-density lipoproteins to oxidation in men. Am J Clin Nutr 1996;63:698–703.
88 Bonamone A, Pagnan A, Biffanti S, et al: Effect of dietary monounsaturated and polyunsaturated fatty acids on the susceptibility of plasma low density lipoproteins to oxidative modification. Arterioscler Thromb 1992;12:529–533.
89 Tsimikas S, Reaven PD: The role of dietary fatty acids in lipoprotein oxidation and atherosclerosis. Curr Opin Lipidol 1998;9:301–307.
90 Mata P, Alonso R, Lopez-Farre A, et al: Effect of dietary fat saturation on LDL and monocyte adhesion to human endothelial cells in vitro. Arterioscler Thromb Vasc Biol 1996;16:1347–1355.
91 Tsimikas S, Philis-Tsimikas A, Alexopoulos S, et al: LDL isolated from Greek subjects on a typical diet or from American subjects on an oleate-supplemented diet induces less monocyte chemotaxis and adhesion when exposed to oxidative stress. Arterioscler Thromb Vasc Biol 1999;19: 122–130.
92 Visioli F, Bellomo G, Montedoro F, et al: Low density lipoprotein oxidation is inhibited in vitro by olive oil constituents. Atherosclerosis 1995;117:25–32.
93 Porkkala-Sarataho EK, Nyyssönen MK, Kaikkonen JE, et al: A randomized single-blind placebo controlled trial of the effects of 200 mg alpha-tocopherol on the oxidation resistance of atherogenic lipoproteins. Am J Clin Nutr 1998;68:134–141.
94 Jialial I, Grundy SM: Effect of combined supplementation with alpha-tocopherol, ascorbate and beta-carotene on low density lipoprotein oxidation. Circulation 1993;88:2780–2786.
95 Siow RC, Sato H, Leake DS, et al: Vitamin C protects human arterial smooth muscle cells against atherogenic lipoproteins. Arterioscler Thromb Vasc Biol 1998;18:1662–1670.

96 Miller III ER, Appel LJ, Risby TH: Effect of dietary patterns on measures of lipid peroxidation: results of a randomized clinical trial. Circulation 1998;98:2390–2395.
97 Felton CV, Crook D, Davies MJ, Oliver MF: Dietary polyunsaturated fatty acids and composition of human aortic plaques. Lancet 1994;344:1195–1196.
98 Rapp JH, Connor WE, Lin DS, Porter JM: Dietary eicosapentanoic acid and docosahexaenoic acid from fish oil: their incorporation into advanced human atherosclerotic plaques. Arterioscler Thromb 1991;11:903–911.
99 Lee TH, Hoover RL, Williams JD, et al: Effect of dietary enrichment with eisosapentaenoic and docosahexaenoic acids on in vitro neutrophil and monocyte leukotriene generation and neutrophile function. N Engl J Med 1985;312:1217–1224.
100 Singer SJ, Nicolson GL: The fluid-mosaic model of the structure of the cell membranes. Science 1972;175:720–731.
101 Stubbs CD, Smith AD: The modification of the mammalian membrane polyunsaturated fatty acid composition in relation to membrane fluidity. Biochim Biophys Acta 1984;779:89–137.
102 Sandker GN, Kromhout D, Aravanis C, et al: Serum cholesteryl ester fatty acids and their relation with serum lipids in elderly men in Crete and Netherlands. Eur J Clin Nutr 1993;47:201–208.
103 Simopoulos AP, Norman HA, Gillapsy JE, Duke JA: Common purslane: a source of omega-3 fatty acids and antioxidants. J Am Coll Nutr 1992;11:374–382.
104 Simopoulos AP, Salem N: n–3 fatty acids in eggs from range-fed Greek chickens. N Engl J Med 1989;321:1412.
105 de Lorgeril M, Salen P: Alpha-linolenic acid and coronary heart disease. Nutr Metab Cardiovasc Dis 2004;14:162–169.
106 Baylin A, Kabagambe EK, Ascherio A, Spiegelman D, Campos H: Adipose tissue alpha-linolenic acid and nonfatal acute myocardial infarction: Costa Rica. Circulation 2003;107:1586–1591.
107 Hu FB, Stampfer MJ, Manson JE, et al: Dietary intake of alpha-linolenic acid and risk of fatal ischemic heart disease among women. Am J Clin Nutr 1999;69:890–897.
108 Djousse L, Pankow JS, Eckfeldt JH, et al: Relation between linolenic acid and coronary artery disease in the national Heart, Lung, and Blood Institute Family Heart Study. Am J Clin Nutr 2001;74:612–619.
109 Albert CM, Kyungwon O, Whang W, Manson JE, Chae CU, Stampfer MJ, Willett WC, Hu F: Dietary alpha-linolenic acid intake and risk of sudden cardiac death and coronary heart disease. Circulation 2005;112:3232–3238.
110 Kromhout D, Bosschieter EB, de Lezenne Coulander C: The inverse relation between fish consumption and 20-year mortality from coronary heart disease. N Engl J Med 1985;312:1205–1209.
111 Kris-Etherton P, Harris W, Appel LJ: Fish consumption, fish oil, omega-3 fatty acids and cardiovascular disease. Circulation 2002;106:2747–2757.
112 Siscovick D, Lemaitre R, Mozaffarian D: The fish story. A diet-heart hypothesis with clinical implications: n–3 polyunsaturated fatty acids, myocardial vulnerability, and sudden death. Circulation 2003;107:2632–2634.
113 Kromhout D: Fish consumption and sudden cardiac death. JAMA 1998;278:65–66.
114 Billman GE, Kang JX, Leaf A: Prevention of sudden cardiac death by dietary pure omega-3 polyunsaturated fatty acids in dogs. Circulation 1999;99:2452–2457.
115 Leaf A, Albert CM, Josephson M, Steinhaus D, Kugler J, Kang JX, Cox B, Zhang H, Schoenfeld D, for the Fatty Acid Antiarrhythmia Trial Investigators: Prevention of fatal arrhythmias in high-risk subjects by fish oil n–3 fatty acid intake. Circulation 2005;112:2762–2768.
116 Emken EA, Adolf RO, Rakoff H, Rohwedder WK: Metabolism of deuterium-labeled linolenic, linoleic, oleic, stearic and palmitic acid in human subjects; in Baillie TA, Jones JR (eds): Synthesis and Applications of Isotopically Labeled Compounds. Amsterdam, Elsevier, 1989, pp 713–716.
117 Serhan CN, Haeggstrom JZ, Leslie CC: Lipid mediator network in cell signaling: update and impact of cytokines. FASEB J 1996;10:1147–1158.
118 Serhan CN: Lipoxin biosynthesis and its impact in inflammatory and vascular events. Biochim Biophys Acta 1994;1212:1–25.
119 Serhan CN, Razen JM: Anti-inflammatory potential of lipoxygenase-derived eicosanoids: molecular switch at 5 and 15 positions? J Clin Invest 1997;99:1147–1148.

120 Kuhn H, Heydeck D, Hugou I, Gniwotta C: In vivo action of 15-lipoxygenase in early stages of human atherogenesis. J Clin Invest 1997;99:888–893.
121 Folcik V, Nivar-Aristy RA, Krajewski LP, Cathcart MK: Lipoxygenase contributes to the oxidation of lipids in human atherosclerotic plaques. J Clin Invest 1995;96:504–510.
122 Wong SCY, Fukuchi M, Melnik P, Rodger I, Giaid A: Induction of cyclooxygenase-2 and activation of nuclear factor-kB in the myocardium of patients with congestive heart failure. Circulation 1998;98:100–107.
123 Morrow JD, Hill KE, Burk RF, et al: A series of prostaglandin F2-like compounds are produced in vivo in humans by a non-cyclooxygenase, free radical-catalyzed mechanism. Proc Natl Acad Sci USA 1990;87:9383–9387.
124 Morrow JD, Roberts LJ: The isoprostanes: unique bioactive products of lipid peroxidation. Prog Lipid Res 1997;36:1–21.
125 Reilly MP, Pratico D, Delanty N, et al: Increased formation of distinct F2 isoprostanes in hypercholesterolemia. Circulation 1998;98:2822–2828.
126 Mallat Z, Philip I, Lebret M, et al: Elevated levels of 8-iso-prostaglandin F2alpha in pericardial fluid of patients with heart failure. Circulation 1998;97:1536–1539.
127 Gniwotta C, Morrow JD, Roberts LJ, Kuhn H: Prostaglandin F2-like compounds, F2-isoprostanes, are present in increased amounts in human atherosclerotic lesions. Arterioscler Thromb Vasc Biol 1997;17:3236–3241.
128 Pratico D, Tangirala RK, Rader DJ, Rokach J, Fitzgerald GA: Vitamin E suppresses isoprostane generation in vivo and reduces atherosclerosis in ApoE-deficient mice. Nat Med 1998;4:1189–1192.
129 Pitsavos C, Panagiotakos DB, Tzima N, et al: Adherence to the Mediterranean diet is associated with total antioxidant capacity in healthy adults. Am J Clin Nutr 2005;82:694–699.
130 Lapointe A, Goulet J, Couillard C, et al: A nutritional intervention promoting the Mediterranean food pattern is associated with a decrease in circulating oxidized LDL particles in healthy women from the Québec City Metropolitan area. J Nutr 2005;135:410–415.
131 Boushey CJ, Beresford SA, Omenn GS, Motulsky AG: A quantitative assessment of plasma homocysteine as a risk factor for vascular disease: probable benefits of increasing folic acid intakes. JAMA 1995;274:1049–1057.
132 Genest JJ, McNamara JR, Salem DR, et al: Plasma homocysteine levels in men with premature coronary artery disease. J Am Coll Cardiol 1990;16:1114–1119.
133 Arnesen E, Refsum H, Bonaa KH, et al: Serum total homocysteine and coronary heart disease. Int J Epidemiol 1995;24:704–709.
134 Malinow MR: Plasma homocysteine: a risk factor for arterial occlusive disease. J Nutr 1996;126:1238S–1243S.
135 Pancharuniti N, Lewis CA, Sauberlich HE, et al: Plasma homocysteine, folate and vitamin B_{12} concentrations and risk for early-onset coronary heart disease. Am J Clin Nutr 1994;59:940–948.
136 Morrison HI, Schaubel D, Desmeules M, Wigle DT: Serum folate and risk of fatal coronary heart disease. JAMA 1996;275:1893–1896.
137 Matthews RG, Kaufman S: Characterisation of the dihydropterin reductase activity of pig liver methylenetetrahydrofolate reductase. J Biol Chem 1980;255:6014–6017.
138 Dusitanond P, Eikelboom JW, Hankey GJ, et al: Homocysteine-lowering treatment with folic acid, cobalamin, and pyridoxine does not reduce blood markers of inflammation, endothelial dysfunction, or hypercoagulability in patients with previous transient ischemic attack or stroke: a randomized substudy of the VITATOPS trial. Stroke 2005;36:144–146.
139 Lange H, Suryapranata H, De Luca G, et al: Folate therapy and in-stent restenosis after coronary stenting. N Engl J Med 2004;350:2673–2681.
140 Schnyder G, Roffi M, Pin R, et al: Decreased rate of coronary restenosis after lowering of plasma homocysteine levels. N Engl J Med 2001;345:1593–1600.
141 Toole JF, Malinow MR, Chambless LE, et al: Lowering homocysteine in patients with ischemic stroke, myocardial infarction, and death: the Vitamin Intervention for Stroke Prevention (VISP) randomized controlled trial. JAMA 2004;291:565–575.
142 Sato Y, Honda Y, Iwamoto J, et al: Effect of folate and mecobalamin on hip fractures in patients with strokes: a randomized controlled trial. JAMA 2005;293:1082–1088.

143 Dedoussis GV, Panagiotakos DB, Chrysohou C, et al: Effect of interaction between adherence to a Mediterranean diet and the methylenetetrahydrofolate reductase 677C-T mutation on homocysteine concentrations in healthy adults: the ATTICA Study. Am J Clin Nutr 2004;80:849–854.
144 Tavani A, La Vecchia C: Fruit and vegetable consumption and cancer risk in a Mediterranean population. Am J Clin Nutr 1995;61(suppl):1374S–1377S.
145 Byers T, Perry G: Dietary carotenes, vitamin C, and vitamin E as protective antioxidants in human cancers. Annu Rev Nutr 1992;12:139–159.
146 Klurfeld DM: Dietary fibre-mediated mechanisms in carcinogenesis. Cancer Res 1991;52:2055S–2059S.
147 MacLennan R, Macrae F, Bain C, et al: Randomized trial of intake of fat, fiber, and beta-carotene to prevent colorectal adenomas: the Australian Polyp Prevention Project. J Natl Cancer Inst 1995;87:1760–1766.
148 Cave WT: Dietary n–3 (omega-3) polyunsaturated fatty acid effects on animal tumorigenesis. FASEB J 1991;5:2160–2166.
149 World Health Organisation: World Health Statistics Annual. Geneva, World Health Organisation, 1992.
150 Block G, Patterson B, Subar A: Fruit, vegetables and cancer prevention: a review of the epidemiological evidence. Nutr Cancer 1992;18:1–29.
151 Steinmetz KA, Potter JD: Vegetables, fruit and cancer: mechanisms. Cancer Causes Control 1991;2:427–442.
152 The Alpha-Tocopherol, Beta Carotene Cancer Prevention Study Group: The effect of vitamin E and beta carotene on the incidence of lung cancer and other cancers in male smokers. N Engl J Med 1994;330:1029–1035.
153 Greenberg ER, Baron JA, Tosteson TD, et al: A clinical trial of antioxidant vitamins to prevent colorectal adenoma. N Engl J Med 1994;331:141–147.
154 Hennekens CH, Buring JE, Manson JE, et al: Lack of effect of long-term supplementation with beta carotene on the incidence of malignant neoplasms and cardiovascular disease. N Engl J Med 1996;334:1145–1149.
155 Omenn GS, Goodman GE, Thornquist MD, et al: Effects of combination of beta carotene and vitamin A on lung cancer and cardiovascular disease. N Engl J Med 1996;334:1150–1155.
156 Yoshizawa K, Willett WC, Morris SJ, et al: Study of prediagnostic selenium level in toenails and the risk of advanced prostate cancer. J Natl Cancer Inst 1998;90:1219–1224.
157 Grffin AC: The chemoprevention role of selenium carcinogenesis; in Arnott MS, van Eys J, Wang Y-M (eds): Molecular Interrelations of Nutrition and Cancer. New York, Raven Press, 1982, pp 401–408.
158 Marnett LJ: Aspirin and the potential role of prostaglandins in colon cancer. Cancer Res 1992;52:5575–5589.
159 Kaminski WE, Jendraschak E, Kiefl R, Von Schacky C: Dietary w–3 fatty acids lower levels of platelet-derived growth factor mRNA in human mononuclear cells. Blood 1993;81:1871–1879.
160 Marcus AJ: Aspirin as prophylaxis against colorectal cancer. N Engl J Med 1995;333:656–658.
161 Michalsen A, Lehmann N, Pithan C, et al: Mediterranean diet has no effect on markers of inflammation and metabolic risk factors in patients with coronary artery disease. Eur J Clin Nutr 2006;60:478–485.
162 Alonso A, Martinez-Gonzales MA: Olive oil consumption and reduced incidence of hypertension: the SUN Study. Lipids 2004;39:1233–1238.
163 Psaltopoulou T, Naska A, Orfanos P, et al: Olive oil, the Mediterranean diet and arterial blood pressure: the Greek European Prospective Investigation into Cancer and Nutrition (EPIC) study. Am J Clin Nutr 2004;80:1012–1018.
164 Schröder H, Marrugat J, Vila M, et al: Adherence to the traditional Mediterranean diet is inversely associated with body mass index and obesity in a Spanish population. J Nutr 2004;134: 3355–3361.
165 Trichopoulou A, Naska A, Orfanos P, Trichopoulos D: Mediterranean diet in relation to body mass index and waist-to-hip ratio: the Greek European Prospective Investigation into cancer and Nutrition study. Am J Clin Nutr 2005;82:935–940.
166 Garaulet M, Pérez-Llamas F, Pérez-Alaya M, et al: Site-specific differences in the fatty acid composition of abdominal adipose tissue in an obese population from a Mediterranean area: relation

with dietary fatty acids, plasma lipid profile, serum insulin, and central obesity. Am J Clin Nutr 2001;74:585–591.
167 Scalbert A, Williamson G: Dietary intake and bioavailability of polyphenols. J Nutr 2000;130: 2073S–2085S.
168 Kroon PA, Clifford MN, Crozier A, et al: How should we assess the effects of exposure to dietary polyphenols in vitro? Am J Clin Nutr 2004;80:15–21.
169 Kühnau J: The flavonoids: a class of semi-essential food components: their role in human nutrition. World Rev Nutr Diet. Basel, Karger, 1976, vol 24, pp 117–191.
170 Donovan JL, Bell JR, Kasin-Karakas S, et al: Catechin is present as metabolites in human plasma after consumption of red wine. J Nutr 1999;129:1662–1668.
171 Cassidy A, Bingham S, Setchell KD: Biological effects of a diet of soy protein rich in isoflavones on the menstrual cycle of premenopausal women. Am J Clin Nutr 1994;60:333–340.
172 Peters U, Poole C, Arab L: Does tea affect cardiovascular disease? A meta-analysis. Am J Epidemiol 2001;154:495–503.
173 Hakim IA, Alsaif MA, Alduwaihy M, et al: Tea consumption and the prevalence of coronary heart disease in Saudi adults: results from a Saudi national Study. Prev Med 2003;36:64–70.
174 Sasazuki S, Kodama H, Yoshimasu K, et al: Relation between green tea consumption and the severity of coronary atherosclerosis among Japanese men and women. Ann Epidemiol 2000;10: 401–408.
175 Yang YC, Lu FH, Wu JS, Chang CJ: The protective effect of habitual tea consumption on hypertension. Arch Intern Med 2004;164:1534–1540.
176 Wu CH, Lu FH, Chang CS, et al: Relationship among habitual tea consumption, percent body fat, and body fat distribution. Obes Res 2003;11:1088–1095.
177 Wu CH, Yang YC, Yao WJ, et al: Epidemiological evidence of increased bone mineral density in habitual tea drinkers. Arch Intern Med 2002;162:1001–1006.
178 Wu AH, Yu MC, Tseng CC, et al: Green tea and risk of breast cancer in Asian Americans. Int J Cancer 2003;106:574 579.
179 Rimm EB, Giovannucci EL, Willett WC, et al: Prospective study of alcohol consumption and risk of coronary disease in men. Lancet 1991;338:464–468.
180 Thun MJ, Peto R, Lopez AD, et al: Alcohol consumption and mortality among middle-aged and elderly US adults. N Engl J Med 1997;337:1705–1714.
181 Gronbaek M, Deis A, Sorensen T, et al: Mortality associated with moderate intakes of wine, beer, or spirits. BMJ 1995;310:1165–1169.
182 Di Castelnuovo A, Rotondo S, Iacoviello L, Donati MB, de Gaetano G: Meta-analysis of wine and beer consumption in relation to vascular risk. Circulation 2002;105:2836–2844.
183 Renaud S, de Lorgeril M: Wine, alcohol, platelet aggregation and the French Paradox for coronary heart disease. Lancet 1992;339:1523–1526.
184 de Lorgeril M, Salen P, Martin JL, et al: Wine drinking and risks of cardiovascular complications after recent acute myocardial infarction. Circulation 2002;106:1465–1469.
185 de Lorgeril M, Salen P, Guiraud A, et al: Resveratrol and non-ethanolic components of wine in experimental cardiology. Nutr Metab Cardiovasc Dis 2003;13:100–103.
186 Hattori R: Pharmacological preconditioning with resveratrol: role of nitric oxide. Am J Physiol Heart Circ Physiol 2002;282:H1988–H1995.
187 Anderson JW, Hanna TJ: Whole grains and protection against coronary heart disease: what are the active components and mechanisms? Am J Clin Nutr 1999;70:307–308.
188 Heinonen S, Nurmi T, Liukkonen K, et al: In vitro metabolism of plant lignans: new precursors of mammalian lignans enterolactone and enterodiol. J Agric Food Chem 2001;49:3178–3186.
189 Vanharanta M, Voutilainen S, Rissanen TH, et al: Risk of cardiovascular disease-related and all-cause death according to serum concentrations of enterolactone: Kuopio Ischaemic Heart Disease Risk Factor Study. Arch Intern Med 2003;163:1099–1104.
190 Vanharanta M, Voutilainen S, Nurmi T, et al: Association between low serum enterolactone and increased plasma F2-isoprostanes, a measure of lipid peroxidation. Atherosclerosis 2002;160: 465–469.
191 Manach C, Scalbert A, Morand C, et al: Polyphenols: food sources and bioavailability. Am J Clin Nutr 2004;79:727–747.

192 National Academy of Sciences, Committee on Diet and Health, National Research Council: Diet and Health: Implications for Reducing Chronic Disease Risk. Washington, National Academy Press, 1989.
193 Hu F: The Mediterranean diet and mortality: olive oil and beyond. N Engl J Med 2003;348:2595–2596.
194 de Lorgeril M, Salen P, Paillard F, et al: Mediterranean diet and the French paradox: two distinct biogeographic concepts for one consolidated scientific theory on the role of nutrition in coronary heart disease. Cardiovasc Res 2003;54:503–515.
195 Simopoulos AP, Visioli F: Mediterranean Diets. World Rev Nutr Diet. Basel, Karger, 2000, vol 87, pp 1–184.
196 Hu F, Willett W: Optimal diet for prevention of coronary heart disease. JAMA 2002;288:2569–2578.
197 Serra-Majem L, Trichopoulou A, Ngo de la Cruz J, et al: Does the definition of the Mediterranean diet to be updated? Publ Health Nutr 2004;7:927–929.
198 Ferro-Luzzi A, James WPT, Kafatos A: The high-fat Greek diet: a recipe for all? Eur J Clin Nutr 2002;56:796–809.
199 Trichopoulos D: In defense of the Mediterranean diet. Eur J Clin Nutr 2002;56:928–929.

Michel de Lorgeril
Nutrition, Vieillissement et Maladies Cardiovasculaires (NVMCV)
UFR de Médecine, Domaine de la Merci
FR–38706 La Tronche Cedex (France)
Tel. +33 476 63 74 71/476 63 71 52, Fax +33 476 63 71 52
E-Mail michel.delorgeril@ujf-grenoble.fr

Endothelial Nitric Oxide Synthase as a Mediator of the Positive Health Effects of Mediterranean Diets and Wine against Metabolic Syndrome

Federico Leighton, Inés Urquiaga

Laboratorio de Nutrición Molecular, Facultad de Ciencias Biológicas, Universidad Católica de Chile, Santiago, Chile

The Mediterranean diet is associated with lower rate of all-causes mortality, coronary heart disease, cardiovascular disease and cancer. The benefits of Mediterranean diets have been attributed to a large consumption of antioxidants, especially polyphenols, provided by fruits, vegetables and wine; and to the type of fat, especially monounsaturated fat from virgin olive oil, and omega-3 polyunsaturated fatty acids (PUFA) from vegetables and fish [1, 2]. In the case of wine, both ethanol and polyphenols are considered the bioactive components with regard to health effects. The targets, on which the study of these effects has concentrated, correspond to cardiovascular risk factors. Four main domains are considered: plasma lipid metabolism, haemostatic mechanisms, endothelial function regulation, and antioxidant defense mechanisms.

Plasma Lipid Metabolism

The Mediterranean diets change the pattern of plasma fatty acids as a result of their food composition. The omega-3 polyunsaturated fatty acid alpha-linolenic acid is a major component of the Mediterranean diets [3] and it has been detected in high concentration in the plasma of the Greek population [4]. Intervention studies have shown that Mediterranean diets increase plasma omega-3 polyunsaturated fatty acids and reduce plasma omega-6/omega-3 ratios [5, 6]. The Lyon Heart Study, for the secondary prevention of coronary heart disease (CHD), showed the positive effect of a Mediterranean-type diet enriched with alpha-linolenic acid [7]. The major effect of omega-3 polyunsaturated fatty acids appears to be anti-arrhythmic in this study. The emphasis is on the dietary ratio of linoleic acid and alpha-linolenic acid, rather than the absolute amounts of alpha-linolenic acid. The competition between these two essential PUFAs for their entry into the elongation and desaturation pathways responsible for the synthesis of eicosanoids is critical for the disease prevention activity of omega-3 fatty acids. The consumption of fish is also associated with a significant reduction in CHD mortality. This effect has been attributed to the cardioprotective effect of long-chain omega-3 polyunsaturated fatty acids, eicosapentaenoic acid (EPA) and docosahexaenoic acid (DHA). The omega-3 polyunsaturated fatty acids in fish oils suppress cardiac arrhythmias and reduce triacylglycerides, but have little effect on low-density lipoprotein (LDL) or high-density lipoprotein (HDL) cholesterol levels [8, 9].

Mediterranean diets are high in monounsaturated fatty acids (MUFA) because of the olive oil. Ecological and prospective cohort studies have shown an inverse association between intake of MUFA and CHD. Oleic acid exerts significant beneficial effects on atherosclerosis and thrombosis. Replacement of saturated or trans unsaturated fats with monounsaturated fats from vegetable oils, leads to a reduction in LDL cholesterol without decreasing the concentration of HDL cholesterol [8, 10].

The ATTICA Study showed that adherence to the traditional Mediterranean diet was associated with a reduction in the triacylglycerides plasma levels ($p = 0.02$) and an increase in the HDL cholesterol levels ($p = 0.03$) [11]. In this investigation, 1,514 men and 1,528 women from Attica in Greece were randomly enrolled. Among several factors, adherence to the Mediterranean diet was assessed by a diet score that incorporated the inherent characteristics of this diet.

Some intervention studies with a Mediterranean-type diet have observed improvements in the plasma lipid profile. In a 3-month intervention study to assess the effect on lipid profiles of a Mediterranean-type diet which was effective for weight loss, a favorable effect on HDL and triacylglycerides levels and a neutral effect on total cholesterol and LDL level were found [12]. In 155 patients, 55 years average age, triacylglycerides level decreased by 31.6% and HDL increased by 9.6%. In 2 years of intervention with a Mediterranean-style diet and a control diet on metabolic syndrome patients, Esposito et al. [13] showed significant decreases in total cholesterol and triacylglycerides, and a significant increase in HDL cholesterol, all of which were greater in the Mediterranean group than those recorded in the control group, with $p < 0.03$ when comparing between groups.

Among plasma lipids, the changes in HDL appear as the most relevant after wine consumption, and higher HDL levels closely correlate with decreased CHD. Ethanol increases HDL levels. In a meta-analysis with data from 36 different studies, Rimm et al. [14] clearly show a dose-dependent relationship among ethanol consumption and plasma levels of HDL, yet the mechanism of the protective effect of elevated HDL levels has not been clearly established. Reverse cholesterol transport is considered an important mechanism, but recently a new paradigm for the cardiovascular effects of HDL and estrogens that involves endothelial nitric oxide synthase (eNOS) has been proposed [15]. These authors conclude that HDL from males, but strikingly more in the case of HDL from pre-menopausal women because of the associated estradiol, stimulate eNOS and vasodilatation in a scavenger receptor class B type I-dependent manner. The scavenger receptor acts as an HDL docking receptor, allowing for estradiol transfer. This finding is consistent with the established fact that women, before menopause, are more protected than men against cardiovascular disease [16]. A transport role for HDL, mediated by scavenger receptor class B type I, has also been shown for vitamin E [17]. Assuming that the stimulation of eNOS is a key mechanism to explain the effects of increased levels of HDL in response to ethanol, it is necessary to consider that the function of eNOS is strictly dependent on the presence of antioxidants that prevent nitric oxide (NO) inactivation by its reaction with superoxide anion and peroxynitrite generation. Also BH4, the eNOS cofactor, requires antioxidant defenses to prevent its oxidation, its deficit leads to eNOS uncoupling with generation of superoxide anion [18]. Therefore, ethanol increases HDL levels, but necessarily requires the presence of effective antioxidant defenses to enhance eNOS activity. As substantiated later, phenolics from fruits, vegetables, virgin olive oil and wine probably contribute to this antioxidant protective role.

Hemostatic Mechanisms

In the process of hemostasis, decreased coagulation and increased fibrinolysis have been detected in relationship with Mediterranean diets, omega-3 polyunsaturated fatty acids and wine or alcohol administration [11, 13, 19–23].

Mediterranean diets and alcohol consumption reduce plasma fibrinogen concentration, thus diminishing the probability of clot formation [11, 13, 14, 21]. Moderate alcohol increases clot lysis in vivo in a mouse model, by increasing the expression of tissue plasminogen activator (t-PA) and urokinase plasminogen activator (u-PA) [24] a response also detected in human monocytes [25]. In contrast to the effect of alcohol and Mediterranean diets, a deficit in eNOS function raises plasma fibrinogen [26, 27].

It has been shown that eNOS plays a key role in the process of thrombosis. In fact, red wine induces a significant reduction of stasis-induced venous thrombosis, but this effect is blunted by the eNOS inhibitor L-NAME [28]. This antithrombotic effect of wine is mainly due to polyphenols, as seen in studies that compared the effect of ethanol, ethanol-free wine and whole red wine [29]. Many studies have investigated the effect of wine or wine phenolics on platelet activation and aggregation. Several observations have demonstrated a significant inhibitory effect of red wine in platelet aggregation [30]. Since NO inhibits platelet aggregation [31] the antiplatelet activity of wine, and of wine phenolics in particular, could be mediated by the direct enhancement of eNOS exerted by these compounds [32–35].

Individuals that consume a Mediterranean diet have longer bleeding time than those that consume a control diet [22]. Also adherence to the traditional Mediterranean diet was associated with a decrease in coagulation and inflammation markers [11] as well as with reduced plasma concentration of inflammation markers [13] as seen too for red wine [36, 37].

omega-3 polyunsaturated fatty acids decrease platelet aggregation, resulting in a modest prolongation of bleeding times [23]. EPA and DHA reduced the endothelial expression of adhesion molecules in stimulated cells and fish oil affects the metabolism of inflammatory mediators like the interleukins and tumor necrosis factor-α (TNF-α) [38, 39].

It has been reported that a fish oil-rich diet upregulates eNOS expression in rat [40]. Okuda et al. [41] showed that EPA induced an increase in NO production by triggering eNOS activation by the Ca^{2+}/calmodulin system in culture human endothelial cells (HVE). High levels of glucose significantly increased endothelial glucose and inhibited NO production; EPA decreased the glucose-mediated inhibition of NO production by HVE.

Also, Omura et al. [42] reported that EPA stimulated NO production in endothelial cell in situ and induced endothelium-dependent relaxation of bovine coronary arteries precontracted with U-46619 (a thromboxane A2 analogue). The stimulation of eNOS activity was independent of increased intracellular Ca^{2+}, but was rather linked to a stimulating effect of EPA on the translocation of eNOS to the cytosol and its dissociation from caveolin, preventing the enzyme inhibition. Other fatty acids such as myristic and to a lesser extent palmitic, but not lauric, stearic, oleic and linoleic, stimulated eNOS in a human microvascular endothelial cell line [43].

It is well documented that insulin increases endothelial NO production by activating eNOS through protein kinase B(Akt)-mediated phosphorylation of serine residue 1179 [44, 45]. Treatment with omega-3 polyunsaturated fatty acids (EPA), but not oleic acid, enhanced insulin-stimulated NO production in porcine pulmonary artery endothelial cells [46].

NO formed by eNOS is responsible for maintaining low vascular tone and preventing leukocytes and platelets from adhering to the vascular wall [47–49]. Endothelium-derived NO has anti-inflammatory properties because it depresses pro-inflammatory cytokine release from the vascular wall and immune system [50, 51]. Nitric oxide may inhibit expression of numerous cytokines in lymphocytes, eosinophils, monocytes and other cell types [50, 52–54]. These include cytokines critical for the development of inflammatory process like interleukin-1β (IL-1β) or TNF-α expression, as well as the expression of IL-6 and interferon-γ (IFN-γ) [55–60].

On the whole, these arguments support the proposition that the effects of Mediterranean diets, omega-3 polyunsaturated fatty acids and wine on haemostatic and inflammatory markers are mediated by eNOS, since they stimulate NO production and NO itself reproduces the effects.

Endothelial Function

The endothelium plays a key role in the regulation of vascular tone and reactivity. Nitric oxide (NO) is the main mediator of vascular relaxation in a process that is inhibited in the presence of free radicals. Superoxide combines with NO and generates peroxynitrite, a reaction which results in inhibition of NO mediated processes and increased oxidative damage by peroxynitrite. Antioxidants are required for eNOS function in order to protect NO, but also to prevent eNOS uncoupling as a consequence of reduced BH4 (tetrahydrobiopterin) levels, a condition associated to increased generation of superoxide by eNOS itself [61]. Endothelin-1, a vasoconstriction mediator synthesized by the endothelium, opposes NO-induced vasodilatation. Red wine enhances the function and in some observations also the expression of eNOS, in a process mediated by wine polyphenols that shows marked differences in activity among the different phenolic compounds [32–35, 61]. Phenolic compounds are characteristically present also in fruits and vegetables that are part of the Mediterranean diets. An additional mechanism to explain the enhancement of endothelial function by red wine phenolics is the inhibition of the secretion of endothelin-1, a vasoconstrictor agent [62].

In addition to the effects of phenols and omega-3 polyunsaturated fatty acids, it has also been reported that ethanol increases endothelial NO production in cells in culture, through modulation of eNOS expression [63], yet ethanol does not seem to increase endothelial function in vivo in humans.

Endothelial function can be evaluated by measuring the flow-dependent vascular reactivity, a noninvasive procedure which has shown that wine, omega-3 fatty acids and Mediterranean diets protect and enhance this eNOS dependent regulatory mechanism [13, 64–66]. The preservation of endothelial function appears in clinical observations as a requisite for cardiovascular health, particularly to prevent atherosclerosis, but the molecular mechanisms responsible for the protective effect have not been established.

Patients with diabetes, insulin resistance, and obesity have augmented levels of circulating free fatty acids [67, 68]. Elevated plasma free fatty acids are one of the first events in the development of metabolic syndrome and are associated with impaired insulin-induced, NO-mediated vasodilation [67, 68]. It was observed in normal subject that the acute elevations of plasma free fatty acids produced by systemic infusion of exogenous fatty acids for 2 h induced insulinopenia and impaired endothelium-dependent vasodilation [67, 68]. Quantitative increases in serum fatty acids may represent an important metabolic variable that contributes to vascular endothelial dysfunction and NO production [46].

Observations in type 2 diabetes patients, suggest a differential effect of specific types of fatty acids on endothelial function, judging from serum and tissue fatty acid profiles [69]. Prolonged feeding with omega-3 fatty acid-rich diets has also shown enhanced eNOS activity in the arterial wall of rats [70], lowered blood pressure [71], and improved endothelium-dependent vasodilation responses in humans [72, 73] strongly suggesting that omega-3 polyunsaturated fatty acids, in contrast to other fatty acyl families, do enhance vascular endothelial NO production and responsiveness.

The present evidence supports the hypothesis that the healthy effects of wine and omega-3 polyunsaturated fatty acids, just as those from Mediterranean diets and polyphenol-rich food, would be mediated, at least in part, via enhancement of eNOS function [74, 75].

Antioxidant Defense Mechanisms

In addition to their eNOS enhancement properties, phenolics are also active as antioxidants in vitro and in vivo. As mentioned before, these two effects are partially related since eNOS function requires the presence of antioxidant activity. The effectiveness of the various phenol antioxidant species in the whole organism, their bioavailability, and the antioxidant activity of their metabolites, are subjects currently under investigation. The apparent target for these natural compounds is eNOS function *via* NO protection and gene expression. The relative contribution of gene expression and antioxidant protection to the stimulatory effect of the various phenolics on eNOS [65, 76], has not been established. The enhancement of endothelial function in response to acute administration of ascorbate and vitamin E [77], but not to spirits or white wine [76] supports the antioxidant contribution of wine phenolics. Strong emphasis was given initially to the prevention of LDL oxidation and subsequent uptake by macrophages, as a key element in the prevention of atherosclerosis by wine antioxidant phenolics. At present, the emphasis on atherosclerosis pathogenesis has shifted to endothelial cell oxidative damage caused by oxidized LDL, cigarette smoke, homocysteine, lipid peroxides, inflammation and others [78–80]. Among the changes observed in endothelial cells after oxidative damage, the decrease in eNOS function apparently plays a central pathogenic role.

Metabolic Syndrome and Its Relationship with Mediterranean Diets and Alcohol Consumption

Since the original proposition by Reaven [81] that dyslipidemia, hypertension, and hyperglycemia commonly cluster together, a systematic analysis of these and other apparently related categories has led to some consensus definitions of metabolic syndrome. The central proposition is that several biochemical and clinical parameters recognized as cardiovascular disease risk factors do cluster together. The definition of metabolic syndrome by the National Cholesterol Education Program's Adult Treatment Panel III (NCEPATP III) report considers the clustering of at least 3 of 5 cardiovascular risk factors, for all of which defined abnormal values are proposed. These five principal risk factors are: waist circumference, plasma triacylglycerol, plasma HDL cholesterol, blood pressure and fasting blood glucose. Similar risk factors have been selected by other organizations such as the World Health Organization (WHO) and the American Association of Clinical Endocrinologists to define the metabolic syndrome [82]. In order to explore the underlying pathophysiological causes for this multivariate condition, several phenotypic characteristics of the metabolic syndrome were evaluated applying multivariate factor analysis; the results show three and four factor domains, classified as obesity, blood pressure, lipids, and central obesity [83]. These authors could account for approximately 60% of the variance in 11 original variables. Their study involved approximately 3,000 subjects included in the Hypertension Genetic Epidemiology Network; metabolic syndrome was present in 34% of black and 39% of white participants. Obesity, with its relationship to lipids and insulin, was found to be the dominant factor in metabolic syndrome.

Research has shown a favorable insulin profile in light-to-moderate alcohol consumers, when compared with nondrinkers and with heavy drinkers. The increased insulin sensitivity associated with light-to-moderate alcohol consumption appears to be the consequence of the body mass index (BMI) and the central adiposity profile in studies of cardiovascular risk factors [84]. For Reaven [85], the key to overcoming metabolic syndrome is an increase in insulin sensitivity. In a study in which alcohol intake and insulin sensitivity, measured by the clamp technique, were correlated, the conclusion was that alcohol consumption was independently and positively associated with insulin-mediated glucose uptake [86]. And in a cross-sectional study in severely obese subjects, it was shown that light-to-moderate alcohol consumption was associated with lower prevalence of type 2 diabetes, together with reduced insulin resistance and a more favorable risk factor profile; the conclusion was that light-to-moderate alcohol consumption should not be discouraged in the severely obese. Also in this study, wine drinkers had lower fasting triacylglycerides, lower insulin and higher HDL cholesterol when compared with spirit drinkers [87]. In a prospective study of 49,324 women, it was shown that light-to-moderate drinking was not associated with weight gain over an 8-year period. However, the result was not so clear for African-American women [88]. In another prospective study done in Denmark with a sample of 2,916 men and 3,970 women, it was found that after 10 years, the moderate consumption of alcohol, beer and spirits, was associated with later high waist circumference, whereas moderate-to-high consumption of wine apparently had the opposite effect [89]. The apparent protective effect of wine on abdominal obesity may be related to our recent finding that wine phenolics interact with Glut-4 glucose transporters in adipocytes and thereby inhibit glucose transport [90]. From studies addressing the relationship among alcohol consumption and the prevalence of metabolic syndrome in Sweden and USA, it can be concluded that moderate alcohol consumption is significantly and inversely associated with metabolic syndrome, a change shown for several components of the metabolic syndrome such as low serum HDL cholesterol, elevated serum triacylglycerides, high waist circumference, hyperinsulinemia and hypertension. Sex differences are observed, and wine drinkers exhibit a more favorable pattern of metabolic and clinical parameters, as well as a better lifestyle, than beer and spirit drinkers [91–93].

Mediterranean diets are associated with a reduced risk of cardiovascular disease and all-cause mortality [94]. The relationship between Mediterranean diets and metabolic syndrome has been investigated in several studies. Some characteristics of this diet have shown a beneficial effect on the development of metabolic syndrome or its components. Indeed, fish and omega-3 polyunsaturated fatty acids intake, which are principal components of the Mediterranean diets, have been associated with a lower risk of cardiovascular disease [95]. Various observations have shown that Mediterranean diets improve blood pressure and lipid profile, decrease risk of thrombosis, improve endothelial function, and insulin resistance, and reduce plasma homocysteine concentration [5, 21, 65, 74, 96, 97]. Pitsavos et al. [98] researched the effect of the consumption of the Mediterranean diet on coronary risk, in subjects with the metabolic syndrome. They studied 848 patients with a first event of an acute coronary syndrome and 1,078 people without any evidence of cardiovascular risk, from all Greek areas, and observed that the adoption of the Mediterranean diet was associated with a 35% reduction of the coronary risk in subjects with the metabolic syndrome. As mentioned, Esposito et al. [13] reported an intervention study in patients with the metabolic syndrome, to assess the effect of a Mediterranean diet on endothelial function and vascular inflammatory markers in this patients. They showed that a Mediterranean diet reduces the prevalence of the metabolic syndrome and its associated cardiovascular risk. At the end of the 2-year follow-up period, 56% of the patients in the Mediterranean group no longer had metabolic syndrome, whereas in the control group the minor decrease in prevalence detected was not statistically significant.

Pathogenesis of the Metabolic Syndrome: A Central Role for Endothelial Nitric Oxide Synthase

In their report on metabolic syndrome, Grundy et al. [82] discuss the present views on its pathogenesis. Obesity, insulin resistance, dyslipidemia and hypertension are all conditions for which pathogenic mechanisms have been extensively explored, and the results from such studies are likely to be relevant when considered in the context of the metabolic syndrome. Endocrine factors, a pro-inflammatory state and the role of the renin-angiotensin system, have also been discussed in relationship with pathogenesis. Oxidative stress has also been considered [99]. Yet, the overall picture does not lead easily into a unifying hypothesis or interpretation, capable of simultaneously explaining the various components that cluster in this highly prevalent syndrome.

That single gene defects may lead to pleiotropic phenotype modifications is a common biological observation. Thus, it is possible that the metabolic syndrome could be the consequence of single gene modifications. There is evidence in support of a central role for defects in NO production in the pathogenesis of many of the cardiovascular risk factors that cluster in the metabolic syndrome. Strikingly, Cook et al. [27] made a very interesting observation in eNOS null mice. These animals present several phenotype changes that mimic the cluster of cardiovascular risk factors that define the human metabolic syndrome including: hypertension, insulin resistance, hypertriacylglyceridemia, elevated fibrinogen, and other changes. The same authors also showed that a high fat diet triggers a marked increase in blood pressure and insulin resistance in eNOS (+/−) mice [100]. Consistent with the findings reported by Cook et al. [27] are reports in humans establishing that eNOS polymorphisms are associated to myocardial infarction [51, 101, 102] and to several signs characteristic of metabolic syndrome including: insulin resistance and type 2 diabetes [103], hypertension [104, 105], inflammatory and oxidative stress markers [106], together with albuminuria, which is another abnormality often found in metabolic syndrome [107]. Also in support of the role played by eNOS in the pathogenesis of metabolic syndrome, it has been found that erectile dysfunction [108] known to arise from decreased NO concentration [109] is associated with the metabolic syndrome.

There are findings that describe other genetic defects associated to metabolic syndrome, but they do not provide, for the moment, arguments as strong as those shown for eNOS. For example, a mutation in a mitochondrial tRNA gene leads to a cluster of metabolic defects partly similar to metabolic syndrome [110]. Also the peroxisome proliferator-activated receptor (PPAR) has been involved in metabolic syndrome pathogenesis [111]. And signs that partly resemble metabolic syndrome have recently been observed in subjects with mutations in PPARγ [112]. Insulin-sensitizing thiazolidinedione-related drugs are PPARγ agonists and are used to decrease insulin resistance. Interestingly, it was demonstrated that PPARγ ligands stimulate NO release from the endothelial cell [113, 114].

Regular physical activity is associated with favorable modification of metabolic syndrome parameters. The mechanism mediating the protective effects of exercise are not clearly defined, but it has been shown that exercise training, in many animal and human studies, augments endothelial function in both large and small vessels [115]. Recent human studies also indicate that exercise training may improve endothelial function by upregulating eNOS protein expression and phosphorylation [116–118]. In another finding suggestive of a central role of eNOS in metabolic syndrome, eNOS null mice were shown to have reduced mitochondrial oxidative capacity in slow-twitch skeletal muscle, and also reduced spontaneous physical activity [119].

Potential Role of Mediterranean Diets, Omega-3 Fatty Acids, Antioxidants and Red Wine, as Endothelial Nitric Oxide Synthase Enhancers, in the Control of the Metabolic Syndrome

We have reviewed the arguments that support a central role for eNOS in the positive health effects of Mediterranean diets and moderate wine consumption, an effect largely attributed to both, omega-3 polyunsaturated fatty acids and polyphenols. Similarly, we review the evidence linking eNOS dysfunction with the cluster of cardiovascular risk factors recognized as metabolic syndrome. The obvious question stemming from the experimental data is to what

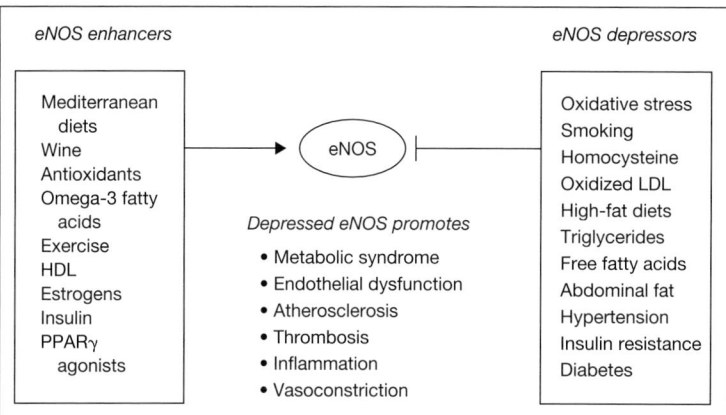

Fig. 1. Factors which are capable of enhancing or depressing eNOS function, via gene expression, enzyme regulation, substrate availability, product stability or others. Decreased eNOS would result in metabolic syndrome, as well as in other biological changes, some of which are indicated.

extent Mediterranean diets and moderate red wine consumption contribute to the control of metabolic syndrome manifestations and its long-term health consequences. In this context, we propose a potential role for Mediterranean diets and red wine, as eNOS enhancers, in the control of the metabolic syndrome. Indirect evidence outlined here, from epidemiological studies that correlate components of the Mediterranean diets, including wine with metabolic syndrome, support our proposition (fig. 1).

On the whole, the evidence linking eNOS with the metabolic syndrome, and with the individual risk factors that characterize it, strongly suggest that the search for a unifying theory to account for the metabolic syndrome should focus systematically on eNOS and its functional role. In fact, Parks and Booyse [80] have emphasized the potential role of eNOS as the 'cardioprotective protein' mediating alcohol and polyphenol cardioprotective activities. Similarly, the relationship among eNOS function, type 2 diabetes, and vascular disease is actively being explored [120].

In the context of atherogenesis, the anti-inflammatory effect of Mediterranean diets and red wine consumption has been characterized; TNF-α-induced adhesion of monocytes to endothelial cells was virtually abolished after red wine consumption [36]. Mediterranean diets also reduce serum concentrations of C-reactive protein (hs-CRP), interleukin-6 (IL-6), IL-7 and IL-18 [13]. Also, red wine decreases IL-1α, hs-CRP, as well as monocyte and endothelial adhesion molecules [37]. Since NO reduces leukocyte adhesion to vascular endothelium,

Mediterranean diet components including wine phenolics, enhance eNOS activity and could thus be involved in these effects. Other interesting relationships among eNOS, metabolic syndrome, endothelial cell inflammation and PPARγ agonists, have recently been described [121].

Additional support for the hypothesis that Mediterranean diets and red wine could contribute to the control of metabolic syndrome, comes from the evidence that metabolic syndrome is associated with oxidative stress. Reduction of oxidative stress might lead not only to decreased oxidative damage to biological structures, but also to changes in signaling pathways responsive to oxidative stress that might be involved in the pathogenesis of the metabolic syndrome [99, 122]. Oxidative stress relates to eNOS because it can lead to superoxide generation when eNOS is uncoupled, and because NO requires antioxidant protection. Thus, malfunction of eNOS might result from oxidative stress affecting NO, or from uncoupled eNOS, generating more superoxide and less NO.

Phenolics from vegetables, fruits and wine enhance eNOS function measured as NO production, they increase eNOS gene expression and also lead to enzyme activation [32, 35, 123–125]. We and others have provided evidence that a Mediterranean-like diet and also red wine consumption, i.e. high phenolic intake conditions, improve endothelial function in human subjects [65]. Wine is a very efficient vehicle to provide antioxidant phenols in human subjects, an effect associated with adherence to Mediterranean diets [13, 74]. So, polyphenols present in red wine and in fruits and vegetables, abundant in Mediterranean diets, as well as exercise and PPARγ agonists, all increase NO release in endothelial cells, improve endothelial function and decrease metabolic syndrome risk factors. Metabolic syndrome unquestionably constitutes a serious challenge for human health today, but perhaps effective therapeutic and preventive measures are already available. The establishment of a pathogenic theory, which we believe needs to be explored in connection with the hypothesis that eNOS function is deficient in metabolic syndrome, would help in unifying criteria for the prevention of the health consequences of this pleiotropic cluster of homeostatic disorders [126].

Acknowledgements

This work was supported by projects FONDEF D03I-1047 and PBMEC-UC 2004–2005.

References

1. Trichopoulou A, Vasilopoulou E, Lagiou A: Mediterranean diet and coronary heart disease: are antioxidants critical? Nutr Rev 1999;57:253–255.
2. Simopoulos AP: The Mediterranean diets: What is so special about the diet of Greece? The scientific evidence. J Nutr 2001;131(suppl):3065S–3073S.

3   Simopoulos AP, Norman HA, Gillaspy JE, Duke JA: Common purslane: a source of omega-3 polyunsaturated fatty acids and antioxidants. J Am Coll Nutr 1992;11:374–382.
4   Sandker GW, Kromhout D, Aravanis A, Bloemberg BP, Mensink RP, Karalias N, Katan MB: Serum cholesteryl ester fatty acids and their relation with serum lipids in elderly men in Crete and The Netherlands. Eur J Clin Nutr 1993;47:201–208.
5   Urquiaga I, Guasch V, Marshall G, San Martin A, Castillo O, Rozowski J, Leighton F: Effect of Mediterranean and Occidental diets, and red wine, on plasma fatty acids in humans: an intervention study. Biol Res 2004;37:253–261.
6   Ambring A, Johansson M, Axelsen M, Gan L, Strandvik B, Friberg P: Mediterranean-inspired diet lowers the ratio of serum phospholipid n–6 to n–3 fatty acids, the number of leukocytes and platelets, and vascular endothelial growth factor in healthy subjects. Am J Clin Nutr 2006;83: 575–581.
7   Renaud S, de Lorgeril M, Delaye J, Guidollet J, Jacquard F, Mamelle N, Martin JL, Monjaud I, Salen P, Toubol P: Cretan Mediterranean diet for prevention of coronary heart disease. Am J Clin Nutr 1995;61(suppl):1360S–1367S.
8   Sacks FM, Katan M: Randomized clinical trials on the effects of dietary fat and carbohydrate on plasma lipoproteins and cardiovascular disease. Am J Med 2002;113(suppl 9B):13S–24S.
9   Christon RA: Mechanisms of action of dietary fatty acids in regulating the activation of vascular endothelial cells during atherogenesis. Nutr Rev 2003;61:272–279.
10 Sanders TA: Olive oil and the Mediterranean diet. Int J Vitam Nutr Res 2001;71:179–184.
11 Chrysohoou C, Panagiotakos DB, Pitsavos C, Das UN, Stefanadis C: Adherence to the Mediterranean diet attenuates inflammation and coagulation process in healthy adults: The ATTICA Study. J Am Coll Cardiol 2004;44:152–158.
12 Flynn G, Colquhoun D: Mediterranean diet improves lipid profiles over three months. Asia Pac J Clin Nutr 2004;13(suppl):S138.
13 Esposito K, Marfella R, Ciotola M, Di Palo C, Giugliano F, Giugliano G, D'Armiento M, D'Andrea F, Giugliano D: Effect of a Mediterranean-style diet on endothelial dysfunction and markers of vascular inflammation in the metabolic syndrome: a randomized trial. JAMA 2004;292: 1440–1446.
14 Rimm EB, Williams P, Fosher K, Criqui M, Stampfer MJ: Moderate alcohol intake and lower risk of coronary heart disease: meta-analysis of effects on lipids and haemostatic factors. BMJ 1999;319:1523–1528.
15 Gong M, Wilson M, Kelly T, Su W, Dressman J, Kincer J, Matveev SV, Guo L, Guerin T, Li XA, et al: HDL-associated estradiol stimulates endothelial NO synthase and vasodilation in an SR-BI-dependent manner. J Clin Invest 2003;111:1579–1587.
16 Matthews KA, Kuller LH, Sutton-Tyrrell K, Chang YF: Changes in cardiovascular risk factors during the perimenopause and postmenopause and carotid artery atherosclerosis in healthy women. Stroke 2001;32:1104–1111.
17 Mardones P, Strobel P, Miranda S, Leighton F, Quinones V, Amigo L, Rozowski J, Krieger M, Rigotti A: Alpha-tocopherol metabolism is abnormal in scavenger receptor class B type I (SR-BI)-deficient mice. J Nutr 2002;132:443–449.
18 Landmesser U, Dikalov S, Price SR, McCann L, Fukai T, Holland SM, Mitch WE, Harrison DG: Oxidation of tetrahydrobiopterin leads to uncoupling of endothelial cell nitric oxide synthase in hypertension. J Clin Invest 2003;111:1201–1209.
19 Renaud S, de Lorgeril M: Wine, alcohol, platelets, and the French paradox for coronary heart disease. Lancet 1992;339:1523–1526.
20 Booyse FM, Parks DA: Moderate wine and alcohol consumption: beneficial effects on cardiovascular disease. Thromb Haemost 2001;86:517–528.
21 Mezzano D, Leighton F, Martinez C, Marshall G, Cuevas A, Castillo O, Panes O, Munoz B, Perez DD, Mizon C, et al: Complementary effects of Mediterranean diet and moderate red wine intake on haemostatic cardiovascular risk factors. Eur J Clin Nutr 2001;55:444–451.
22 Mezzano D, Leighton F, Strobel P, Martinez C, Marshall G, Cuevas A, Castillo O, Panes O, Munoz B, Rozowski J, et al: Mediterranean diet, but not red wine, is associated with beneficial changes in primary haemostasis. Eur J Clin Nutr 2003;57:439–446.

23 Kris-Etherton PM, Harris WS, Appel LJ: Fish consumption, fish oil, omega-3 polyunsaturated fatty acids, and cardiovascular disease. Arterioscler Thromb Vasc Biol 2003;23:e20–e30.
24 Tabengwa EM, Grenett HE, Parks DA, Booyse FM: Moderate alcohol increases clot lysis in vivo in a mouse model by increasing t-PA and u-PA and decreasing PAI-1 expression. American Heart Association Scientific Sessions Orlando, 2003.
25 Tabengwa EM, Wheeler CG, Yancey DA, Grenett HE, Booyse FM: Alcohol-induced up-regulation of fibrinolytic activity and plasminogen activators in human monocytes. Alcohol Clin Exp Res 2002;26:1121–1127.
26 Pinelli A, Trivulzio S, Tomasoni L, Bertolini B, Brenna S, Bonacina E, Accinni R: Drugs modifying nitric oxide metabolism affect plasma cholesterol levels, coagulation parameters, blood pressure values and the appearance of plasma myocardial necrosis markers in rabbits: opposite effects of L-NAME and nitroglycerine. Cardiovasc Drugs Ther 2003;17:15–23.
27 Cook S, Hugli O, Egli M, Vollenweider P, Burcelin R, Nicod P, Thorens B, Scherrer U: Clustering of cardiovascular risk factors mimicking the human metabolic syndrome X in eNOS null mice. Swiss Med Wkly 2003;133:360–363.
28 de Gaetano G, De Curtis A, di Castelnuovo A, Donati MB, Iacoviello L, Rotondo S: Antithrombotic effect of polyphenols in experimental models: a mechanism of reduced vascular risk by moderate wine consumption. Ann NY Acad Sci 2002;957:174–188.
29 Wollny T, Aiello L, Di Tommaso D, Bellavia V, Rotilio D, Donati MB, de Gaetano G, Iacoviello L: Modulation of haemostatic function and prevention of experimental thrombosis by red wine in rats: a role for increased nitric oxide production. Br J Pharmacol 1999;127:747–755.
30 Ruf JC: Alcohol, wine and platelet function. Biol Res 2004;37:209–215.
31 Danielewski O, Schultess J, Smolenski A: The NO/cGMP pathway inhibits Rap 1 activation in human platelets via cGMP-dependent protein kinase I. Thromb Haemost 2005;93:319–325.
32 Leikert JF, Rathel TR, Wohlfart P, Cheynier V, Vollmar AM, Dirsch VM: Red wine polyphenols enhance endothelial nitric oxide synthase expression and subsequent nitric oxide release from endothelial cells. Circulation 2002;106:1614–1617.
33 Wallerath T, Deckert G, Ternes T, Anderson H, Li H, Witte K, Forstermann U: Resveratrol, a polyphenolic phytoalexin present in red wine, enhances expression and activity of endothelial nitric oxide synthase. Circulation 2002;106:1652–1658.
34 Martin S, Andriambeloson E, Takeda K, Andriantsitohaina R: Red wine polyphenols increase calcium in bovine aortic endothelial cells: a basis to elucidate signalling pathways leading to nitric oxide production. Br J Pharmacol 2002;135:1579–1587.
35 Wallerath T, Li H, Godtel-Ambrust U, Schwarz PM, Forstermann U: A blend of polyphenolic compounds explains the stimulatory effect of red wine on human endothelial NO synthase. Nitric Oxide 2005;12:97–104.
36 Badia E, Sacanella E, Fernandez-Sola J, Nicolas JM, Antunez E, Rotilio D, de Gaetano G, Urbano-Marquez A, Estruch R: Decreased tumor necrosis factor-p0induced adhesion of human monocytes to endothelial cells after moderate alcohol consumption. Am J Clin Nutr 2004;80: 225–230.
37 Estruch R, Sacanella E, Badia E, Antunez E, Nicolas JM, Fernandez-Sola J, Rotilio D, de Gaetano G, Rubin E, Urbano-Marquez A: Different effects of red wine and gin consumption on inflammatory biomarkers of atherosclerosis: a prospective randomized crossover trial. Effects of wine on inflammatory markers. Atherosclerosis 2004;175:117–123.
38 De Caterina R, Cybulsky MI, Clinton SK, Gimbrone MA Jr, Libby P: The omega-3 fatty acid docosahexaenoate reduces cytokine-induced expression of proatherogenic and proinflammatory proteins in human endothelial cells. Arterioscler Thromb 1994;14:1829–1836.
39 De Caterina R, Liao JK, Libby P: Fatty acid modulation of endothelial activation. Am J Clin Nutr 2000;71(suppl):213S–223S.
40 Lopez D, Orta X, Casos K, Saiz MP, Puig-Parellada P, Farriol M, Mitjavila MT: Upregulation of endothelial nitric oxide synthase in rat aorta after ingestion of fish oil-rich diet. Am J Physiol Heart Circ Physiol 2004;287:H567–H572.
41 Okuda Y, Kawashima K, Sawada T, Tsurumaru K, Asano M, Suzuki S, Soma M, Nakajima T, Yamashita K: Eicosapentaenoic acid enhances nitric oxide production by cultured human endothelial cells. Biochem Biophys Res Commun 1997;232:487–491.

42 Omura M, Kobayashi S, Mizukami Y, Mogami K, Todoroki-Ikeda N, Miyake T, Matsuzaki M: Eicosapentaenoic acid (EPA) induces Ca(2+)-independent activation and translocation of endothelial nitric oxide synthase and endothelium-dependent vasorelaxation. FEBS Lett 2001;487: 361–366.
43 Zhu W, Smart EJ: Myristic acid stimulates endothelial nitric-oxide synthase in a CD36- and an AMP kinase-dependent manner. J Biol Chem 2005;280:29543–29550.
44 Montagnani M, Chen H, Barr VA, Quon MJ: Insulin-stimulated activation of eNOS is independent of Ca^{2+} but requires phosphorylation by Akt at Ser(1179). J Biol Chem 2001;276: 30392–30398.
45 Konopatskaya O, Whatmore JL, Tooke JE, Shore AC: Insulin and lysophosphatidylcholine synergistically stimulate NO-dependent cGMP production in human endothelial cells. Diabet Med 2003;20:838–845.
46 Lynn MA, Rupnow HL, Kleinhenz DJ, Kanner WA, Dudley SC, Hart CM: Fatty acids differentially modulate insulin-stimulated endothelial nitric oxide production by an Akt-independent pathway. J Invest Med 2004;52:129–136.
47 Lowenstein CJ, Dinerman JL, Snyder SH: Nitric oxide: a physiologic messenger. Ann Intern Med 1994;120:227–237.
48 Lugnier C, Keravis T, Eckly-Michel A: Cross talk between NO and cyclic nucleotide phosphodiesterases in the modulation of signal transduction in blood vessel. J Physiol Pharmacol 1999;50: 639–652.
49 Ignarro LJ: Nitric oxide as a unique signaling molecule in the vascular system: a historical overview. J Physiol Pharmacol 2002;53:503–514.
50 Giustizieri ML, Albanesi C, Scarponi C, De Pita O, Girolomoni G: Nitric oxide donors suppress chemokine production by keratinocytes in vitro and in vivo. Am J Pathol 2002;161: 1409–1418.
51 Antoniades C, Tousoulis D, Vasiliadou C, Pitsavos C, Chrysochoou C, Panagiotakos D, Tentolouris C, Marinou K, Koumallos N, Stefanadis C: Genetic polymorphism on endothelial nitric oxide synthase affects endothelial activation and inflammatory response during the acute phase of myocardial infarction. J Am Coll Cardiol 2005;46:1101–1109.
52 Marcinkiewicz J, Chain BM: Differential regulation of cytokine production by nitric oxide. Immunology 1993;80:146–150.
53 Marcinkiewicz J, Grabowska A, Chain BM: Is there a role for nitric oxide in regulation of T cell secretion of IL-2? J Immunol 1996;156:4617–4621.
54 Marcinkiewicz J: Regulation of cytokine production by eicosanoids and nitric oxide. Arch Immunol Ther Exp (Warsz) 1997;45:163–167.
55 Guzik TJ, Korbut R, Adamek-Guzik T: Nitric oxide and superoxide in inflammation and immune regulation. J Physiol Pharmacol 2003;54:469–487.
56 Spiecker M, Darius H, Kaboth K, Hubner F, Liao JK: Differential regulation of endothelial cell adhesion molecule expression by nitric oxide donors and antioxidants. J Leukoc Biol 1998;63:732–739.
57 Lindemann S, Sharafi M, Spiecker M, Buerke M, Fisch A, Grosser T, Veit K, Gierer C, Ibe W, Meyer J, et al: NO reduces PMN adhesion to human vascular endothelial cells due to downregulation of ICAM-1 mRNA and surface expression. Thromb Res 2000;97:113–123.
58 Takahashi M, Ikeda U, Masuyama J, Funayama H, Kano S, Shimada K: Nitric oxide attenuates adhesion molecule expression in human endothelial cells. Cytokine 1996;8:817–821.
59 De Caterina R, Libby P, Peng HB, Thannickal VJ, Rajavashisth TB, Gimbrone MA Jr, Shin WS, Liao JK: Nitric oxide decreases cytokine-induced endothelial activation. Nitric oxide selectively reduces endothelial expression of adhesion molecules and proinflammatory cytokines. J Clin Invest 1995;96:60–68.
60 Bogdan C: Nitric oxide and the regulation of gene expression. Trends Cell Biol 2001;11:66–75.
61 Kawashima S: The two faces of endothelial nitric oxide synthase in the pathophysiology of atherosclerosis. Endothelium 2004;11:99–107.
62 Corder R, Douthwaite JA, Lees DM, Khan NQ, Viseu Dos Santos AC, Wood EG, Carrier MJ: Endothelin-1 synthesis reduced by red wine. Nature 2001;414:863–864.
63 Venkov CD, Myers PR, Tanner MA, Su M, Vaughan DE: Ethanol increases endothelial nitric oxide production through modulation of nitric oxide synthase expression. Thromb Haemost 1999;81: 638–642.

64 Goode GK, Garcia S, Heagerty AM: Dietary supplementation with marine fish oil improves in vitro small artery endothelial function in hypercholesterolemic patients: a double-blind placebo-controlled study. Circulation 1997;96:2802–2807.
65 Cuevas AM, Guasch V, Castillo O, Irribarra V, Mizon C, San Martin A, Strobel P, Perez D, Germain AM, Leighton F: A high-fat diet induces and red wine counteracts endothelial dysfunction in human volunteers. Lipids 2000;35:143–148.
66 Goodfellow J, Bellamy MF, Ramsey MW, Jones CJ, Lewis MJ: Dietary supplementation with marine omega-3 polyunsaturated fatty acids improve systemic large artery endothelial function in subjects with hypercholesterolemia. J Am Coll Cardiol 2000;35:265–270.
67 Steinberg HO, Tarshoby M, Monestel R, Hook G, Cronin J, Johnson A, Bayazeed B, Baron AD: Elevated circulating free fatty acid levels impair endothelium-dependent vasodilation. J Clin Invest 1997;100:1230–1239.
68 Steinberg HO, Paradisi G, Hook G, Crowder K, Cronin J, Baron AD: Free fatty acid elevation impairs insulin-mediated vasodilation and nitric oxide production. Diabetes 2000;49:1231–1238.
69 Folsom AR, Ma J, McGovern PG, Eckfeldt H: Relation between plasma phospholipid saturated fatty acids and hyperinsulinemia. Metabolism 1996;45:223–228.
70 Boutard V, Fouqueray B, Philippe C, Perez J, Baud L: Fish oil supplementation and essential fatty acid deficiency reduce nitric oxide synthesis by rat macrophages. Kidney Int 1994;46:1280–1286.
71 Joly GA, Schini VB, Hughes H, Vanhoutte PM: Potentiation of the hyporeactivity induced by in vivo endothelial injury in the rat carotid artery by chronic treatment with fish oil. Br J Pharmacol 1995;115:255–260.
72 McVeigh GE, Brennan GM, Johnston GD, McDermott BJ, McGrath LT, Henry WR, Andrews JW, Hayes JR: Dietary fish oil augments nitric oxide production or release in patients with type 2 (non-insulin-dependent) diabetes mellitus. Diabetologia 1993;36:33–38.
73 Chin JP, Kaye DM, Hurlston RM, Angus JA, Jennings GL, Dart AM: Effects of dietary marine oil supplementation on reactivity of human buttock subcutaneous arteries and forearm veins in vitro. Br J Pharmacol 1994;112:566–570.
74 Leighton F, Cuevas A, Guasch V, Perez DD, Strobel P, San Martin A, Urzua U, Diez MS, Foncea R, Castillo O, et al: Plasma polyphenols and antioxidants, oxidative DNA damage and endothelial function in a diet and wine intervention study in humans. Drugs Exp Clin Res 1999;25:133–141.
75 Sies H, Schewe T, Heiss C, Kelm M: Cocoa polyphenols and inflammatory mediators. Am J Clin Nutr 2005;81(suppl):304S–312S.
76 Shimada K, Watanabe H, Hosoda K, Takeuchi K, Yoshikawa J: Effect of red wine on coronary flow-velocity reserve. Lancet 1999;354:1002.
77 Plotnick GD, Corretti MC, Vogel RA: Effect of antioxidant vitamins on the transient impairment of endothelium-dependent brachial artery vasoactivity following a single high-fat meal. JAMA 1997;278:1682–1686.
78 Stocker R, Keaney JF Jr: Role of oxidative modifications in atherosclerosis. Physiol Rev 2004;84:1381–1478.
79 De Caterina R: Endothelial dysfunctions: common denominators in vascular disease. Curr Opin Lipidol 2000;11:9–23.
80 Parks DA, Booyse FM: Cardiovascular protection by alcohol and polyphenols: role of nitric oxide. Ann NY Acad Sci 2002;957:115–121.
81 Reaven GM: Banting lecture 1988. Role of insulin resistance in human disease. Diabetes 1988;37:1595–1607.
82 Grundy SM, Brewer HB Jr, Cleeman JI, Smith SC Jr, Lenfant C: Definition of metabolic syndrome: Report of the National Heart, Lung, and Blood Institute/American Heart Association conference on scientific issues related to definition. Circulation 2004;109:433–438.
83 Kraja AT, Hunt SC, Pankow JS, Myers RH, Heiss G, Lewis CE, Rao D, Province MA: An evaluation of the metabolic syndrome in the HyperGEN study. Nutr Metab (Lond) 2005;2:2.
84 Bell RA, Mayer-Davis EJ, Martin MA, D'Agostino RB Jr, Haffner SM: Associations between alcohol consumption and insulin sensitivity and cardiovascular disease risk factors: the Insulin Resistance and Atherosclerosis Study. Diabetes Care 2000;23:1630–1636.

85 Reaven G: Why syndrome X? Fro Harold Himsworth to insulin resistance syndrome. Cell Metabol 2005;1:9–14.
86 Goude D, Fagerberg B, Hulthe J: Alcohol consumption, the metabolic syndrome and insulin resistance in 58-year-old clinically healthy men (AIR study). Clin Sci (Lond) 2002;102:345–352.
87 Dixon JB, Dixon ME, O'Brien PE: Alcohol consumption in the severely obese: relationship with the metabolic syndrome. Obes Res 2002;10:245–252.
88 Wannamethee SG, Field AE, Colditz GA, Rimm EB: Alcohol intake and 8-year weight gain in women: a prospective study. Obes Res 2004;12:1386–1396.
89 Vadstrup ES, Petersen L, Sorensen TI, Gronbaek M: Waist circumference in relation to history of amount and type of alcohol: results from the Copenhagen City Heart Study. Int J Obes Relat Metab Disord 2003;27:238–246.
90 Strobel P, Allard C, Perez-Acle T, Calderon R, Aldunate R, Leighton F: Myricetin, quercetin and catechin-gallate inhibit glucose uptake in isolated rat adipocytes. Biochem J 2005;386:471–478.
91 Rosell M, De Faire U, Hellenius ML: Low prevalence of the metabolic syndrome in wine drinkers – is it the alcohol beverage or the lifestyle? Eur J Clin Nutr 2003;57:227–234.
92 Djousse L, Arnett DK, Eckfeldt JH, Province MA, Singer MR, Ellison RC: Alcohol consumption and metabolic syndrome: does the type of beverage matter? Obes Res 2004;12:1375–1385.
93 Freiberg MS, Cabral HJ, Heeren TC, Vasan RS, Curtis Ellison R: Alcohol consumption and the prevalence of the Metabolic Syndrome in the US: a cross-sectional analysis of data from the Third National Health and Nutrition Examination Survey. Diabetes Care 2004;27:2954–2959.
94 Trichopoulou A, Naska A: European food availability databank based on household budget surveys: the Data Food Networking initiative. Eur J Public Health 2003;13(suppl):24–28.
95 Kris-Etherton PM, Harris WS, Appel LJ: Fish consumption, fish oil, omega-3 polyunsaturated fatty acids, and cardiovascular disease. Circulation 2002;106:2747–2757.
96 Psaltopoulou T, Naska A, Orfanos P, Trichopoulos D, Mountokalakis T, Trichopoulou A: Olive oil, the Mediterranean diet, and arterial blood pressure: the Greek European Prospective Investigation into Cancer and Nutrition (EPIC) study. Am J Clin Nutr 2004;80:1012–1018.
97 Panagiotakos DB, Polychronopoulos E: The role of Mediterranean diet in the epidemiology of metabolic syndrome: converting epidemiology to clinical practice. Lipids Health Dis 2005;4:7.
98 Pitsavos C, Panagiotakos DB, Chrysohoou C, Papaioannou I, Papadimitriou L, Tousoulis D, Stefanadis C, Toutouzas P: The adoption of Mediterranean diet attenuates the development of acute coronary syndromes in people with the metabolic syndrome. Nutr J 2003;2:1.
99 Furukawa S, Fujita T, Shimabukuro M, Iwaki M, Yamada Y, Nakajima Y, Nakayama O, Makishima M, Matsuda M, Shimomura I: Increased oxidative stress in obesity and its impact on metabolic syndrome. J Clin Invest 2004;114:1752–1761.
100 Cook S, Hugli O, Egli M, Menard B, Thalmann S, Sartori C, Perrin C, Nicod P, Thorens B, Vollenweider P, et al: Partial gene deletion of endothelial nitric oxide synthase predisposes to exaggerated high-fat diet-induced insulin resistance and arterial hypertension. Diabetes 2004;53:2067–2072.
101 Shimasaki Y, Yasue H, Yoshimura M, Nakayama M, Kugiyama K, Ogawa H, Harada E, Masuda T, Koyama W, Saito Y, et al: Association of the missense Glu298Asp variant of the endothelial nitric oxide synthase gene with myocardial infarction. J Am Coll Cardiol 1998;31:1506–1510.
102 Hingorani AD, Liang CF, Fatibene J, Lyon A, Monteith S, Parsons A, Haydock S, Hopper RV, Stephens NG, O'Shaughnessy KM, et al: A common variant of the endothelial nitric oxide synthase (Glu298→Asp) is a major risk factor for coronary artery disease in the UK. Circulation 1999;100:1515–1520.
103 Monti LD, Barlassina C, Citterio L, Galluccio E, Berzuini C, Setola E, Valsecchi G, Lucotti P, Pozza G, Bernardinelli L, et al: Endothelial nitric oxide synthase polymorphisms are associated with type 2 diabetes and the insulin resistance syndrome. Diabetes 2003;52:1270–1275.
104 Fernandez ML, Ruiz R, Gonzalez MA, Ramirez-Lorca R, Couto C, Ramos A, Gutierrez-Tous R, Rivera JM, Ruiz A, Real LM, et al: Association of NOS3 gene with metabolic syndrome in hypertensive patients. Thromb Haemost 2004;92:413–418.

105 Pereira AC, Sposito AC, Mota GF, Cunha RS, Herkenhoff FL, Mill JG, Krieger JE: Endothelial nitric oxide synthase gene variant modulates the relationship between serum cholesterol levels and blood pressure in the general population: new evidence for a direct effect of lipids in arterial blood pressure. Atherosclerosis 2006;184:193–200.

106 Chrysohoou C, Panagiotakos DB, Pitsavos C, Antoniades C, Skoumas J, Brown M, Stefanadis C: Evidence for association between endothelial nitric oxide synthase gene polymorphism (G894T) and inflammatory markers: the ATTICA study. Am Heart J 2004;148:733–738.

107 Liu Y, Burdon KP, Langefeld CD, Beck SR, Wagenknecht LE, Rich SS, Bowden DW, Freedman BI: T-786C polymorphism of the endothelial nitric oxide synthase gene is associated with albuminuria in the diabetes heart study. J Am Soc Nephrol 2005;16:1085–1090.

108 Matfin G, Jawa A, Fonseca VA: Erectile dysfunction: interrelationship with the metabolic syndrome. Curr Diab Rep 2005;5:64–69.

109 Bivalacqua TJ, Champion HC, Hellstrom WJ, Kadowitz PJ: Pharmacotherapy for erectile dysfunction. Trends Pharmacol Sci 2000;21:484–489.

110 Wilson FH, Hariri A, Farhi A, Zhao H, Petersen KF, Toka HR, Nelson-Williams C, Raja KM, Kashgarian M, Shulman GI, et al: A cluster of metabolic defects caused by mutation in a mitochondrial tRNA. Science 2004;306:1190–1194.

111 Gurnell M, Savage DB, Chatterjee VK, O'Rahilly S: The metabolic syndrome: peroxisome proliferator-activated receptor gamma and its therapeutic modulation. J Clin Endocrinol Metab 2003;88: 2412–2421.

112 Hegele RA: Lessons from human mutations in PPARgamma. Int J Obes Relat Metab Disord 2005;29(suppl 1):S31–S35.

113 Calnek DS, Mazzella L, Roser S, Roman J, Hart CM: Peroxisome proliferator-activated receptor gamma ligands increase release of nitric oxide from endothelial cells. Arterioscler Thromb Vasc Biol 2003;23:52–57.

114 Cho DH, Choi YJ, Jo SA, Jo I: Nitric oxide production and regulation of endothelial nitric-oxide synthase phosphorylation by prolonged treatment with troglitazone: evidence for involvement of peroxisome proliferator-activated receptor (PPAR) gamma-dependent and PPARgamma-independent signaling pathways. J Biol Chem 2004;279:2499–2506.

115 Green DJ, Maiorana A, O'Driscoll G, Taylor R: Effect of exercise training on endothelium-derived nitric oxide function in humans. J Physiol 2004;561:1–25.

116 Fukai T, Siegfried MR, Ushio-Fukai M, Cheng Y, Kojda G, Harrison DG: Regulation of the vascular extracellular superoxide dismutase by nitric oxide and exercise training. J Clin Invest 2000;105: 1631–1639.

117 Dimmeler S, Zeiher AM: Exercise and cardiovascular health: get active to 'AKTivate' your endothelial nitric oxide synthase. Circulation 2003;107:3118–3120.

118 Hambrecht R, Adams V, Erbs S, Linke A, Krankel N, Shu Y, Baither Y, Gielen S, Thiele H, Gummert JF, et al: Regular physical activity improves endothelial function in patients with coronary artery disease by increasing phosphorylation of endothelial nitric oxide synthase. Circulation 2003;107:3152–3158.

119 Momken I, Lechene P, Ventura-Clapier R, Veksler V: Voluntary physical activity alterations in endothelial nitric oxide synthase knockout mice. Am J Physiol Heart Circ Physiol 2004;287: H914–H920.

120 Hayden MR, Tyagi SC: Is type 2 diabetes mellitus a vascular disease (atheroscleropathy) with hyperglycemia a late manifestation? The role of NOS, NO, and redox stress. Cardiovasc Diabetol 2003;2:2.

121 Sjoholm A, Nystrom T: Endothelial inflammation in insulin resistance. Lancet 2005;365: 610–612.

122 Urakawa H, Katsuki A, Sumida Y, Gabazza EC, Murashima S, Morioka K, Maruyama N, Kitagawa N, Tanaka T, Hori Y, et al: Oxidative stress is associated with adiposity and insulin resistance in men. J Clin Endocrinol Metab 2003;88:4673–4676.

123 Stoclet JC, Kleschyov A, Andriambeloson E, Diebolt M, Andriantsitohaina R: Endothelial NO release caused by red wine polyphenols. J Physiol Pharmacol 1999;50:535–540.

124 Benito S, Lopez D, Saiz MP, Buxaderas S, Sanchez J, Puig-Parellada P, Mitjavila MT: A flavonoid-rich diet increases nitric oxide production in rat aorta. Br J Pharmacol 2002;135:910–916.
125 Hollenberg NK: Red wine polyphenols enhance endothelial nitric oxide synthase expression and subsequent nitric oxide release from endothelial cells. Curr Hypertens Rep 2003;5:287–288.
126 Leighton F, Miranda-Rottmann S, Urquiaga I: A central role of eNOS in the protective effect of wine against metabolic syndrome. Cell Biochem Funct 2005.

Dr. Federico Leighton
Facultad de Ciencias Biológicas
Universidad Católica de Chile, Casilla 114-D
Santiago (Chile)
Tel./Fax +56 2 222 2577, E-Mail fleighton@bio.puc.cl

Effects of an Omega-3-Enriched Mediterranean Diet (Modified Diet of Crete) versus a Swedish Diet

Peter Friberg, Mats Johansson

Department of Metabolism and Cardiovascular Research/Clinical Physiology, Sahlgrenska Academy/Sahlgrenska University Hospital, Göteborg, Sweden

Cardiovascular diseases involve dysfunction of the heart and blood vessels leading to coronary heart disease, stroke and heart failure, which are the most important causes of premature death and morbidity worldwide. Atherosclerosis, which to a large extent is the common denominator for cardiovascular disease, starts very early in life and involves an inflammatory process of the vessel wall [1, 2]. We need to focus more strongly on modifiable risk factors in early life to be able to reduce the incidence of cardiovascular disease. Diet is essential for preventing cardiovascular disease [3] and recent data demonstrate reduced mortality in people adhering to a Mediterranean diet [4].

Components of a Mediterranean Diet

The term 'Mediterranean diet' represents the dietary patterns of many countries around the Mediterranean area and was put into more scientific focus several decades ago. The Mediterranean diet food characteristics, as agreed from the literature [5], comprise: abundant plants minimally processed, seasonally fresh and locally grown plant foods; fresh fruits as the typical daily dessert, with sweets (based on nuts, olive oil and concentrated sugars or honey) consumed during feast days; olive oil as the principal source of dietary lipids; dairy products – mainly cheese and yogurts consumed in low-to-moderate amounts; red meat consumed in low frequency and amounts; and finally wine consumed in moderate amounts. This definition of a 'Mediterranean diet' can of course be discussed. No doubt, however, a Mediterranean-style diet is very popular among people. In addition, many studies have focused on the type of fat intake. Besides the frequent use of olive oil in the Mediterranean diets, also polyunsaturated fatty acids are favoured in the media and put under scientific scrutiny.

There are three classes of naturally occurring fats, which are characterized by the number of double bonds present in their fatty acid side chains. These are saturated (SFA), monounsaturated (MUFA), and polyunsaturated (PUFA) fatty acids. PUFAs can then be further classified into 2 groups due to the position of the first double bond; omega-3 fatty acids and omega-6 fatty acids. Two of the most common omega-6 fatty acids are arachidonic acid (AA) and linoleic acid (LA). Fish is a rich source of omega-3 fatty acids, containing eicosapentaenoic acid (EPA) and docosahexaenoic acid (DHA). Nuts, seeds and vegetable oils contain the essential omega-3 alpha-linolenic acid (ALA). Importantly, ALA can be converted to EPA and then to DHA by the same competitively enzymatic reaction that converts LA to AA, hence producing omega-6 PUFAs. It appears more relevant, however, from a beneficial cardiovascular point of view, to stimulate and promote the conversion of ALA to EPA.

As pointed out by Willett [6], 30–40 years ago the USA and several other countries moved to replace SFA with PUFA, which subsequently meant a substantial decline in rates of coronary heart disease. One likely factor that explains this reduction of coronary disease is the increase in PUFA intake. Hence, a successful strategy to reduce complications in patients with cardiovascular disease, and possibly to have some primary prevention effect as well, should be to use a Mediterranean diet rich in omega-3 PUFAs as well as in MUFAs.

One may also surmise that a high ratio between omega-6 and omega-3, reflecting increased and decreased consumption of omega-6 and omega-3 fatty acids, respectively, in the industrialised world, reaching levels of around 15–20/1, may be associated with developing overweight and obesity and consequently with cardiovascular disease. These values should then be compared with omega-6/omega-3 ratios of 1–5/1 mirroring earlier day's diet and also associated with lower degree of cardiovascular disease [7]. The presently relative high intake of omega-6 fatty acids and thus the potential increase of prostaglandins, thromboxane and leukotrienes, is likely to contribute to a more pro-thrombotic, pro-aggregatory and pro-inflammatory state, not only in patients but also in healthy subjects. Thus, it must be a goal to try to aim for achieving levels of omega-6/omega-3 ratio of 2–3/1 by using a Mediterranean style diet, as demonstrated by Ambring et al. [8].

Epidemiology and Mediterranean Diets

The link between a Mediterranean-style diet and greater longevity and reduced cardiovascular morbidity has been established and has also been proposed for other diseases, e.g. various forms of cancers. However, much of the evidence for a beneficial effect on cardiovascular morbidity by a Mediterranean diet is sustained by observational studies and personal reviews as importantly pointed out by Serra-Majem et al. [5]. However, there are recent data obtained from randomized trials to support the contention of a Mediterranean diet being a healthy diet beneficially affecting health [9].

Another important longitudinal study involving diet and lifestyle in the elderly is the HALE study collecting data from 11 European countries [10]. During a 10-year follow-up period, men and women between 70 and 90 years of age, who had adhered to a Mediterranean diet, were nonsmokers, physically active and had a modest alcohol intake, had less than half the mortality rate from all causes, cardiovascular disease and cancer than those who did not comply to this diet. Moreover, in a multicenter, prospective study involving 9 European countries, a dietary score that assessed adherence to a modified Mediterranean diet, rich in plant foods and unsaturated lipids, was associated with a longer life expectancy in apparently healthy elderly people, even when adjusted for various confounders such as socio-economic situations and physical activity [11]. In one of these European countries, Greece, further evidence was found that a Mediterranean diet in the general population seems to improve survival of patients with coronary heart disease [12].

Type of Diet and Unsaturated Fatty Acids and Blood Components/Inflammation

The mechanisms underlying the cardiovascular benefits of Mediterranean-style diets are not fully understood. These diets are associated with a lower level of low-density lipoprotein (LDL) oxidation, due both to a higher presence of MUFA [13] and a less pro-inflammatory state. Omega-3 PUFAs are potentially considered as being anti-atherogenic and anti-inflammatory compounds. In this context it is important to stress that atherosclerosis and inflammation have, to some extent, similar mechanistic pathways in their early stage, in particular the interactions between the vascular wall (endothelium) and blood components (leukocytes and platelets).

Fat intake has been blamed for being unhealthy, but more importantly, focus should be on the type of fat in the diet. For quite some time 'fat-free' food products have been promoted, which, interestingly enough coincides with recent years' dramatic increase in overweight and obesity.

Dietary interventions, like a Mediterranean-style diet or a diet high in plant sterols, soy protein, and fiber, effectively reduce LDL-cholesterol and apolipoprotein B concentrations in both normo- and hypercholesterolemic healthy subjects [14, 15]. Jenkins et al. [15] could demonstrate that besides dietary lowering of LDL-cholesterol, C-reactive protein (CRP) concentrations were also lowered. Moreover, there is sparse information as to whether leukocytes and vascular endothelial growth factor (VEGF), the latter also being released by neutrophils and platelets [16, 17], are affected by dietary intervention. In the Lyon Diet Heart Study, being a secondary prevention trial, the amount of leukocytes was shown to be linked to cardiovascular risk [18, 19].

In 1997, the Swedish National Food Administration evaluated the eating habits of the Swedish population [20], which formed the base for the Swedish diet used in the study by Ambring et al. [8, 14]. This survey demonstrated macronutrient composition to be: 16: 48: 34: 2% of energy from protein, carbohydrates, fat, and alcohol, dietary fatty acids 15: 13: 5: 1% of energy from saturated, mono-unsaturated, omega-6 polyunsaturated and omega-3 polyunsaturated, dietary cholesterol (321 g) and fiber (17 g). In this study subjects were subjected to a 7-day food diary. This included one cooked meal/day with a rotational 7-day menu. The composition of the Mediterranean-inspired diet, in contrast with the Swedish diet, contained twice the amount of fiber, 4–9 times more antioxidants, three times the amount of omega-3 PUFA, less than half the amount of SFA, almost three times less cholesterol and a 35% decrease in the glycemic index. In addition, sterol esters (2 g/day) were given as an ingredient in margarine. The daily intake of calories, protein, carbohydrate and total amount of fat was intended to be similar in the two diets. The amount of alcohol was also aimed to be constant in the two diet periods; however, consumption of beer was preferable during the Swedish diet and wine during the Mediterranean-inspired diet. The amount of alcohol intake was restricted to 10 g of alcohol/day and to be consumed evenly throughout the week. Compliance, as well as the self-selected foods, was assessed by use of three unannounced telephone interviews (24-hour recalls)/period and nutritional composition calculated (table 1).

By switching from the Swedish diet to the more favorable Mediterranean-style diet in low risk healthy subjects caused substantial lowering of plasma lipids and lipoproteins, a clear reduction in the number of leukocytes, involving monocytes, neutrophils, and lymphocytes, as well as in the number of platelets after only a 4-week period. These hematological alterations occurred probably as a result of a decrease in the omega-6/omega-3 PUFA ratio of 45% [8, 14] (fig. 1). This change in hematology pattern suggests a lower inflammatory activity.

Not only fish should be included in the diet, but also green leafy vegetables, flaxseed, rapeseed and walnuts should be part of regular meals, given their high content of ALA, which ultimately generates higher concentrations of omega-3 fatty acids (EPA, DHA). For example, eggs from chickens that choose their own food instead of being grain-fed are very different relative to the ratio of omega-6/omega-3 PUFA, close to 1:1, for the natural chicken eggs compared with

Table 1. Average dietary intakes from three 24-hour recalls during either the Swedish or Mediterranean-inspired diets [1]

Energy and food components	Swedish diet	Mediterranean-inspired diet
Energy, kcal	2,090 ± 87	1,869 ± 80*
Protein, E %	15 ± 0.3	16 ± 0.3
Carbohydrates, E %	48 ± 0.5	48 ± 0.7
Fat, E %	36 ± 0.5	34 ± 0.7*
SFA, E %	17 ± 0.3	8 ± 0.3*
MFA, E %	12 ± 0.2	14 ± 0.3*
Omega-3 FA, E %	1 ± 0	2 ± 0.1*
Dietary fiber, g	19 ± 1	40 ± 1*

Values are means ± SEM. *$p < 0.05$. E % = percentage energy from dietary component. SFA and MFA indicate saturated fatty acids and monounsaturated fatty acids, respectively.

approximately 20:1 for the grain-fed chicken eggs [21]. Hence, it seems important to aim consistently and effectively to reduce the omega-6/omega-3 PUFA ratio in our diet. Clearly, it can be done, as shown in the study by Ambring et al. [8, 14], who demonstrated marked reduction of the omega-6/omega-3 ratio.

Furthermore, the aforementioned study [8] showed a consistent fall in VEGF concentrations, suggesting less need for endothelial cell repair processes. Collectively, these alterations may be linked to the higher omega-3 PUFA intake, which favors the synthesis of less inflammatory eicosanoids. Hence, the favorable serum fatty acid pattern evident in this study, reflected as a substantially lower omega-6/omega-3 ratio, and/or higher antioxidant influence by means of the augmented fruit intake as part of this beneficial Mediterranean-style diet, would both beneficially affect the number of blood cells and VEGF concentrations. Lower VEGF concentrations may confer a more optimal milieu for the vascular endothelium and hence requiring less need for angiogenesis, mirrored as lowered VEGF production.

The phospholipid fatty acids are essential components of membrane constituents which influence the physical properties of cell membrane function. Fatty acids and their metabolites also interfere with many steps of inflammation, such as vascular contraction, chemotaxis, cell adhesion and diapedesis, and cell activation. Fatty acids can directly or indirectly, via the eicosanoids, modulate leukocyte function, and hence control proliferation and production of cytokines and adhesion molecules [22].

It is established that both MUFA, and PUFA of the omega-3 series, have anti-inflammatory actions that may contribute to their beneficial effects on LDL fatty

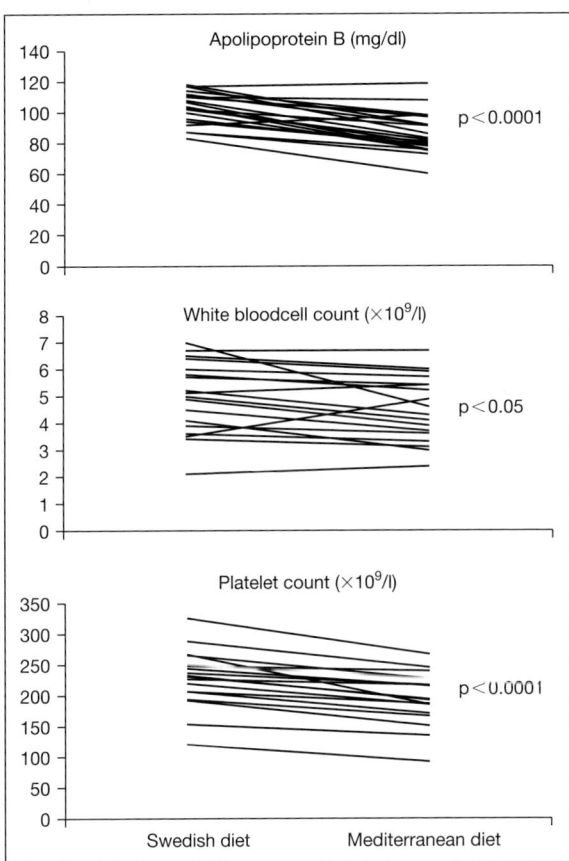

Fig. 1. Individual values depicting the changes of apolipoprotein B (top panel), white blood cell count (middle panel) and the number of platelets (lower panel) when diet was altered, in a randomized cross-over design, from a Swedish to a Mediterranean style diet for 4 weeks in healthy subjects without cardiovascular risk factors (modified from [8] and [14]).

acid composition [23] and endothelial function [24, 25]. Besides findings of lower LDL-cholesterol and apolipoproteins-B (apo-B) plasma concentrations in the study by Ambring et al. [8, 14] (fig. 1), there was a reduction of SFA intake in combination with a more than tripled amount of MUFA and PUFA in subjects eating the Mediterranean-style diet compared to the traditional Swedish diet. This is in good agreement with the results demonstrating a lower total amount of SFA serum concentrations, lower arachidonic acid concentrations and substantially higher amount of omega-3 PUFA concentrations yielding a much lower omega-6/omega-3 ratio following the Mediterranean diet regimen than the Swedish one.

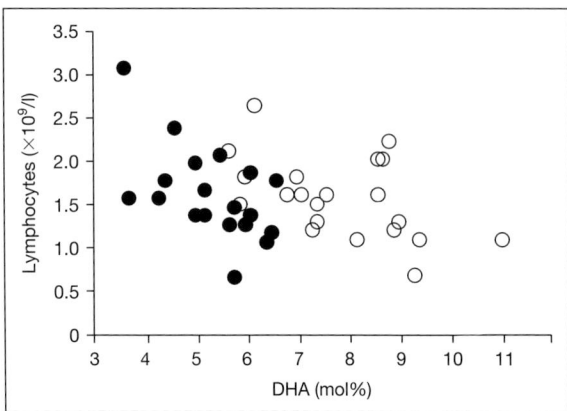

Fig. 2. Number of lymphocytes in relation to increasing concentrations of docosahexaenoic acid (DHA) after the Swedish (●) and Mediterranean (○) style diets. Significance for Pearson correlation coefficient (r = −0.54, p = 0.006) was assessed by permutation. Reproduced with permission from Ambring et al. [8].

Fat fish and flaxseed, which contain omega-3 fatty acids, were used during the Mediterranean diet period. It has been shown that fatty acids and mediators derived from them also can regulate the expression of adhesion proteins in both leukocytes and endothelial cells [26]. A cross-sectional study concerning habitual dietary intake of fatty acids (omega-3 and omega-6) and the relation to inflammatory markers has confirmed these beneficial effects [27]. Moreover, in the study by Ambring et al. [8], an inverse relationship was found between the number of lymphocytes and the concentrations of DHA (fig. 2). Taken together, findings of a lower leukocyte in adjunct to reduction of the amount of platelet count during Mediterranean-style diet [8] (fig. 1) might reflect a lower inflammatory state, and possibly influencing the activity of the platelet pool, which might confer a protective effect against atherogenesis even in healthy subjects.

Mediterranean Diet and Blood Vessels

Ample evidence suggests that inflammation has an essential role in the development and progression of atherosclerosis [2, 28]. Raised concentrations of inflammatory mediators, such as CRP and interleukin-6 (IL-6), may reflect inflammation and expression of adhesion molecules in the arterial wall which would allow leukocytes to adhere. Moreover, high blood cholesterol is associated with endothelial dysfunction both in adults and in the young [29]. In terms of vascular repairing and regenerating proteins, VEGF, an angiogenic growth factor, is elevated in patients who are at elevated cardiovascular risk, such as hypertensives with three or more clinical risk factors [30], indicating an increased need for vascular repair.

In humans with evidence of cardiovascular disease or demonstrating cardiovascular risk factors, dietary supplementation with omega-3 fatty acids is associated with beneficial influence on endothelial cells, reflected by improved endothelium-dependent vasodilatation in the forearm vasculature [31]. In the study by Ambring et al. [14], it was not possible to demonstrate enhanced vasodilatory responses in healthy subjects in response to a 4-week Mediterranean-style diet, probably because of their lack of cardiovascular risk factors. Corollary, Leeson et al. [32] were unable to show a relation between plasma omega-3 fatty acid concentrations and vascular function in a large group of young adults. However, in a subgroup consisting of individuals with increased cardiovascular risk, such as smoking, higher fasting insulin, glucose or triglyceride concentrations, omega-3 fatty acid levels were positively associated with flow-mediated dilatation [32]. Similarly, patients with the metabolic syndrome who, in a randomized single-blind study, received a Mediterranean-style diet improved their endothelial function and reduced markers of systemic vascular inflammation in adjunct to a reduction in the number of components of the syndrome [33]. Hence, it appears that increased cardiovascular risk, which usually is linked to endothelial dysfunction, has to be present in order to demonstrate improved arterial vasodilatory function by a Mediterranean diet.

Omega-3 PUFAs may also constitute beneficial vascular effects other than upon the endothelium. In patients with established atherosclerotic plaques, awaiting carotid endarterectomy, it was elegantly shown that those who received fish oil capsules (omega-3) incorporated these fatty acids into the plaque compared with patients receiving sunflower oil (omega-6) [34]. Intriguingly, it was further demonstrated that plaques from the omega-3 group of patients were less infiltrated with macrophages and presented with a well-formed fibrous cap, suggesting a lower degree of plaque inflammatory status. Altogether, these findings support the contention that fish oil supplementation to atherosclerotic patients create more stable plaques, which may confer less risk of rupture, and these changes can occur rapidly after dietary change. Along the same lines, Djousse et al. [35] were able to demonstrate that increased consumption of dietary ALA (omega-3) was associated with lower prevalence of calcified atherosclerotic plaque in the coronary arteries measured by cardiac computerized tomography.

Collectively, higher intake of omega-3 PUFAs appears to slow down the atherogenic process, perhaps by promoting anti-inflammatory action, which is of great relevance both in early stages of atherosclerotic development as well as in situations where plaques have already developed.

Mediterranean Diet and Unsaturated Fatty Acids and Their Importance for Metabolic and Blood Pressure Control

Unsaturated fatty acids, and omega-3 PUFA in particular, as important components of a Mediterranean-style diet, have also been documented to exercise beneficial effects on metabolism and cardiovascular hemodynamic factors. It becomes important to stress that positive effects can be obtained in early life, even during pregnancy. This has been demonstrated in elegant studies from Finland in the STRIP study [36]. Healthy 7-month-old infants and their families were subjected to low-saturated fat counseling long-term, which, 9 years later, resulted in a positive effect on insulin resistance index compared with a control group.

There is clear evidence that early, perinatal omega-3 status markedly affects adult cardiovascular physiology and metabolism. Experimentally, Weisinger et al. [37] reported exciting data showing that rats raised with early omega-3 PUFA deficiency showed increased blood pressure later in life compared with controls. Moreover, in animals with adequate omega-3 PUFA supply at an early age, where a switch to deficient omega-3 status occurred late postnatally, protected against the blood pressure elevation. These data by Weisinger et al. [37] support observations that overweight and symptoms related to the metabolic syndrome in the adult animal can be programmed by modulating the essential fatty acids (EFA) in the perinatal period [38–40], suggesting that obesity per se may be associated with a disturbed omega-6/omega-3 PUFA balance in the maternal diet during pregnancy, lactation and early childhood. These experimental findings have also been extended into the human situation. In an elegant, multicenter, randomized controlled trial, Forsyth et al. [41] investigated whether supplementation of infant formula milk with long chain PUFA influenced blood pressure in later childhood. The study revealed that PUFA supplementation was associated with lower blood pressure at 6 years of age versus the control group. Given that blood pressure tracks from childhood into adult life [42] and the observed increase in blood pressure over time in 9- to 17-year-olds [43], early exposure to dietary long chain PUFA, as in the Mediterranean diet or by dietary supplementation, may prevent or minimize cardiovascular risk and events in adulthood.

There are adult studies reporting on monounsaturated fatty acids and blood pressure, as nicely reviewed by Alonso et al. [44]. Many studies lack, however, a proper design. In contrast, Alonso and Martinez-Gonzales [45], in their prospectively designed SUN Study, demonstrated an inverse relationship between olive oil consumption and the risk of developing hypertension. This association, however, was found only in men. Further support for a blood pressure reducing effect by omega-3 PUFA has been obtained previously by Bonaa et al. [46] and recently by Djousse et al. [47]. The latter study demonstrated convincingly that dietary ALA was associated with both a lower prevalence of hypertension and lower resting systolic blood pressure in both men and women.

Mechanistically, it is interesting to speculate that a change of fatty acids in favor of MUFA (and PUFA) modifies membrane phospholipids that may alter blood pressure control, endothelial function and ion channels. In addition, given that a diet rich in omega-3 fatty acids promote production of vasodilatory prostaglandins, through competitive enzymatic kinetics (desaturase), and suppress vasoconstrictor influence, such as with thromboxane A2 [48], one has to consider also that the nonlipid fraction may contain beneficial and important factors, e.g. antioxidants. Further research is needed here to discern what compounds are responsible for the positive effects.

Taken together, although there are studies showing varying results in terms of MUFAs' influence on blood pressure, it appears that the majority of evidence demonstrates that MUFA from vegetable sources, particularly from olive oil in the context of Mediterranean-style diets and dietary intake of ALA, can be favorable both in the management of high blood pressure and, importantly, play a role in a public health perspective in preventing hypertension.

Mediterranean Diet, Unsaturated Fatty Acids and Overweight/Obesity

Given the importance to keep cardiovascular risk at a minimum, the emerging idea is to stress the essential point to promote a well-balanced and nutritious diet already from childhood. Today, with the high prevalence of overweight and obesity among children and adolescents, Mediterranean-style food and omega-3 PUFA intake are rather low, also reflected as a high omega-6/omega-3 ratio. Klein-Platat et al. [49] showed that a low ratio between PUFA and SFA and low long-chain omega-3 PUFA concentrations were associated with the metabolic syndrome and inflammation in overweight but otherwise healthy adolescents. No such relationships could be found in normal-weight adolescents. This pattern corroborates recent findings from our research group inasmuch that obese children and adolescents presented with lower serum phospholipid PUFA levels vs. lean subjects [50]. Notably, correlations were found between omega-3 fatty acids and total, superficial and deep subcutaneous adipose tissue, as determined by magnetic resonance imaging (MRI) [50]. One may speculate that low-long chain omega-3 PUFA levels in these young subjects, and in overweight and obese children and adolescents in general, have been prevailing for a long time, probably most of their lives, which might constitute but one factor contributing to increasing levels of blood pressure and its consequences, such as increased left ventricular mass and reduced blood pressure dipping responses observed in these groups [51, 52]. Thus, strong emphasis must be made in promoting a diet to young children, which is rich in fish and vegetables, has a Mediterranean profile, and possibly also by supplementing long-chain omega-3 PUFAs.

Mediterranean Diet and Heart Rate

Not only blood pressure is associated with increased cardiovascular risk and mortality but it is now also well established that both higher resting heart rate and an abnormal heart rate profile during exercise and recovery is predictive for sudden death [53]. Although old and established knowledge of the huge importance of the autonomic nervous system (ANS) for maintaining cardiovascular control [54], strong links exist between pathophysiological changes within the ANS and death from myocardial infarction and heart failure [55–57]. Hence, autonomic imbalance, i.e. a relative or absolute decrease in vagal tone, or an increase in activity in the sympathetic division, needs to be considered when addressing issues of cardiovascular risk. In the context of ANS it is most interesting to note that fatty fish and fish oil intake, yielding a low omega-6/omega-3 ratio, is associated with lower risk of cardiac arrhythmias, including sudden death, arrhythmic coronary heart disease death, and atrial fibrillation [for refs, cf. 58]. Given the increased cardiovascular risk and risk for sudden death due to elevated heart rate, it would be favorable if increased intake of omega-3 PUFA, preferably long-chain omega-3 PUFA could lead to a slowing of resting heart rate and perhaps to a more beneficial heart rate profile during exercise. Indeed, in the recently published meta-analysis of randomized, double-blind, placebo-controlled clinical trials, fish oil reduced heart rate, particularly in patients with higher resting heart rate or longer duration of fish oil supplementation (>3 months) [58]. Although the exact mechanisms for these beneficial effects on heart rate are not fully understood, one may surmise that this is due to the incorporation of omega-3 fatty acids into myocyte membranes which in turn may influence both ion channels and various receptor functions. Besides direct effect of fish oils on cardiac electrophysiological properties, one has also to consider direct effects on vagal and sympathetic neurons, as for example reflected by improved heart rate variability [59]. Collectively, the results from the meta-analysis by Mozzafarian et al. [58] provide solid evidence that marine fish oil creates beneficial effects on the heart by reducing heart rate through mechanisms, which may be further investigated but are likely to include both direct cardiac electrophysiological effects as well as positive effect on the ANS.

Conclusions

A Mediterranean-style diet favors an increased intake of polyunsaturated fatty acids of the omega-3 series, and particularly a lowering of the omega-6/omega-3 ratio, of course in adjunct to a substantial intake of vegetables and fruit.

The propensity for favorably affecting and reducing cardiovascular risk by having adequate dietary omega-3 PUFA, as in a Mediterranean-style diet is obvious. Although there is solid evidence suggesting that much of the cardioprotection is based on omega-3 fatty acids, the role of antioxidant power, which may prevail in the nonlipid part of the Mediterranean style diet, remains to be elucidated.

Child and adolescent obesity has increased remarkably during quite a short time in Western societies. Evidence that major health problems among adults may be preventable or at least greatly diminished by early interventions provides the rational for thinking even more creatively about an adequate diet to young children and adolescents, not to mention promoting more physical activity. No doubt, child health in general, and food and activity are important parts of their lives and health has such profound effects on adult life health. Investment in health must begin in our children and it needs to be iterated that optimal diet habits, such as a Mediterranean-style diet involving more fish and ALA-rich vegetables, should be introduced and even emphasized more in early childhood.

Acknowledgements

The authors thank Gun Bodehed-Berg, Anneli Ambring, Mette Axelsen, Magdalena Laffrenzen, Birgitta Strandvik and Li-Ming Gan for providing valuable help.

This study was supported by grants from the Swedish Heart and Lung Foundation and the Sahlgrenska Academy at Göteborg University, Sahlgrenska University Hospital.

References

1 Li S, Chen W, Srinivasan SR, Bond MG, Tang R, Urbina EM, Berenson GS: Childhood cardiovascular risk factors and carotid vascular changes in adulthood: the Bogalusa Heart Study. JAMA 2003;290:2271–2276.
2 Libby P: Inflammation in atherosclerosis. Nature 2002;420:868–874.
3 Kris-Etherton P, Eckel RH, Howard BV, St Jeor S, Bazzarre TL: AHA Science Advisory: Lyon Diet Heart Study. Benefits of a Mediterranean-style, National Cholesterol Education Program/American Heart Association Step I Dietary Pattern on Cardiovascular Disease. Circulation 2001;1031823–1825.
4 Trichopoulou A, Costacou T, Bamia C, Trichopoulos D: Adherence to a Mediterranean diet and survival in a Greek population. N Engl J Med 2003;348:2599–2608.
5 Serra-Majem L, Roman B, Estruch R: Scientific evidence of interventions using the Mediterranean diet: A systematic review. Nutr Rev 2006;64:s27–s47.

6 Willett WC: The Mediterranean diet: science and practice. Publ Health Nutr 2006;9:105–110.
7 Simopoulos AP: Importance of the ratio of omega-6/omega-3 essential fatty acids: evolutionary aspects; in Simopoulos AP, Cleland LG (eds): omega-6/omega-3 Essential Fatty Acid Ratio: The Scientific Evidence. World Rev Nutr Diet. Basel, Karger, 2003, vol 92, pp 1–22.
8 Ambring A, Johansson M, Axelsen M, Gan L, Strandvik B, Friberg P: Mediterranean-inspired diet lowers the ratio of serum phospholipid n–6 to n–3 fatty acids, the number of leukocytes and platelets, and vascular endothelial growth factor in healthy subjects. Am J Clin Nutr 2006;83: 575–581.
9 de Lorgeril M, Salen P: The Mediterranean-style diet for the prevention of cardiovascular diseases. Publ Health Nutr 2006;9:118–123.
10 Knoops KTB, de Groot LCPGM, Kromhout D, Perrin A-E, Moreiras-Varela O, Menotti A, van Staveren WA: Mediterranean diet, lifestyle factors, and 10-year mortality in elderly European men and women. JAMA 2004;292:1433–1439.
11 Trichopoulou A, Orfanus P, Norat T, et al: Modified Mediterranean diet and survival: EPIC-elderly prospective cohort study. BMJ 2005;330:991.
12 Trichopoulou A, Bamia C, Trichopoulous D: Mediterranean diet and survival among patients with coronary heart disease in Greece. Arch Intern Med 2005;165:929–935.
13 Reaven PD, Witztum JL: Oxidized low density lipoproteins in atherogenesis: role of dietary modification. Annu Rev Nutr 1996;16:51–71.
14 Ambring A, Friberg P, Axelsen M, Laffrenzen M, Taskinen MR, Basu S, et al: Effects of Mediterranean inspired diet on blood lipids, vascular function and oxidative stress in healthy subjects. Clin Sci (Lond) 2004;106:519–525.
15 Jenkins DJ, Kendall CW, Marchie A, Faulkner DA, Wong JM, de Souza R, et al: Effects of a dietary portfolio of cholesterol-lowering foods vs. lovastatin on serum lipids and C-reactive protein. JAMA 2003;290:502–510.
16 Webb NJA, Myers CR, Watson CJ, Bottomley MJ, Brenchley PEC: Activated human neutrophils express vascular endothelial growth factor (VEGF). Cytokine 1998;10:254–257.
17 Mohle R, Green D, Moore MAS, Nachman RL, Rafii S: Constitutive production and thrombin-induced release of vascular endothelial growth factor by human megakaryocytes and platelets. Proc Natl Acad Sci USA 1997;94:663–668.
18 de Lorgeril M, Salen P, Martin JL, Monjaud I, Delaye J, Mamelle N: Mediterranean diet, traditional risk factors, and the rate of cardiovascular complications after myocardial infarction: final report of the Lyon Diet Heart Study. Circulation 1999;99:779–785.
19 Renaud S, de Lorgeril M: Dietary lipids and their relation to ischaemic heart disease: from epidemiology to prevention. J Intern Med Suppl 1989;731:39–46.
20 Becker W: Riksmaten 1997–1998. Vår Föda 1999;1:24–26.
21 Simopoulos AP, Salem N Jr: [n–3] Fatty acids in eggs from range-fed Greek chickens. N Engl J Med 1989;321:1412.
22 Pompeia C, Lopes LR, Miyasaka CK, Procopio J, Sannomiya P, Curi R: Effect of fatty acids on leukocyte function. Braz J Med Biol Res 2000;33:1255–1268.
23 Tsimikas S, Philis-Tsimikas A, Alexopoulos S, Sigari F, Lee C, Reaven PD: LDL isolated from Greek subjects on a typical diet or from American subjects on an oleate-supplemented diet induces less monocyte chemotaxis and adhesion when exposed to oxidative stress. Arterioscler Thromb Vasc Biol 1999;19:122–130.
24 Carluccio MA, Massaro M, Bonfrate C, Siculella L, Maffia M, Nicolardi G, et al: Oleic acid inhibits endothelial activation: a direct vascular antiatherogenic mechanism of a nutritional component in the Mediterranean diet. Arterioscler Thromb Vasc Biol 1999;19:220–228.
25 Carluccio MA, Siculella L, Ancora MA, Massaro M, Scoditti E, Storelli C, et al: Olive oil and red wine antioxidant polyphenols inhibit endothelial activation: antiatherogenic properties of Mediterranean diet phytochemicals. Arterioscler Thromb Vasc Biol 2003;23:622–629.
26 Seljeflot I, Arnesen H, Brude IR, Nenseter MS, Drevon CA, Hjermann I: Effects of omega-3 fatty acids and/or antioxidants on endothelial cell markers. Eur J Clin Invest 1998;28:629–635.
27 Pischon T, Hankinson SE, Hotamisligil GS, Rifai N, Willett WC, Rimm EB: Habitual dietary intake of n–3 and n–6 fatty acids in relation to inflammatory markers among US men and women. Circulation 2003;108:155–160.

28 Ross R: The pathogenesis of atherosclerosis: a perspective for the 1990s. Nature 1993;362: 801–809.
29 Sorensen KE, Celermajer DS, Georgakopoulos D, Hatcher G, Betteridge DJ, Deanfield JE: Impairment of endothelium-dependent dilation is an early event in children with familial hypercholesterolemia and is related to the lipoprotein[a] level. J Clin Invest 1994;93:50–55.
30 Felmeden DC, Spencer CGC, Belgore FM, Blann AD, Beevers DG, Lip GYH: Endothelial damage and angiogenesis in hypertensive patients: relationship to cardiovascular risk factors and risk factor management. Am J Hypertens 2003;16:11–20.
31 Chin JP, Gust AP, Nestel PJ, Dart AM: Marine oils dose-dependently inhibit vasoconstriction of forearm resistance vessels in humans. Hypertension 1993;21:22–28.
32 Leeson CPM, Mann A, Kattenhorn M, Deanfield JE, Lucas A, Muller DPR: Relationship between circulating n–3 fatty acid concentrations and endothelial function in early adulthood. Eur Heart J 2002;23:216–222.
33 Esposito K, Marfella R, Ciotola M, Di Palo C, Giugliano F, Giugliano G, D'Armiento M, D'Andrea F, Giugliano D: Effect of a Mediterranean-style diet on endothelial dysfunction and markers of vascular inflammation in the metabolic syndrome: a randomized trial. JAMA 2004;292:1440–1446.
34 Thies F, Garry JMC, Yaqoob P, Rerkasem K, Williams J, Shearman CP, Gallagher PJ, Calder PC, Grimble RF: Association of n–3 polyunsaturated fatty acids with stability of atherosclerotic plaques: a randomised controlled trial. Lancet 2003;361:477–485.
35 Djousse L, Arnett DK, Carr JJ, Eckfeldt JH, Hopkins PN, Province MA, Ellison RC: Dietary linolenic acid is inversely associated with calcified atherosclerotic plaque in the coronary arteries. Circulation 2005;111:2921–2926.
36 Kaitosaari T, Rönnemaa T, Viikari J, et al: Low-saturated fat dietary counselling starting in infancy improves insulin sensitivity in 9-year-old healthy children. Diabetes Care 2006;29:781–785.
37 Weisinger HS, Armitage JA, Sinclair AJ, Vingrys AJ, Burns PL, Weisinger RS: Perinatal omega-3 fatty acid deficiency affects blood pressure later in life. Nat Med 2001;7:258–259.
38 Korotkova M, Gabrielsson B, Holmäng A, Larsson B-M, Hansson LÅ, Strandvik B: Gender related long-term effects in adult rats by perinatal dietary ratio of n 6/n–3 fatty acids. Am J Physiol Regul Integr Comp Physiol 2005;288:R575–579.
39 Korotkova M, Ohlsson C, Gabrielsson B, Hanson, LÅ, Strandvik B: Perinatal essential fatty acid deficiency affects weight and bone growth and mineralization in adult male rats. Br J Nutr 2004;92:643–648.
40 Ailhaud G, Guesnet P: Fatty acid composition of fats is an early determinant of childhood obesity: a short review and an opinion. Obes Rev 2004;5:21–26.
41 Forsyth JS, Willatts P, Agostoni C, Bissenden J, Casaer P, Boehm G: Long chain polyunsaturated fatty acid supplementation in infant formula and blood pressure in later childhood: follow up of a randomised controlled trial. BMJ 2003;326:953.
42 Srinivasan SR, Myers L, Berenson GS: Changes in metabolic syndrome variables since childhood in prehypertensive and hypertensive subjects: the Bogalusa Heart Study. Hypertension 2006;48:33–39.
43 Muntner P, He J, Cutler JA, Wildman RP, Whelton PK: Trends in blood pressure among children and adolescents. JAMA 2004;291:2107–2113.
44 Alonso A, Ruiz-Gutierrez V, Martinez-Gonzalez MA: Monounsaturated fatty acids, olive oil and blood pressure: epidemiological, clinical and experimental evidence. Publ Health Nutr 2006;9:251–257.
45 Alonso A, Martinez-Gonzalez MA: Olive oil consumption and reduced incidence of hypertension: the SUN study. Lipids 2004;39:1233–1238.
46 Bonaa KH, Bjerve KS, Straume B, Gram IT, Thelle D: Effect of eicosapentaenoic and docosahexaenoic acids on blood pressure in hypertension: a population-based intervention trial from the Tromso study. N Engl J Med 1990;322:795–801.
47 Djousse L, Arnett DK, Pankow JS, Hopkins PN, Province MA, Ellison RC: Dietary linolenic acid is associated with a lower prevalence of hypertension in the NHLBI Family Heart Study. Hypertension 2005;45:368–373.
48 Salonen R, Nikkari T, Seppanen K, Venalainen JM, Ihanainen M, Rissanen V, Rauramaa R, Salonen JT: Effects of omega-3 fatty acid supplementation on platelet aggregability and platelet produced thromboxane. Thromb Haemost 1987;57:269–272.

49 Klein-Platat C, Drai J, Oujaa M, Schlienger JL, Simon C: Plasma fatty acid composition is associated with the metabolic syndrome and low-grade inflammation in overweight adolescents. Am J Clin Nutr 2005;821:178–184.
50 Karlsson M, Mårild S, Brandberg J, Lönn L, Friberg P, Strandvik B: Serum phospholipid fatty acids, adipose tissue and metabolic markers in obese adolescents. Int J Obesity 2006;in press.
51 Friberg P, Allansdotter-Johnsson A, Ambring A, Ahl R, Arheden H, Framme J, Johansson A, Holmgren D, Wahlander H, Marild S: Increased left ventricular mass in obese adolescents. Eur Heart J 2004;25:987–992.
52 Framme J, Dangardt F, Marild S, Osika W, Wahrborg P, Friberg P: 24-h Systolic blood pressure and heart rate recordings in lean and obese adolescents. Clin Physiol Funct Imaging 2006;26:235–239.
53 Jouven X, Empana JP, Schwartz PJ, Desnos M, Courbon D, Ducimetiere P: Heart-rate profile during exercise as a predictor of sudden death. N Engl J Med 2005;352:1951–1958.
54 Folkow B: Physiological aspects of primary hypertension (review). Physiol Rev 1982;62:347–504.
55 Schwartz PJ: The autonomic nervous system and sudden death. Eur Heart J 1998;19(suppl F):F72–F80.
56 La Rovere MT, Bigger JT Jr, Marcus FI, Mortara A, Schwartz PJ: Baroreflex sensitivity and heart-rate variability in prediction of total cardiac mortality after myocardial infarction. Lancet 1998;351: 478–484.
57 Petersson M, Friberg P, Eisenhofer G, Lambert G, Rundqvist B: Long-term outcome in relation to renal sympathetic activity in patients with chronic heart failure. Eur Heart J 2005;26:906–913.
58 Mozaffarian D, Geelen A, Brouwer IA, Geleijnse JM, Zock PL, Katan MB: Effect of fish oil on heart rate in humans: a meta-analysis of randomized controlled trials. Circulation 2005;112: 1945–1952.
59 Christensen JH, Gustenhoff P, Korup E, Aaroe J, Toft E, Moller J, Rasmussen K, Dyerberg J, Schmidt EB: Effect of fish oil on heart rate variability in survivors of myocardial infarction: a double blind randomised controlled trial. BMJ 1996;312:677–678.

Prof. Peter Friberg
Department of Clinical Physiology
Sahlgrenska University Hospital
SE–413 45 Göteborg (Sweden)
Tel. +46 31 342 15 96, Fax +46 31 82 76 14, E-Mail peter.friberg@mednet.gu.se

Dietary Fat Intake of European Countries in the Mediterranean Area: An Update

Franca Marangoni, Antonella Martiello, Claudio Galli

Department of Pharmacological Sciences, University of Milan, Milan, Italy

The pattern of the diet which was typical during the early 1960s in countries in the Mediterranean basin has been extensively described in several meetings and publications, and the complexity of the topic has recently raised the issue of updating the definition of this diet [1]. In essence, the main points are:
(1) Countries bordering the Mediterranean belong to three different continents (Europe, Asia and Africa) making a total of 21 (European: Gibraltar, Spain, France, Monaco, Italy, Slovenia, Croatia, Bosnia and Herzegovina, Albania, Greece; Asian: Turkey, Cyprus, Syria, Israel, Lebanon; African: Egypt, Libya, Malta, Tunisia, Algeria, Morocco).

The most relevant contribution to the concept of the Mediterranean diet arises from the features of the diets, which were most extensively studied, i.e. those in typical Southern European countries (e.g. Greece, Cyprus, Malta) and in the Mediterranean regions of Spain, Italy and France. The contributions of diets in the major North African countries, predominantly located along the Mediterranean Coast (Egypt, Libya, Algeria, Tunisia), and also from the diet of countries on the Eastern shores of the Mediterranean are relevant although less studied. Significant differences occur also in the diet of different areas in the same country (e.g. Southern vs. Northern Italy). As a general consideration, differences in dietary habits are related to the availability of food items, especially of plant origin, in relation to specific characteristics of climates, environmental features, cultures, etc.
(2) There were certain common characteristics in the various diets throughout the different countries, deriving from the features of local food production and consumption, as a combination of the agricultural traditions and of the consumption of wild foods obtained from noncultivated plants and wild, unbred animals. Common features of the diets in the Mediterranean basin can be summarized as follows [2, 3]:

- High consumption of fresh fruits, vegetables, legumes, herbs and garlic, bread and other cereals, potatoes, nuts and seeds.
- Olive oil is the key fat source, rich in monounsaturated fatty acids.
- Dairy products, fish and poultry are consumed in low-to-moderate amounts.
- Little red meat is eaten, from different sources, with an appreciable contribution from grass-fed animals, e.g. sheep and goat meat, and their milk and derived products.
- Eggs are eaten zero to four times a week.
- Wine is drunk in moderate (or low) amounts daily.

A general concept that can be applied in considering the Mediterranean diet is that there is a prevalence of unprocessed or natural foods. Consumption of natural, unprocessed foods implies the ingestion of parts (cells, tissues, organs) of plants and animal organisms that spontaneously and actively adapted to local environmental conditions, rather than the intakes of separated or extracted molecules. In these types of foods, a physiological balance between various components of biological (structural and functional) relevance has been reached through adaptive processes and these complex mixtures of structured ingredients, which would include bioactive components, is then transferred to the organism that is ingesting the food. This process has naturally taken place throughout the course of evolution of animal species, including humans (hunters and gatherers), before the appearance and development of agriculture. The ingestion of natural foods involves also dilution of their components into a relatively high food mass and this would increase their bioavailability.

In addition, a certain level of physical exercise associated with working activities completed the life style profile in the Mediterranean countries.

Major differences between the features of the diets in North African countries and Southern European countries concern the type of carbohydrates, e.g. pasta, rice and polenta (cornmeal) in European countries, couscous (a semolina grain) in North Africa and rice, bulgur and chick peas in Eastern Mediterranean.

(3) Significant changes in the traditional dietary patterns occurred during the last decades in Mediterranean countries and these should be taken into consideration when evaluating the present situation. However, the growing evidence that the association of several components of the Mediterranean diet leads to protective effects vs. various pathologies requires more detailed assessments of the quantitative aspects, i.e. the contents of specific nutrients, in this case, types of fatty acids, in the various food items that are representative of the diet. This is an essential information in order to design complex meals that will provide the optimal intakes of the nutrients that have been shown to be protective by various studies, and to formulate practical recommendations.

(4) In the above perspective, this chapter is specifically devoted to selectively consider fats in the Mediterranean diet, updating the data presented in the previous volume of the series on the same topic [4], to the latest available information. In essence, focus will be on the contribution of various components of the diets in European Mediterranean countries to the overall fat consumption. More specifically, the following dietary components will be considered in selected Mediterranean countries versus Northern European countries:

1 Total fat consumption, animal versus vegetable.
2 Visible fats used for cooking or dressing, of animal versus vegetable origin.
3 Consumption of plant foods, e.g. vegetables and legumes, widely consumed in the Mediterranean diet, including some consideration to selected vegetable foods particularly rich in certain fatty acids.
4 Consumption of various animal foods: fish, bovine meat and dairy products, and other relevant animal foods, including consideration to some locally consumed wild animals, e.g. snails, frogs.
5 Fatty acid composition of invisible fats in major foods. In addition, data on the quantitative and qualitative aspects of the contribution to fat intakes by minor sources will be presented.

Further, the protective effects of the consumption of a fatty acid typical of Mediterranean diets, namely oleic acid in olive oil, and of selected fatty acids, such as the omega-3 fatty acids, with special attention to the land based alpha-linolenic acid (ALA), and their interactions, will be discussed.

Finally, practical recommendations will be provided on how to formulate menus providing certain amounts of health promoting fatty acids, based on the quantitative and qualitative data, and conclusions will be drawn.

Fats in the Mediterranean Diet

The consumption of fats in 2002, subdivided into total, vegetable and animal, in various European countries, comparing selected Northern European (NE) countries with Southern European (SE), North African (NA) and Eastern Mediterranean (EM), are shown in figure 1. It appears that the total fat consumption of SE populations tend to be higher than those of the other population groups, especially those in NA, reflecting somehow the generally higher use of visible fats for salad dressings and cooking, that contributes significantly to total fat consumption.

As to the proportions between vegetable and animal fat consumption (fig. 1; table 1) the ratios of vegetable versus animal fats are higher in SE, being generally higher than 1.0 with the exception of France, than in NE countries

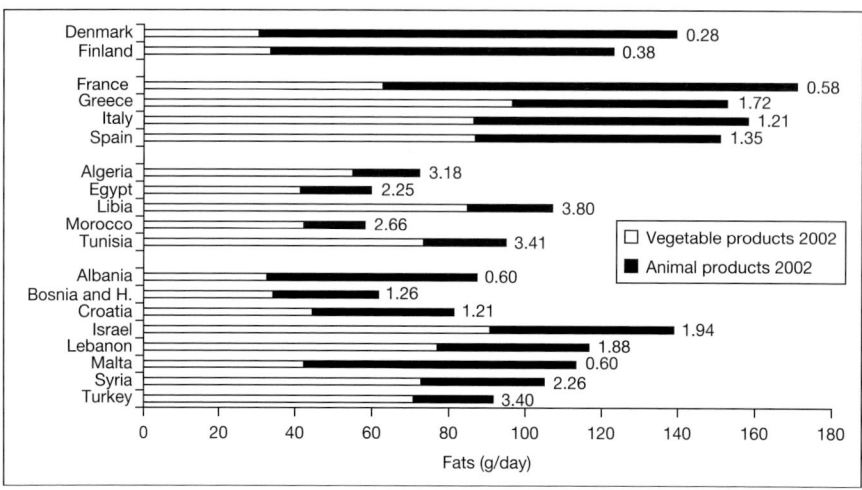

Fig. 1. Total fat intake (g/day per person), from animal and vegetable products, in Mediterranean countries and, as comparison, in Denmark and in Finland. Values at the right side of the bars represent the vegetable/animal fat ratios. Data from FAOSTAT 2002.

under consideration (less than 0.4). In France, the Southern part of the country, with expected significant dietary differences versus the Northern part, contributes only partly to the overall national situation. In the NA and EM areas the ratios are quite different, being rather high in NA (>2), mainly due to the lower animal fat intakes, and ranging between 0.6 (Albania and Malta) and over 3 (Turkey) in EM. No major changes in the vegetable/animal (V/A) fat ratios occurred between the periods 1990–1998, 1998–2002 and the year 2002.

Vegetable Fats

Visible

When the consumption of visible fats are considered in NE, SE, and EM countries (table 2), it appears that the intakes of all types of vegetable oils are higher in SE. In these countries, as previously mentioned, oils are widely used for salad dressing and similar applications, and this results in relatively high consumption rates, assessed as disappearance data, than in NE. Olive oil is by far the most abundant in Greece, Italy and Spain, but appreciable consumption of other vegetable oils also takes place in certain SE countries, e.g. sunflower oil in France and Spain, corn oil in Greece, soybean oil in Italy and Spain.

Table 1. Total fat intake (g/day per person) from vegetable and animal products in North Europe (NE), South Europe (SE), North Africa (NA) and the Eastern Mediterranean (EM): data from FAOSTAT

Countries		Products		Value (vegetable/animal fat ratios)		
		vegetable 2002	animal 2002	2002	1998–2002	1990–1998
NE	Denmark	30.6	108.9	0.3	0.3	0.2
	Finland	33.7	89.3	0.4	0.4	0.3
SE	France	62.8	108.1	0.6	0.5	0.5
	Greece	96.5	56.2	1.7	1.6	1.8
	Italy	86.4	71.7	1.2	1.2	1.1
	Spain	86.8	64.1	1.3	1.4	1.5
NA	Algeria	55.0	17.3	3.2	3.1	3.7
	Egypt	41.4	18.4	2.2	2.2	2.9
	Libya	84.8	22.3	3.8	3.2	4.9
	Morocco	42.3	15.9	2.7	3.0	3.6
	Tunisia	73.4	21.5	3.4	3.7	4.0
EM	Albania	32.8	54.5	0.6	0.7	0.5
	Bosnia and Herzegovina	34.4	27.3	1.3	1.0	0.9
	Croatia	44.5	36.8	1.2	1.0	0.9
	Israel	90.7	48.3	1.9	2.0	1.9
	Lebanon	77.0	39.7	1.9	2.1	1.8
	Malta	42.3	71.0	0.6	0.6	0.6
	Syria	72.8	32.2	2.3	2.4	2.1
	Turkey	70.8	20.8	3.4	2.8	2.8

Appreciable consumption of olive oil occurs also in other Mediterranean countries, such as Cyprus. Consumption of olive oil in Greece, Italy and Spain in 2002, was similar to that in the period 1990–1998, i.e. 50, 36 and 31 g/person/day in 2002 versus 54, 31 and 31, respectively, in 1990–1998. Some increment over time occurred instead in France, from 2 to 4 g/person/day. The high consumption of olive oil in SE is responsible to the high intakes of oleic acid in these countries, a fatty acid which by itself appears to exert favorable effects on various parameters.

Animal fat consumption, mainly butter, is still quite lower in the typical SE Greece and Spain, than in the NE, but in the whole of Italy it is comparable to, and in France it is even higher than in the NE, reflecting the contributions of

Table 2. Daily intakes (g/person) of visible vegetable (a) and animal (b) fats: data from FAOSTAT 2002

Products	North Europe		South Europe				North Africa		Eastern Mediterranean	
	Denmark	Finland	France	Greece	Italy	Spain	Algeria	Egypt	Israel	Turkey
(a)										
Olive oil	1.4	0.5	4.4	50.1	36.2	30.9	4.1	0.0	1.1	1.1
Corn oil	1.5	0.0	1.6	9.0	4.6	0.8	0.0	0.5	1.8	5.3
Soybean oil	2.2	8.4	4.5	1.4	10.7	11.1	2.2	4.5	13.6	6.8
Sunflower seed oil	0.2	2.7	19.8	12.2	12.6	26.7	12.5	6.6	1.6	12.9
Palm oil	0.0	2.6	1.4	0.0	1.9	0.0	7.9	0.0	3.0	9.6
Coconut oil	0.0	2.4	0.0	0.0	1.6	2.1	0.0	0.3	0.1	0.5
(b)										
Butter	3.7	7.2	18.6	2.3	6.6	1.9	1.2	4.7	0.7	3.6

dietary habits of the Northern parts of these two countries. They are instead very low in NA and EM. Changes between 1998 and 2002 are rather small.

Food Consumption as Sources of Invisible Fats

Data are presented concerning only NE, SE and selected NA and EE countries.

Consumption of Plant Foods

Plant foods in various forms (green vegetables, legumes, cereals, dry fruits, etc.) represent a significant portion of the diet in most Mediterranean countries. Therefore, although the fat content in most vegetables and plant foods is rather low, the appreciable proportions of certain fatty acids, e.g. ALA, and the high vegetable consumption may contribute to significant overall intakes of nutritionally relevant and health promoting fatty acids.

The detailed consumption of major vegetables and plant foods in NE, SE, NA and EM countries is shown in table 3. Consumption of beans and pulses are higher in SE (and in EM) than in NE while peas are not very relevant components of the Mediterranean diet. Wheat consumption is highest in Italy and Greece, being very high also in NA and EM, while in France and Spain it is comparable to that in NE. In SE, with the exception of Italy, potatoes are consumed in amounts comparable to those in NE. The consumption of walnuts is higher in SE than in the other areas, and is also appreciable in absolute terms. Fat content in walnuts is rather high and of interest are the relevant proportions of ALA, 18:3ω3 [6].

Table 3. Annual consumption (kg/year) per capita of vegetable foods in different European countries: data from FAOSTAT 2002

Products	North Europe		South Europe				North Africa		Eastern Mediterranean	
	Denmark	Finland	France	Greece	Italy	Spain	Algeria	Egypt	Israel	Turkey
Beans	0.2	0.0	0.9	2.9	1.7	1.5	1.6	0.3	1.9	3.5
Peas	0.7	1.2	0.5	0.0	1.3	0.1	0.5	0.1	0.7	0.1
Pulses	1.0	1.2	2.0	4.8	5.6	5.7	6.1	9.9	6.2	14.2
Wheat	109.7	77.9	98.6	135.5	151.3	88.2	184.8	130.4	127.4	193.6
Vegetables	108.2	70.8	137.8	245.5	151.0	147.7	87.1	174.4	227.8	224.3
Potatoes	77.4	69.9	66.2	67.1	39.4	80.3	41.1	18.2	47.9	60.7
Nuts	4.0	1.0	4.1	11.3	6.7	8.1	1.3	0.6	5.6	6.1

Table 4. Annual consumption (kg/year) per capita of animal foods in different European countries: data from FAOSTAT 2002

Products	North Europe		South Europe				North Africa		Eastern Mediterranean	
	Denmark	Finland	France	Greece	Italy	Spain	Algeria	Egypt	Israel	Turkey
Meat										
Beef	27.5	18.0	28.2	19.2	24.0	15.2	4.3	9.8	22.2	4.7
Lamb and Goat	0.5	0.3	3.4	12.4	1.5	5.9	5.8	1.5	1.3	4.7
Pork	64.7	33.5	37.2	32.6	42.9	67.4	0.0	0.0	2.6	0.0
Poultry	20.3	14.6	27.7	17.7	17.9	26.4	7.8	9.1	71.9	9.8
Fish										
Freshwater fish	3.6	8.8	3.5	2.4	1.9	2.2	0.0	7.1	3.3	0.8
Seafood	24.3	32.6	31.3	23.3	26.2	47.5	3.5	15.0	22.0	7.3
Animal products										
Whole milk	460.0	128.8	62.1	71.4	32.8	90.9	74.1	15.2	77.5	75.5
Cheese	21.0	15.5	24.6	25.6	22.5	6.7	0.7	7.1	16.9	1.7
Eggs	16.4	8.9	15.3	9.0	11.8	14.3	3.0	2.3	10.7	6.9

Consumption of Animal Foods

Consumption of animal foods, providing invisible fats, in the various countries are shown in table 4. Comparisons between SE and NE countries, reveal that: in SE the consumption of beef is comparable, with the exception of Spain where it is lower; that of lamb and goat, mainly as free living animals, is quite higher, especially in Greece and Spain; that of pork is intermediate between those in Denmark and in Finland, in SE countries being highest in Spain and lowest in Greece; poultry consumption is generally higher than in NE, especially in the case of France and Spain. As to seafood intake, it ranges from 23 (Greece) to 47 (Spain) kg/year in SE versus 24 and 32 in the two NE countries, Denmark and Finland. The consumption of fresh water fish tends to be lower in SE than in NE. Fish consumption is a strict determinant of the intake of long chain PUFA of the omega-3 series, such as eicosapentaenoic acid (EPA) and docosahexaenoic acid (DHA), fatty acids that are certainly present in higher amounts, however, in marine fish, especially from cold water than in fresh water fish.

Among the animal products, whole milk, cheese and eggs in SE vs. NE countries, the consumption of whole milk is markedly lower, while that of cheese is higher in three out of four countries (France, Greece and Italy, being lower in Spain). The types of cheese (data not reported) may also be somewhat different among SE countries (e.g. from cow's or goat's milk). The consumption of eggs in SE and in NE is comparable, somewhat in contrast with the definition of the Mediterranean diet. There are, however, some differences within SE countries, with egg consumption being higher in France and Spain than in Italy and Greece.

No reliable data are available on the intake of locally available wild animals, consumed by local, generally small, communities as part of local traditional knowledge, in certain areas of SE. As an example, snails are part of the traditional dietary habits in Crete [5] and frogs in certain areas in Italy. These local foods, consumed on a small scale, have an interesting fatty acid composition from the point of view of nutrition, as will be discussed later.

As a general consideration, in certain Mediterranean countries, such as Italy, Spain and especially France, the dietary habits in the Mediterranean part of the country, i.e. Southern Italy and Provence (France), are rather different from those in the continental part. Previous data on the regional differences between Northern and Southern Italy, in 1953 and 1983, showing also changes of dietary patterns in the South in the indicated period, have not however been updated. On the other hand, a rather recent publication on the nutritional characteristics of the population of Ventimiglia di Sicilia, a rural community in Sicily, indicates that although the typical features of the Mediterranean diet were maintained, the high total caloric intake in association with other changes in lifestyle may be responsible for the large prevalence of overweight and obesity in this community [7].

Composition of Selected Foods (Fatty Acid Profile and Content): Animal and Vegetable

The total fat content per 100 g of food and, in some instances also per portion, along with the proportions of major fatty acid classes in selected foods are reported in table 5. Data are obtained from the United States Department of

Table 5. Fatty acid composition and levels: data from USDA and our laboratory

Food	Total fats		SFA		MUFA		PUFA		Omega-3		Omega-6	
	g/100 g	g/portion	g/100 g	g/portion	g/100 g	g/portion	g/100 g	g/portion	g/100 g	g/portion	g/100 g	g/portion
Visible fats												
Vegetable												
Corn oil	100.0	10.0[a]	12.9	1.3[a]	27.5	2.7[a]	54.6	5.5[a]	n.d.	n.d.	n.d.	n.d.
Margarine	80.4	8.0[a]	12.9	1.3[a]	36.0	3.6[a]	27.8	2.8[a]	n.d.	n.d.	n.d.	n.d.
Olive oil	100.0	10.0[a]	13.8	1.4[a]	72.9	7.3[a]	10.5	1.0[a]	0.7	0.1	9.7	1.0
Animal												
Butter	81.1	8.1[a]	51.4	5.1[a]	21.0	2.1[a]	3.0	0.3[a]	0.2	0.02[a]	2.7	0.3[a]
Lard	100.0	10.0[a]	39.0	3.9[a]	45.1	4.5[a]	11.2	1.1[a]	1.0	0.1[a]	10.2	1.0[a]
Hidden fats												
Vegetable												
Beans (white)	0.8	1.1[f]	0.2	0.3[f]	0.07	0.09[f]	0.4	0.5[f]	n.d.	n.d.	n.d.	n.d.
Nuts (South Italy)	47.3	7.0[b]	4.7	0.7[b]	5.4	0.8[b]	26.0	3.9[b]	5.3	0.8[b]	20.7	3.1[b]
Animal												
Beef, loaf cooked	14.3	17.2[e]	5.4	6.5[e]	6.1	7.3[e]	0.4	0.5[e]	0.1	0.1[e]	0.4	0.5[e]
Chicken, roasted	3.6	4.3[e]	1.0	1.2[e]	1.2	1.4[e]	0.5	0.6[e]	0.1	0.1[e]	0.5	0.6[e]
Goat, raw	2.3	2.8[e]	0.7	8.4[e]	1.0	1.2[e]	0.2	0.2[e]	n.d.	n.d.	n.d.	n.d.
Pork, raw	26.5	3.2[e]	9.8	11.8[e]	12.2	14.6[e]	2.4	0.3[e]	n.d.	n.d.	n.d.	n.d.
Turkey	4.9	5.9[e]	1.6	19.2[e]	1.0	1.2[e]	1.4	0.2[e]	n.d.	n.d.	n.d.	n.d.
Frogs*	0.9	0.9[d]	0.2	0.2[d]	0.1	0.1[d]	0.2	0.2[d]	0.04	0.04[d]	0.2	0.2[d]
Snails*	1.8	1.8[d]	0.1	0.1[d]	0.1	0.1[d]	0.3	0.3[d]	0.06	0.06[d]	0.1	0.1[d]

Table 5. (continued)

Food	Total fats		SFA		MUFA		PUFA		Omega-3		Omega-6	
	g/100 g	g/portion	g/100 g	g/portion	g/100 g	g/portion	g/100 g	g/portion	g/100 g	g/portion	g/100 g	g/portion
Fish, Tuna Salmon	9.3	11.2[e]	1.5	1.8[e]	2.9	3.4[e]	4.1	4.9[e]	1.0	1.2[e]	4.1	4.9[e]
Chinook	4.3	5.2[e]	0.9	10.8[e]	2.0	2.4[e]	1.0	1.2[e]	0.5	0.6[e]	0.5	0.6[e]
Trout, raw	3.5	4.2[e]	0.7	8.4[e]	1.1	1.3[e]	1.2	1.4[e]	0.7	0.8[e]	0.5	0.6[e]
Mozzarella	22.3	26.8[d]	13.1	13.1[d]	6.5	6.5[d]	0.5	0.5[d]	0.3	0.3[d]	0.3	0.3[d]
Parmesan	25.8	12.9[c]	16.4	8.2[c]	7.5	3.7[c]	0.4	0.2[c]	0.2	0.1[c]	0.2	0.1[c]
Goat's cheese	35.6	17.8[c]	24.6	12.3[c]	8.1	4.0[c]	0.6	0.3[c]	–	–	0.6	0.3[c]

[a]Portion = 10 g; [b] portion = 15 g; [c] portion = 50 g; [d] portion = 100 g; [e] portion = 120 g; [f] portion = 135 g.
*Our data.
n.d. = Not detectable.

Agriculture (USDA, www.ars.usda.gov/fnic/foodcomp/search/ updated to 2005), but also data resulting from analyses carried out in our lab are included. The relative fatty acid (FA) composition of visible fats is obviously different comparing animal versus vegetable sources, with SFA prevailing in animal fats and PUFA in vegetable fats, including margarines, where however, depending upon the processing for their preparation, some *trans* FA are also present. The overall consumption of *trans* FA in Mediterranean Countries is however rather low, and is mainly confined to naturally occurring *trans* products, such as those, e.g. conjugated linoleic acid (CLA) derived from biohydrogenation of PUFAs in ruminants [8]. PUFA levels are quite higher in vegetable oils than in animal fats, with the exception of olive oil with a relatively low PUFA and very high MUFA (oleic acid) content, while, among animal fats, lard contains appreciable amounts of PUFA (practically almost exclusively omega-6) comparable to those in olive oil.

As to the invisible fats in various types of meat, the highest content is in pork, followed by beef, with markedly lower levels in the other animal foods. Both beef, a ruminant, and pork supply appreciable amounts of SFA, but pork is also very rich in MUFA and contains appreciable amounts of PUFA (mainly omega-6), reflecting the present patterns of animal feed. Goats and poultry contain less fat, with significant proportions of MUFA and PUFA. Various health benefits have been pointed out for grass-fed livestock. According to various research studies, meat and milk from grass-fed ruminants contains more CLA [9], vitamin E, omega-3 fatty acids, beta-carotene, and vitamin A than the meat and milk from grain-fed animals. CLA and omega-3 fatty acids are *good fats* with anti-cancer, anti-diabetes, and anti-obesity properties.

Of interest is the fatty acid content of snails and frogs, the first for the appreciable content of PUFA, with almost 50% represented by the omega-3 fatty acids (mainly ALA).

The composition of fats (SFA, MUFA and PUFA omega-6 and omega-3) consumed by populations in SE and in NE countries are shown in figure 2. Data have been calculated on the basis of the amounts of fat (animal and vegetable, visible and invisible) consumed by the populations, and the fatty acid composition of the food items considered in table 5. It appears that consumption of SFA is highest in Denmark and France, and the lowest in Greece and Spain, while MUFA are consumed at about the same levels in SE, the highest consumption occurring, however, in Denmark. PUFAs are consumed at the highest level in Spain, followed by Italy, Greece and Denmark, with France and Finland at the lowest levels. The high levels of SFA intake in Denmark and France can be explained on the basis of the high consumption of bovine meat, the high intake of MUFA in typical SE countries is related to olive oil intake, while in Denmark possibly to pork consumption. The higher PUFA intake in SE may be due to

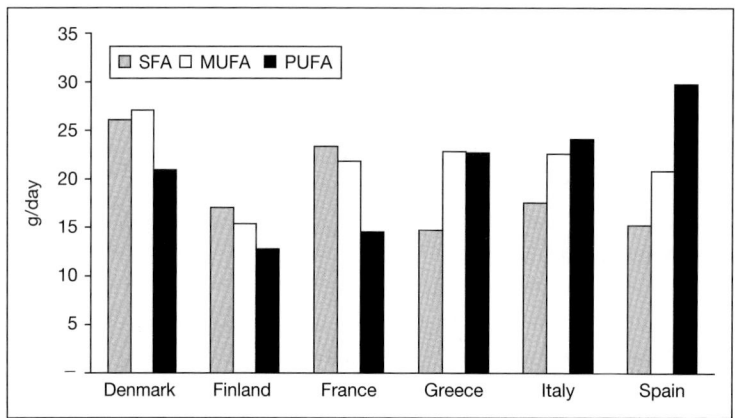

Fig. 2. Intakes of SFA, MUFA and PUFA (g/day per person) from visible (seasonings) and hidden (vegetables, and animal products) fats. In particular, the consumed food items which were considered were the following: Visible fats: coconut, cottonseed, corn, palm, rapeseed, sesame seed, soybean, sunflower and olive oils, butter. Hidden fats: beans, maize, nuts, potatoes, wheat, eggs, mutton, goat's meat, beef, pork, poultry, whole and skimmed milk, cheese, seafood and freshwater fish. Data from USDA and FAOSTAT 2002.

both vegetable fats and fish, and in Denmark, possibly mainly in relation to the fish intake. In general, the relative proportion of the three fatty acid classes in the diets of various countries indicate that in the typical SE countries there is a progressive increment from SFA to MUFA and PUFA, while in Denmark, Finland and also France there is an opposite trend.

Relevant Fatty Acids in the Mediterranean Diets (Content and Health Properties): Oleic Acid and Omega-3

Oleic acid: This fatty acid, the major component of olive oil and therefore the major fatty acid in the typical diets of SE Countries, has some characteristic features, from a chemical and a biological points of view, with respect to other fatty acids, that create a unique profile for this fatty acid in living systems and in nutrition. Oleic acid has intermediate physicochemical properties, such as the 'molecular shape' with a kink in the middle, with respect to SFA and PUFA. Therefore, it represents a transition element in terms of melting point and of the features of biomembranes (e.g. fluidity) enriched in this fatty acid; it is also the most abundant fatty acid in most organisms, being efficiently biosynthesized. Finally, when consumed with olive oil, rather than as a component of, for example, various types of meats, such as pork, it is mainly used raw for salad dressing, i.e. in association with healthy foods, such as vegetables and legumes.

A vast literature has been produced on the health-promoting effects of MUFA, in particular oleic acid, that has been reviewed by Perez-Jimenez et al. [10]. The consumption of diets enriched in monounsaturated fat, replacing SFA, has been in fact related to a lower rate of coronary heart disease, through, for example, decrease of plasma LDL-cholesterol levels. However, nonlipid effects of this monounsaturated fat have also been shown: starting with its influence on other cardiovascular risk factors, such as carbohydrate metabolism and blood pressure. Sub[...]turated fat has been provide[...]enefits beyond cholesterol, s[...]nd modulation of coagulatio[...]

Olive oi[...] also contains appreciable a[...] nature, especially the orth[...] for this is that the oil is obta[...] the seed, as in the case of m[...]y compounds, such as pheno[...] that are characterized by a[...]em to interact with various [...]ophilic antioxidants. Oliv[...]of the typical organoleptic f[...]peroxidation, but have been[...]rocesses [11]. In fact, pheno[...]protective in LDL oxidatio[...] increase the plasma antioxidant capacity and decrease the urinary excretion of isoprostanes (biomarkers of in vivo lipid peroxidation) in animals and humans. In addition, they modulate cell functions (e.g. platelets, leukocytes), by inhibiting lipoxygenases responsible for the production of the proaggregatory and proinflammatory eicosanoids, thromboxanes and leukotrienes, respectively, in vitro, in the isolated cells. Finally, after ingestion even in relatively low amounts (i.e. about 7–8 mg) in humans, olive oil phenols (as components of virgin olive oil) markedly reduce serum levels of the above eicosanoids [12].

New Findings about Omega-9 MUFA

Another feature of oleic acid concerns the type of interaction that this fatty acid appears to establish with other unsaturated fatty acids for esterification into lipids, as assessed through the evaluation of the relationships between their relative concentration in plasma total lipids. Analyses of the fatty acid profiles of plasma lipids of over 75 subjects [13] revealed that there is a strong negative correlation beween levels of oleic acid and those of the omega-6 fatty acids, ($y = -0.882 x + 61.253$, $R^2 = 0.585$, $p = 0.0001$) but not between oleic acid and levels of the omega-3 fatty acids ($y = -0.019 x + 4.12$, $R^2 = 0.007$). The reciprocal replacement of omega-9 and omega-6 fatty acids, implies that high oleic acid intake would reduce the omega-6 fatty acids, that are considered endowed of potential proinflammatory and prothrombotic actions.

Although the mechanisms underlying the above findings are a matter of speculation, the chemical and metabolic features of the fatty acids involved may provide an explanation. Under our dietary conditions, the high intake of fats (>100 g/day) tend to overload the fatty acid transport system in plasma. In fact, the total amount of fatty acids, mainly as glycerol and cholesterol esters, in the whole plasma compartment, evaluated by quantitative gas chromatography is of the order of about 10 g. Under these conditions, it is predictable that competition among fatty acids for esterification into lipid classes, a quantitatively and qualitatively limiting process, will arise. Since all unsaturated fatty acids are almost exclusively esterified in the *sn* position 2 of glycerol, this implies that the two major classes of unsaturated fatty acids, MUFA and omega-6 PUFA will compete, replacing each other. In contrast, the omega-3 fatty acids not only are a minor fraction of total PUFA, but in addition they, especially DHA which is normally the most abundant of the omega-3 fatty acids in plasma, do not appear to be effectively released from glycerolipids by phospholipases, at difference from the omega-6 fatty acids [14].

The overall significance of the above findings is that diets rich in both oleic and omega-3 fatty acids, i.e. dietary conditions reflecting those of typical Mediterranean countries, would represent an optimal strategy for health and prevention of disease.

Omega-3 fatty acids: Intake of the long-chain PUFA of the omega-3 series, typically present in fish and derivatives in the Mediterranean area are relevant but not generally higher, except in Spain, than in Northern European countries, and especially in Norway for example (not shown). In addition, levels of omega-3 long-chain PUFA are generally higher in fish from cold waters, such as the Atlantic ocean and Northern European areas, than from warm waters such as the Mediterranean sea. However, it should be pointed out that Mediterranean diets are rather rich in ALA, present in a large number of plant-derived foods.

A number of studies have indeed shown that increments in the intakes of ALA, in the range of 1–2 g/day, exert protective effects [15–17]. It is, however, still under debate whether the beneficial effects of ALA may be related to the FA itself or to the LCP derivatives that may be generated from this FA, considering that the production of the major 22 C compound, DHA has been shown not to be very efficient in terrestrial animals [18]. On the other hand, the advantage of ALA consumption rather than, or in addition to that of the omega-3 long-chain PUFA, is that sources are practically inexhaustible due to the abundance of this fatty acid in plant sources.

Table 6. TL and ALA contents of various foods: data from USDA or from INRAN (A) and from our laboratory (B).

Foods	g TL/100 g		mg ALA/portion (average values)		Portions, g[1]
	A	B	A	B	
Legumes					
Bean	1.4 (white)	1.0 (eyed)	n.d.	290	135
Lentils	1.1	1.1	147	185	135
Chickpeas	6.0	2.4 (dry)	136	161	135
Red lentils	n.d.	0.9	n.d.	139	135
Lupins	2.9	2.6	134	100	100
Green lentils	1.0	0.8	135	77	135
Peas	0.4	1.1	47	64	135
Meat					
Beef	5.0	4.1	120	116	120
Snail	1.7	1.8	n.d.	28	100
Frogs	0.3	0.9	10	29	100
Pork	1.2	1.4	12	47	120
Chicken (breast)	2.5	1.5	12	17	120
Veal	8.0	5.4	12	12	120
Vegetable					
Spinach	0.4	0.7	345	475	250
Lettuce	0.2	0.3	46	64	80
Various dry fruits					
South Italy, nuts	57.7	47.3	n.d.	792	15
Pine seed (Naples)	n.d.	40.6	n.d.	24	15
Pine seed (Liguria)	n.d.	25.8	n.d.	15	15
Peanuts	47.6	36.1	1	1	15

[1]Portion sizes adapted from USDA Food Composition Tables: http://www.nal.usda.

ALA Content in Mediterranean Foods

The content of ALA expressed as g/portion in some major components of the Mediterranean diet as well as in conventional meals, obtained from (a) data of the USDA and the Istituto Nazionale per la Ricerca Agricola e Nutrizionale (Rome, Italy) or (b) assessed in the lab through lipid extraction and quantitative FA analysis by GLC are shown in table 6.

Although the total fat content of vegetables and legumes is rather low, their relative richness in ALA, associated with the large size of the average portions and the high rates of consumption, result in appreciable levels of intake. A regular portion of spinach and beans e.g. provide significant amounts of this omega-3 fatty acid – over 400 mg ALA from spinach and almost 300 mg ALA from beans – about 25 and 15% of the recommended daily intakes (1–2 g).

Even higher relative proportions of ALA are found in various edible plants growing in the Mediterranean basin, especially in the wild state [19], and purslane (*Portulaca oleracea*), a plant that grows mainly in the wild state in SE countries such as Greece, has a relatively high relative content of ALA [20] although information on the general consumption rates (possibly high in certain communities) is limited.

Dry fruits, such as nuts, provide very high amounts of ALA even in relatively low amounts, due to both the high fat content and the high proportion of ALA (over 1 g in about 20 g of nuts corresponding to 4 nuts). This level of nut consumption over a 3-week period of time results in significant elevations not only of ALA but also EPA in whole blood lipids in healthy subjects [21]. Instead, other types of dry fruits are rather low in this omega-3 fatty acid.

Among animal foods, frogs and snails provide appreciable amounts of ALA, at least compared to other meats, although they are negligible when compared to plant foods.

Menus for Optimal Intakes of ALA

On the basis of the analytical data from the laboratory on the actual content of ALA in various foods of plant origin, it is possible to formulate menus that would provide the recommended intake (>2 g/day) of the land-based omega-3 fatty acid ALA. Examples of such combinations of food items are shown in table 7. It appears, for example, that a meal consisting of a combination of appetizers based on few nuts, a soup (beans or spelt and beans), rabbit and a side dish of spinach, or in association perhaps with a course of fish, ending with a cake containing walnuts, would be an appropriate approach to this end.

Conclusions

The types of fat in the diets of the Mediterranean countries still retain some of the original features, i.e. low SFA, relatively high intakes of MUFA and PUFA, but attention should be paid to avoid the changes that are presently taking place in large segments of the population, concerning food intake. These are related to changes in the availability of certain food items rather than others on the market, changes in lifestyle, e.g. working hours and environment, involving to a large extent also eating habits, e.g. eating out, reduced physical activity. As an example, fat intake was the most expensive part of the diet and the least accessible to populations of developing countries (Africa, certain parts of Asia),

Table 7. Optimal ALA intakes (>2 g/day) can be obtained through selection of typical foods in the Southern Italy tradition

Appetizers	
Three nuts	280 mg
First dishes	
Beans soup	640 mg
Soup of spelt and beans	520 mg
Chickpea soup	145 mg
Pine seed with pasta 'pesto'	25 mg
Side dishes	
Spinach	450 mg
Lettuce	64 mg
Main dishes	
Rabbit, roasted	320 mg
Tuna salad	330 mg
Dessert	
Nuts and cocoa pie	1,070 mg
Chestnut cake	35 mg

due to the difficulty of local production and provision (climatic conditions, costs of importation) [22]. Today fat intake is a less expensive component of the diet, to such an extent that certain vegetable fats, produced on a very large scale, are even used as fuels or lubricants in the automotive field. On the other hand, the major type of oil that is produced and consumed in SE countries, i.e. olive oil, is substantially more expensive than most vegetable oils.

Therefore, it becomes mandatory that strategies are proposed at the national and international levels with the aim of defining and promoting the consumption of foods typical of the Mediterranean diet, known to provide the type of fat that has been shown to be protective in the diet. In addition, practical and large scale projects should be activated, aimed at designing menus that can be followed both for home family-based meals, and in the preparation of meals for communities or restaurants.

References

1   Serra-Majem L, Trichopoulou A, Ngo de la Cruz J, Cervera P, Alvarez AG, La Vecchia C, Lemtouni A, Trichopoulos D, on behalf of the International task Force on the Mediterranean Diet: Does the definition of the Mediterranean diet need to be updated? Publ Health Nutr 2004;7: 927–929.
2   Simopoulos AP: The Mediterranean diet: what is so special about the diet of Greece? The scientific evidence. J Nutr 2001;131:3065S–3073S.
3   Trichopoulou A, Cistacou T, Bamia C, Trichopoulos D: Adherence to a Mediterranean diet and survival in a Greek population. N Engl J Med 2003;348:2599–2608.
4   Marangoni F, Galli C: Dietary fats of European countries in the Mediterranean area; in Simopoulos AP, Visioli F (eds): Mediterranean Diets. World Rev Nutr Diet. Basel, Karger, 2000, vol 87, pp 78–89.

5   Moschandreas J, Kafatos A: Food and nutrient intakes of Greek (Cretan) adults. Recent data for food-based dietary guidelines in Greece. Br J Nutr 1999;81(suppl 2):S71–S76.
6   Feldman EB: The scientific evidence for a beneficial health relationship between walnuts and coronary heart disease. J Nutr 2002;132:1062S–1101S.
7   Barbagallo CM, Cavera G, Sapienza M, Noto D, Cefalù AB, Polizzi F, Onorato F, Rini GB, Di Fede G, Pagano M, Montalto G, Rizzo M, Descovich GC, Nortarbartolo A, Averna MR: Nutritional characteristics of a rural southern Italy population: the Ventimiglia di Sicilia project. Am Coll Nutr 2002;21:523–529.
8   Hulshof KF, van Erp-Baart MA, Anttolainen M, Becker W, Church SM, Couet C, Hermann-Kunz E, Kesteloot H, Leth T, Martins I, Moreiras O, Moschandreas J, Pizzoferrato I, Rimestad AH, Thorgeirsdottir H, van Amelsvoort JMM, Aro A, Kafatos AG, Lanzmann-Petithory D, van Poppel G: Intake of fatty acids in western Europe with emphasis on *trans* fatty acids: The TRANSFAIR study. Eur J Clin Nutr 1999;53:143–157.
9   Khanal RC and Olson KC: Conjugated linoleic acid (CLA) contents in milk. meat and eggs: a review. Pakistan J Nutr 2004;3:82–98.
10 Perez-Jimenez F, Lopez-Miranda J, Mata P: Protective effect of dietary monounsaturated fat on arteriosclerosis: beyond cholesterol. Atherosclerosis. 2002;163:385–398.
11 Visioli F, Galli C: Biological properties of olive oil phytochemicals. Crit Rev Food Sci Nutr 2002;42:209–221.
12 Visioli F, Caruso D, Grande S, Bosisio R, Villa M, Galli G, Sirtori C, Galli C: Virgin Olive Oil Study (VOLOS): vasoprotective potential of extra virgin olive oil in mildly dyslipidemic patients. Eur J Nutr 2004;44:121–127.
13 Risè P, Marangoni F, Visioli F, Galli C: Fatty acid profiles and interactions in circulating lipids in defining strategies for dietary studies in population groups. Abstr Present. 2nd Int Symp on Triglycerides and High Density Lipoproteins, New York, 2005.
14 Shikano M, Masuzawa Y, Yazawa K, Takayama K, Kudo I, Inoue K: Complete discrimination of docosahexaenoate from arachidonate by 85 kDa cytosolic phospholipase A2 during the hydrolysis of diacyl- and alkenylacylglycerophosphoethanolamine. Biochim Biophys Acta 1994;1212:211–216.
15 Harris WS: Alpha linolenic acid a gift from the land? Circulation 2005;111:2872–2874.
16 De Lorgeril M, Salen P, Martin JL, Monjaud I, Delaye J, Mamelle N: Mediterranean diet, traditional risk factors, and the rate of cardiovascular complications after myocardial infarction: final report of the Lyon Diet Heart Study. Circulation 1999;99:779–786.
17 Djousse L, Arnett DK, Carr JJ, Eckfeldt JH, Hopkins PN, Province MA, Ellison RC, Investigators of the NHLBI FHS: Dietary linolenic acid is inversely associated with calcified atherosclerotic plaque in the coronary arteries: the National Heart, Lung, and Blood Institute Family Heart Study. Circulation 2005;111:2921–2926.
18 Burdge G: Alpha-linolenic acid metabolism in men and women: nutritional and biological implications. Curr Opin Clin Nutr Metab Care 2004;7:137–144.
19 Simopoulos AP: Omega 3 fatty acids and antioxidants in edible plants. Biol Res 2004;37:263–277.
20 Simopoulos AP: Purslane: a plant source of omega-3 fatty acids and melatonin. J Pineal Res 2005;39:331–332.
21 Marangoni F, Colombo C, Martiello A, Poli A, Paoletti R, Galli C: Levels of the n-3 fatty acid eicosapentaenoic acid in addition to those of alpha-linolenic acid are significantly raised in blood lipids by the intake of four walnuts a day in humans. Nutr Metab Cardiovasc Dis 2006 Sep 25; [Epub ahead of print].
22 Fats and Oils in Human Nutrition. Report of a Joint Expert Consultation. FAO Food and Nutrition Paper 57. Chapter 4. Global Trends in the Availability of Edible Fats and Oils, 1994, pp 25–33.

Prof. Claudio Galli, MD
Department of Pharmacological Sciences
University of Milano, Via Balzaretti, 9
IT–20133 Milano (Italy)
Tel. +39 (02) 5031 8309/7, Fax +39 (02) 5031 8384, E-Mail Claudio.Galli@unimi.it

The Mediterranean Diet in Italy: An Update

P. Rubba[a], F.P. Mancini[b,c], M. Gentile[a], M. Mancini[a]

Departments of [a]Clinical and Experimental Medicine and [b]Biochemistry and Medical Biotechnologies, Federico II University, Naples, and [c]Department of Biological and Environmental Sciences, University of Sannio, Benevento, Italy

The interest in the Mediterranean diet stems from the finding that coronary heart disease (CHD) mortality is lower in Southern Europe (in the countries bordering the Mediterranean Sea) than in Northern Europe. This benefit seems to be largely due to the relatively safe and even protective dietary habits of these regions [1–5], which consist of cereals, legumes, vegetables, fresh and dried fruit, fish and more rarely meat, olive oil, and wine consumed only with meals. Ancel Keys for the first time indicated that the dietary habits of people living along the Mediterranean Sea was very healthy and he termed it 'Mediterranean diet' [6].

Progenitors of this diet can be traced back to the time of the ancient Greeks, whose diet can be regarded as very similar to today's Mediterranean diet [7]. The diet of the ancient Romans was also close to the Mediterranean one, although mainly during the time of the Republic, but not during the Empire. In Italy, during the Middle Ages, most people ate frugally, both because of shortage of food supply and, more interestingly, because of rules and suggestions from the Church. It is remarkable what is written about meals in the Order of St. Benedict, which date back to the 6th century: frugality was the rule, except for some additions when work was heavier than usual, abstaining from eating the meat of four-footed animals except for sick and weak people, drinking wine with moderation although 'those to whom God gives the strength to abstain must know that they will earn their own reward' [7].

In the 1950s, Italian society began to change from an ancient, rural, and agriculture-based system to a modern, urban, and industrialized one [8]. This had a strong impact on the eating habits of Italians, particularly in southern regions, with the consequent progressive dilution of the original healthy Mediterranean dietary traditions with new eating styles imported from the rest

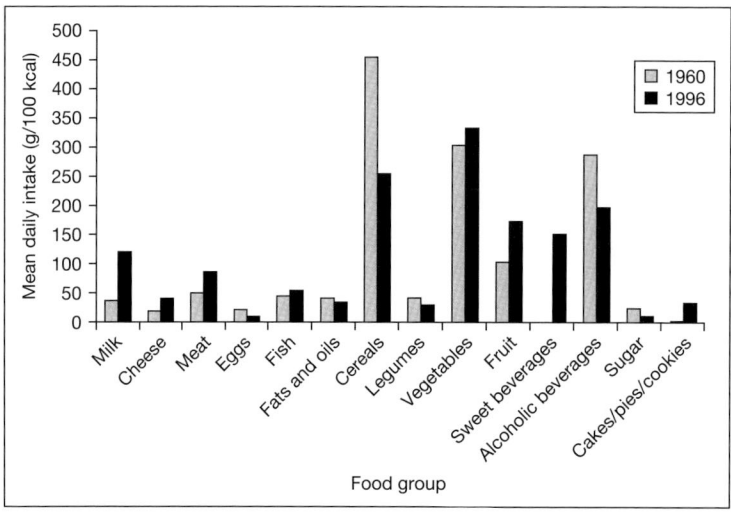

Fig. 1. Dietary habits of Italians.

of the industrialized world. In fact, over the last four decades the dietary habits of most Italians have undergone marked modifications (fig. 1), thus losing many of the health benefits of the Mediterranean diet [9, 10].

From the 1950s to the 1980s, the consumption of meat and fats in Italy increased almost four and three folds, respectively; a much smaller increase was reported for sugar, milk, fruit and vegetables (less than twofold), while no change in cereal consumption was detected [11]. Most of this revolution was nearly completed by the 1980s. From then on, advertising has become the main force leading nutritional preferences. However, some positive trends have begun to take place in more recent times, as reflected by national surveys conducted in 1980–1984 and 1994–1996 [12–14]. By comparing data from the two surveys using the food group approach of the market basket, and by measuring the contribution of the main food groups to the individual food intake, it appears that in about 10 years the contribution of oil and fats has almost halved and the intake of cholesterol-rich foods like meat and eggs has also decreased, although to a lesser extent.

These studies also detected a significant increase in the intake of fish and seafood. Fish consumption is a well-known feature of the Mediterranean diet and has been associated with improved cardiovascular prognosis. However, its availability is decreasing and the cost progressively increasing. Furthermore, pollution of the Mediterranean might discourage fish consumption [15]. In relation to cardiovascular protection, it would be of public health interest to evaluate whether polyunsaturated fatty acids of vegetable origin might replace, to some extent, polyunsaturated fatty acid from seafood. Moreover, a marked increase in sweetened beverages has been reported [16]. This might affect caloric balance and promote obesity.

Dietary habits differ among the various regional areas in Italy [17]. This observation has also been supported by the already mentioned national survey of food consumption patterns in Italy [13], carried out in 1994–1996, on adolescents, adults, and the elderly. Nutritional data were analyzed by several criteria, including a geographical division of Italy into four areas: Northwest, Northeast, Central, and South. Although some degree of similarity of food habits was found between the Northern regional areas as well as between Central and Southern ones, an overall North to South gradient in the adherence to the Mediterranean diet was observed, with the Southern people still having more traditional Mediterranean dietary habits. In fact, data show higher consumption of cereals (bread, pizza, and pasta), legumes, tomatoes and seafood in Central and Southern regions as compared to the Northern ones. It is also interesting to note a higher olive oil and lower butter consumption in Southern regions. Very recently, Pala et al. [18] analyzed the dietary behavior of elderly Italians participating in the European Prospective Investigation into Cancer and Nutrition (EPIC). In the southern cohorts of Naples and Ragusa – two cities by the sea –, they found higher consumption of cooked vegetables, legumes, cabbage, fish and fresh fruit as compared to the Northern cohort of Varese, a city near the Alps. Added fats are mainly vegetable oils in Italy with a high preference for extra virgin olive oil, produced along the coastline almost everywhere in Italy, although it may be replaced by or rather mixed with, the less expensive seed oil in some families of low socioeconomic status [18]. Higher consumption of foods rich in saturated fats, particularly red meat, appears to be related to poorly educated males, while pasta, polenta, rice and other grains are still consumed widely by the Italian EPIC cohort [18]. Young people in general, but in particular less educated ones living in the South of Italy, tend to consume less fruit and vegetables [19].

In the past, major emphasis was put on the low saturated fat content of the Mediterranean diet, while more recent evidence has underlined the importance of plant foods (including carbohydrate and nondigestible fiber), and of a regular use of olive oil.

The aim of this review is to update the evidence on consumption of macronutrients (dietary fat and plant foods, carbohydrate and fiber) and some vitamins in Italy, mainly in view of an impact of dietary habits on CHD risk. However, there is also increasing interest in its potential benefit in relation to cancer protection.

Dietary Scores

Nutritional epidemiology has relied mostly upon studies on the relationship between diseases and a single or few nutrients or foods. Valuable as it may be, this methodology, however, does not take into account that people eat a variety of foods containing multiple nutrients with potential interactive effects. Although the single nutrient approach is ideal when evaluating conditions linked to a single dietary factor, like vitamin deficiencies, it may be inadequate when a disease has been associated with many dietary factors. In the case of CHD, for instance, the effect of a single nutrient may be too small to be detected, but the cumulative effect of multiple nutrients may become large enough. For these reasons, and also to characterize the dietary pattern of an individual or a group of people, especially in longitudinal studies, nutritionists have set up a complementary strategy, which is to analyze overall dietary patterns including the combination of the various foods and nutrients from the diet. Dietary patterns can be defined in several ways [20]. The approach mostly used to evaluate the Mediterranean dietary pattern is to elaborate dietary scores or indices that incorporate the food composition of the Mediterranean diet. Two major features of these scores are: the possibility to evaluate the intake of a set of different types of foods altogether rather than the intake of single components, and the possibility to establish the adherence of the group's or individual's diet to a particular dietary pattern, i.e. Western, Asian, Mediterranean, etc. The study of the overall food intake, instead of the single nutrient intake, has been advocated because of the synergistic or antagonistic effects that a single food can display. However, two major requirements have to be satisfied in order to obtain an accurate and valid nutritional methodology: a precise definition of the Mediterranean diet, and the validation of the dietary score by means of biomarkers. Various authors have identified different strategies to calculate the indices.

Alberti-Fidanza and co-workers have proposed the Mediterranean Adequacy Index (MAI), an overall indicator that characterizes a diet in comparison to a Reference Mediterranean Diet (RMD) [21, 22]. The MAI can be computed in two ways: (a) 18 food groups are considered, 10 typical of the RMD (bread, cereals, legumes, potatoes, vegetables, fruit, nuts, fish, red wine, vegetable oils) and 8 nontypical of the RMD (milk, dairy products, meat, eggs, animal fat and margarine, sweet beverages, cakes/pies/cookies, sugar); the sum of the percentages of the energy content of the intake of food groups typical of the RMD relative to the total energy intake, and the sum of the percentages of the energy content of the intake of food groups distant from the RMD relative to the total energy intake are calculated; the MAI equals to the ratio between the two values obtained; (b) the same 18 food groups are considered and the relative intakes are expressed as g/day, g/1,000 kcal, or g/MJ; the MAI is equal to the ratio between the sum of one of the three measurement units of the 10 typical Mediterranean food groups and the sum of the eight nontypical Mediterranean food groups. In both ways, the higher the MAI value of the diet analyzed, the closer that diet is to a RMD. Most importantly, the MAI of random samples of men surveyed for their dietary habits in the 16 cohorts of the Seven Countries Study was inversely related to the 25-year death rates [23].

Trichopoulou et al. [24–26] worked out a Mediterranean Diet Score (MDS) that estimates the adherence to a traditional Greek Mediterranean diet. Nine food items were identified: vegetables, legumes, fruits, cereals, fish, monounsaturated lipids (or the sum of mono- and polyunsaturated lipids in the modified Mediterranean dietary score), meat, dairy products and ethanol. In particular lipids were evaluated as the ratio between monounsaturates (or the sum of monounsaturates and polyunsaturates) and saturates. A value of zero was assigned to each of the nine components specified, if the food considered was presumed to be beneficial and its individual consumption is below the sex-specific median consumption of that food in the individuals studied. A value of one was assigned if the same item is consumed in larger amounts compared to the same median value. The opposite procedure was applied to presumed detrimental components (meat and dairy products). For ethanol, a value of one was attributed to men consuming from 10 to 50 g of ethanol/day and to women consuming from 5 to 25 g of ethanol/day. The score is calculated by adding up the values obtained, and can range from zero (minimal adherence to the Mediterranean diet) to nine (maximal adherence). The authors found that a closer adherence to the Mediterranean diet was associated with a lower total mortality risk in Greek adults [27].

Huijbregts et al. [28] analyzed dietary patterns by means of the Healthy Diet Indicator (HDI), an indicator similar to that of Trichopoulou's group. Also in this case, nine items (either nutrients or food groups) were considered: saturated fatty acids, polyunsaturated fatty acids, protein, complex carbohydrates, dietary fiber, fruits and vegetables, pulses (plus nuts and seeds), cholesterol. Similarly to the MDS, values of zero or one were assigned to each item. The value of one was assigned if the consumption of that item was in the range recommended by the World Health Organization, otherwise the value was zero. The HDI was the sum of the nine values obtained and could vary from 0 to 10. The authors found an inverse significant association between HDI and 20-year all-causes mortality in elderly men from Finland, the Netherlands, and Italy.

More recently, Panagiotakos et al. [29] formulated a Mediterranean diet score by considering 11 main components of the Mediterranean diet including nonrefined cereals, fruits, vegetables, legumes, olive oil, fish, red meat, poultry; a score from 0 to 5 was assigned to each food group according to the frequency these items were consumed, and a total score, ranging from 0 to 55, was obtained by adding them up. The higher the total score, the closer the eating pattern is to the Mediterranean diet. Also in this case, the Mediterranean diet score resulted directly related to the monounsaturated fat intake, the monounsaturated to saturated fat intake ratio, and inversely related to serum lipids, blood pressure, markers of inflammation and coagulation, and the risk of acute coronary syndromes.

Other authors have calculated more generic dietary scores that quantify how rich is a given diet in some components, with reasonable evidence supporting their beneficial effects on coronary artery disease [30] or that take into account a limited number of foods typical of the Mediterranean diet [31]. In the former work, a dietary pattern with a high heart-protecting score was associated with a reduced risk of peripheral arterial disease in Italian patients with type 2 diabetes. In the latter study, people who had suffered from myocardial infarction and were in the best dietary score quarter, presented a substantial reduction in the risk of early death compared to people in the worst score quarter.

Because the relationship among different dietary indices and all-causes mortality in the same population had never been investigated before, Knoops et al. [32] compared the MDS, MAI, and HDI scores in elderly men and women from 10 European countries in the HALE population. The authors concluded that all the three indices were inversely correlated with mortality to the same extent.

These approaches to quantify the nutritional changes of population groups simplify the understanding of the 'nutritional transition', a slight but continuous change occurring in human dietary habits worldwide.

Macronutrients and Coronary Heart Disease

The relationship between dietary fatty acids (FA) and coronary heart disease has been known for over 30 years [33–36], following the pioneering evidence from the Seven Countries Study, started in the 1960s. In general, a more frequent consumption of foods high in saturated FA (SFA) was associated with higher plasma cholesterol, glucose and blood pressure [35]. In these studies, the dietary surveys were performed by using recall methods whose limitations are well known. In particular, these methods rely upon human memory and are seldom representative of an individual's usual long-term diet [37]. A major progress has therefore been the evaluation of the dietary intake of FA by a more objective and accurate methodology. This is represented by the chemical analysis of adipose tissue or plasma cholesteryl esters FA by gas-chromatographic technique [38–40].

Table 1. Dietary and adipose tissue FA in 4 European countries with different CHD mortality in middle-aged men (mean values)

Country	n	Diet P/S	AT P/S	CHD deaths/100,000
Italy (SA)	74	0.40	0.58	43
Italy (NA)	73	0.51	–	55
Sweden	77	0.29	0.44	67
Scotland	131	0.24–0.32	0.30	140
SW Finland	83	–	0.26	146
N. Karelia	102	0.27	0.27	212

Three surveys were done in countries with different CHD mortality, and included a dietary interview and adipose tissue or plasma cholesteryl esters analysis. One of them compared middle-aged men from Southern Italy, Finland and Scotland with regard to adipose tissue composition [39]. In another study middle-aged men from Naples, Southern Italy and Stockholm, were compared for diet composition and fatty acid spectrum in plasma cholesteryl esters [40]. Information was also available on adipose tissue FA in Sweden as compared to Scotland [38]. The results of the dietary interviews, which were published in separate reports [41–43], are summarized in table 1. These findings show that the polyunsaturated/saturated FA ratio (P/S ratio) in the adipose tissue correlates well with the CHD mortality gradient in different European populations, even better than the dietary P/S ratio (table 1). Adipose tissue composition reflected dietary FA consumed over a relatively long period of time (2–3 years). It was also likely to represent the FA spectrum the tissues were actually exposed to. The relative difference in polyunsaturated FA (PUFA) was mainly accounted for by differences in omega-6 FA, while no difference in adipose tissue omega-3 fatty acid was detectable across population samples. In particular, both adipose tissue and plasma cholesteryl esters analysis demonstrated that the proportion of arachidonic acid ($20:4\omega6$) was consistently higher in Italy as compared to Northern Europe [41, 42]. However, adipose tissue provides information only on relative proportions and no substitute of dietary survey methods is available to estimate the absolute amount of FA in the diet. Even with their shortcomings, dietary survey data indicate [17, 43, 44] that high P/S ratio in Italy (an area from Southern Europe with relatively low CHD mortality) is mainly due to a relatively low intake of saturated FA and a higher consumption of monounsaturated FA (MUFA), with only minor differences in PUFAs (table 2). In this respect there is agreement between older surveys [33, 34] and more recent ones.

The importance of monounsaturated FA in relation to CHD risk has received attention in more recent years. There is now evidence that regular

Table 2. Dietary fatty acids in population samples from European countries (middle-aged men; mean values)

Country	Energy kcal	Total fat g/day	SFA g/day	MUFA g/day	PUFA g/day
Italy[1] (n = 32)	2,995	105	29	66	10
Scotland[2] (n = 47)	2,660	116	50	41	16
N. Karelia[3] (n = 35)	2,490	108	55	36	13

[1] Nonmanual.
[2] Nonsmokers, nonmanual.
[3] Free-living families.

consumption of olive oil (rich in monounsaturated FA) has a significant beneficial influence on serum lipids and blood pressure; this appears to be true both among and within populations [17, 44]. In Italy the main source of monounsaturated FA is olive oil. The mechanisms of the vasculoprotective effects associated with olive oil consumption have been reviewed [45]. The importance of the relative proportions of unsaturated and saturated FA is indirectly supported by the findings in the Women Health Initiative in USA [46], where 50,000 women reduced their total fat intake, without changes in the relative proportion of unsaturated and saturated FA. In this large intervention study, despite the total fat reduction, minimal changes were observed in plasma cholesterol and blood pressure, with no impact on cardiovascular morbidity and mortality.

The plasma lipid profile is influenced by dietary composition during the second half of infancy as reported in a comparison between infants in Sweden and Italy weaned with different foods in first 2 years of life. Children weaned according to Mediterranean dietary habits (vegetable soup, milk soup and pasta) in which olive oil replaces animal fats as the main source of fat, seem to develop, once breastfeeding and milk formulas are ceased, a lipid profile with lower total cholesterol and apo B levels than Swedish children. This difference also depends on the duration of breastfeeding and possible difference in the composition of maternal milk. A mean intake of energy from fat in Mediterranean children is 28% which is slightly lower than European pediatric recommendation, but this lower intake was not found to have defined adverse effects on growth. Further studies are required to assess the importance of these factors, including the occurrence of long-term effects on growth [47].

In adolescents from southern European countries, nutritional habits have lost two important characteristics of the Mediterranean diet, a low consumption of saturated fatty acids and a high intake of complex carbohydrates, in favor of

Table 3. Dietary carbohydrate (CHO) and fiber in population samples from European countries (middle-aged men)

Country	n	Energy kcal	CHO g/day	Fiber g/day
Italy (SA)				
Manual	26	4,048	444	83
Nonmanual	32	2,995	329	56
Scotland (nonsmokers)				
Manual	38	2,742	315	20
Nonmanual	47	2,660	292	22

a large increase in the consumption of meat and dairies. A relatively high consumption of olive oil and a high intake of vegetable and fruit still persist. The nutrient pattern is as rich in total fat as in the USA, and slightly lower than in Northern Europe; these habits may explain the rise of total plasma cholesterol. Adolescents observed in the last two decades have plasma cholesterol levels similar to those reported in the USA. Adolescents in Southern Europe prefer to have three to four main meals, with a high consumption of fat- and sugar-rich foods; however, snacking is less frequent than in other industrialized countries.

Controlled clinical trials have consistently demonstrated a lipid lowering effect of complex carbohydrates and nonabsorbable fiber. Nevertheless, a high intake of bread and pasta should be avoided because, with a sedentary life style it might be associated with overweight, obesity and insulin resistance [48].

Less information is available on dietary carbohydrates and fiber in Italian men as compared to other European populations with differing CHD mortalities. However, data taken from the above mentioned dietary surveys in Scotland and Italy [42, 43] clearly indicate that in the Mediterranean area there is a remarkably higher consumption of fiber, while the differences in total carbohydrate intake are only minimal (table 3). A case-control study lends some support to the hypothesis of cardiovascular protection from high intake of dietary fiber [49]. Thus, in addition to saturated fatty acid intake and olive oil consumption, also dietary fiber is expected to contribute to the cross cultural differences in serum lipids and lipoproteins seen in Europe.

The overall result of these dietary influences on plasma lipids can be summarized as follows (table 4):
(a) A gradient in total cholesterol concentration, from southern to northern Europe, closely following the P/S gradient.
(b) No marked differences in triglyceride concentrations or total/high-density lipoprotein (HDL)-cholesterol ratio, because of the relatively lower

Table 4. Serum lipids (mmol/l) in four European countries with different CHD mortalities in middle-aged men (mean values)

Country	n	Total cholesterol	TG	HDL-CHOL	CHD deaths/100,000
Italy (SA)	74	5.37	2.04	1.22	43
Italy (NA)	73	5.47	1.52	1.25	55
Sweden	77	6.23	1.55	1.40	67
Scotland	131	5.79	1.70	1.35	140
SW Finland	83	6.40	1.57	1.36	146
N. Karelia	102	6.65	1.80	1.43	212

HDL-cholesterol concentration in Italy. Thus, the most consistent lipoprotein effect of cross-cultural differences in dietary intake of FA and fiber is on low-density lipoprotein (LDL)-cholesterol concentrations [38–40].

Nutrition, Hypertension and Stroke in Italy

The habitual low intake of saturated FA typical of the Mediterranean diet has relevant effects also on the heart and the circulation, such as a reduction in blood pressure levels. This was observed already by Puska et al. [41] and by Strazzullo et al. [50] and subsequently confirmed by Trevisan et al. [17]. More recently, the Dash Study has reinforced the concept that the substitution of saturated with unsaturated FA in the diet of hypertensive patients helps maintain lower blood pressure values [51]. However, despite the optimal profile in terms of FA composition of the Italian diet, stroke, particularly ischemic stroke, has a major impact on public health due to its high incidence, prevalence and rate of subsequent disability in Italy as in most industrialized countries. Many nutrition-related factors, such as salt intake, obesity, alcohol abuse, hyperhomocysteinemia and smoking have been recognized as playing a role in the pathogenesis of this disease. Nevertheless, unequivocal evidence of a protective or adverse role of single foods and nutrients against the risk of stroke has been difficult to achieve due to confounding biological variability. In several cases, causal relationships could be inferred from case-control and cohort studies in the presence of plausible and reproducible associations, evidence of dose-dependent effects and consistency in the results of different studies. In two recent Italian papers [52, 53], the present knowledge and future perspectives about the role of nutrition in the prevention of ischemic stroke has been reviewed. Overall, it seems that differences in nutritional risk factors for stroke in European populations are so balanced that no significant gradient in stroke mortality is detectable.

Vitamins

Circulating LDL rapidly accumulate in human atherosclerotic plaque and accumulation is prevented by oral administration of the natural antioxidant vitamin E [54]. Experimental studies and observational epidemiological data have suggested that individuals with high dietary intake of antioxidant vitamins, such as those living in the Mediterranean area or those taking antioxidant supplements, have a somewhat lower-than-average risk of cardiovascular disease [55–58]. However, controlled clinical trials using antioxidant vitamin supplements have yielded negative findings [59–61].

A possible explanation for these discrepant results has been suggested by cohort studies on early signs of atherosclerosis, as detected by noninvasive ultrasound methodology [62–65]. A cohort of free-living women from Naples (Southern Italy) was evaluated by noninvasive ultrasound to detect early signs of carotid atherosclerosis [66]. Quantitative B-mode imaging was performed on carotid arteries in all women and intima-media thickness (IMT) was evaluated. Intima-media thickening and atherosclerotic plaques were detected [66] in association with relatively higher titers of antibodies against oxidized LDL, and in association with higher levels of lipid peroxides (TBARS). The associations of these oxidation markers with early carotid lesions were independent of LDL- or HDL-cholesterol concentrations, smoking habit or blood pressure. These data are consistent with other ultrasound data supporting the association of oxidation markers with evidence of arterial wall damage. Furthermore, carotid wall abnormalities were found associated [67] with relatively low intake and plasma levels of vitamin E. Protection from oxidative stress might be particularly important in the early stages of atherosclerosis and in people with inadequate intake of antioxidants. Therefore, a possible explanation for the disappointing findings from controlled clinical trials might be a poor identification of patients who might gain true benefit from antioxidant treatment [68].

There is scientific and public health interest in the possibility that antioxidant vitamins, in particular alpha-tocopherol (vitamin E), might represent a safe means to prevent lipoprotein oxidation and antagonize the atherosclerotic process. Antioxidant vitamins or other antioxidants seem to inhibit the oxidative modification of LDL into a particularly atherogenic form and thus preserve endothelial function. The preservation of endothelium-dependent regulation of blood flow in the coronary circulation through antioxidants is likely to be extremely important in conditions of acute ischemia or disturbed blood flow such as angina pectoris or myocardial infarction: better adaptability to impaired perfusion might preserve myocardial tissue from irreversible necrotic changes or, in cases of severe ischemia, reduce infarct size [69, 70].

So far, it has been impossible to exclude that the benefits presently associated with antioxidants are due to other, unmeasured differences in lifestyle or diet composition. There is also evidence that plasma concentration of vitamin E and plasma antioxidant activity in response to oral supplementation are markedly affected by food intake [71]. Yet, it is worth considering that the mixture of natural antioxidants of the Mediterranean diet has been safely consumed for centuries, and its potential protective effect on cardiovascular risk could be applicable also to other populations.

The Mediterranean diet is relatively rich in folic acid and vitamin B_6, which are known to lower plasma homocysteine. A meta-analysis of the prospective studies on serum homocysteine concentration and cardiovascular disease [72] showed a consistent association between hyperhomocysteinemia and the rate of cardiovascular disease. The association was attenuated when the risk from high blood pressure and cigarette smoking was taken into account; however, an independent and significant predictive role for serum homocysteine concentration has been confirmed, independently of traditional cardiovascular risk factors. On the basis of these data, it is possible to estimate that a decrease in serum homocysteine by 3 µmol/l would be associated with an approximately 20% reduction in the risk of cardiovascular disease. Such a decrease can be achieved by supplementation of folic acid and vitamins B_{12} and B_6, which modulate homocysteine levels by acting on methionine metabolism [53]. This goal is difficult to achieve by dietary intervention alone: enrichment of the habitual diet with folate-rich foods is associated with a plasma homocysteine reduction of approximately 10% (1.0–1.5 µmol/l). This is in agreement with data indicating that an increase in daily folate intake in the range of 100–300 µg/day (achieved with dietary intervention) is associated with a plasma homocysteine reduction of less than 20%.

In summary, dietary changes in the direction of a Mediterranean diet, i.e. increasing fruit and vegetables consumption, are effective in decreasing plasma homocysteine concentration and in increasing other nutrients with a favorable impact on cardiovascular prevention. However, supplements are also probably needed, in order to produce a detectable impact on vascular damage.

Randomized controlled trials [73–75] have so far failed to conclusively demonstrate the beneficial effect of these supplements on cardiovascular events.

It is possible that the strength of the association between homocysteine and the risk of cardiovascular disease is weaker than previously believed. Extending the duration of intervention, or starting supplementation of vitamin B treatment in an earlier stage would possibly allow the detection of the significant effects associated with differences in homocysteine concentration [73].

Mediterranean Diet and Obesity

Obesity and its related metabolic abnormalities (dyslipidemia, hypertension, insulin resistance and impaired glucose tolerance) commonly appear during childhood and adolescence and persist frequently into adulthood, increasing the risk of cardiovascular disease.

Overweight in adolescence is a more powerful predictor of cardiovascular risk than in adulthood. As already mentioned, Southern Europe has lower cardiovascular and total mortality rates from coronary diseases than Nordic countries, but these favorable prerogatives can change if trends in dietary habits and physical activity will continue to worsen in the forthcoming years [76].

Prevalence of obesity is increasing in Europe, the trend being higher in the Mediterranean countries. This is particularly evident in Italy where a progressive increase of the population's average body weight has been observed in recent years: of the 60 million inhabitants nearly 16,000,000 adults are overweight (BMI 25–30) and 4,000,000 are typically obese (BMI >30) with some regional differences [77]. In North-Western Italy 30% of adults are overweight and 7.8% obese, in the North-East 32.1 and 8.0%, in Central Italy 32.8 and 8.0% and in the South 37.9 and 11.3%, respectively.

There is a high prevalence of overweight and obesity in young generations in Italy [78]. 36% of Italian boys and girls, aged 7–11 years, are overweight or obese. This is the highest value in Europe for this age group, followed by 35% in Malta, 34% in Spain and 31% in Greece. North Europe is much lower with 21% in United Kingdom, 18% in Sweden and 15% in Denmark [79].

An epidemiological study conducted in rural free-living Sicilian schoolchildren (Ventimiglia Study) [80] demonstrated that about one third of the study population had a diet that was higher in total calories, monounsaturated fatty acid and fiber, and lower in saturated fatty acid and cholesterol, than an all-Italy sample of schoolchildren. 13% of these children had LDL-cholesterol levels above 130 mg/dl and 11% had HDL-cholesterol below 35 mg/dl. These data suggest that prevention campaigns that including behavioral education in schools may be useful to reduce the incidence of obesity in young people.

Epidemiological surveys demonstrate that 38% of the obese children living in southern Italy meet the definition of the metabolic syndrome (MS) proposed by de Ferranti et al. [81]; they suggested parameters as a fasting glucose level >110 mg/dl; a fasting triglyceride serum concentration >100 mg/dl; a fasting high-density lipoprotein cholesterol concentration <50 mg/dl for females and <45 mg/dl for males; a waist circumference >75th percentile for age and gender; and a systolic or diastolic blood pressure >90th percentile for age, gender, and height. Children who met ≥3 of the above-mentioned criteria qualified as having the MS.

Obesity in children may lead to insulin resistance and impaired glucose regulation over time. Insulin resistance was found in southern Italy in 41% of the obese children and adolescents but only 4% of them had impaired glucose tolerance [82]. Overweight and obesity have been associated with increased carotid intima-media thickness and stiffness in adults and children. Increased stiffness of the common carotid artery represents an early marker of impaired vascular health [83]. Overweight and obesity have been associated with an increased prevalence of MS also in this study.

Common carotid arterial stiffness was significantly higher in the group of obese children with the MS compared with those without. Obese girls with insulin resistance had increased aortic stiffness compared to obese girls with low insulin resistance, even after adjustment for traditional cardiovascular risk factors [84].

The globalization process nowadays is modifying foods markets and foodstuff availability, affecting the lifestyle habits – including eating habits – of younger generations all across Europe. Despite this cultural change, consumption of dairy products and snacks seem to be less frequent in Mediterranean counties.

It is particularly intriguing that obesity is so prevalent in the European areas, where diet is still of the Mediterranean type. Could the high consumption of bread, pasta, pizza, olive oil and wine facilitate adiposity? However, the high fiber content of green vegetables, legumes and fresh fruit, typical of the Mediterranean diet, reinforces satiety, a strong anti-obesity element. Epidemiological evidence has shown an increase in sedentary lifestyle in the Mediterranean countries, which certainly contributes to the higher obesity prevalence in this part of Europe [85]. The description of 'uncomplicated obesity' in nearly a third of the Italian obese population [86] reinforces the possibility of a protective role against cardiovascular and neoplastic complications of a Mediterranean dietary pattern even in obese people. Obesity is always due to a positive energy balance, with food intake higher than energy expenditure. This appears to be the case of the observed high prevalence of obesity today in the Mediterranean regions. In order to keep these benefits and to counteract the increasing prevalence of obesity, the typical Mediterranean eating culture should be reinforced and balanced by adequate and regular physical activity.

Mediterranean Diet and Cancer in Italy

The fundamental observation of Doll and Peto [87], who suggested that at least 35% of all cancers could be prevented by diet, has been confirmed by epidemiological studies showing that differences in dietary habits influence the risk of several types of cancer [88]. Cancer mortality rates are lower in the Mediterranean areas than in northern Europe [89]. It has been estimated that eating the Mediterranean way could prevent up to 25% of colorectal, 15% of breast and 10% of prostate, pancreas and endometrial cancers [90]. Several studies have shown a reduced risk of developing cancer of the upper aerodigestive tract at higher levels of Mediterranean score: odds ratios for subjects with a Mediterranean score of six or more were 0.40 for oral and pharyngeal neoplasm, 0.26 for esophageal, and 0.23 for laryngeal cancer [91, 92].

In general, the abundance of fruit and vegetables is regarded as a major contributor to the protective effect from cancer exerted by the Mediterranean diet. Numerous studies have been designed to evaluate the relationship between the frequency of consumption of vegetables, fruit and associated micronutrients, and the risk of cancer. Mediterranean populations, Italians in particular, who consume large amounts of vegetables and fruit, displayed a lower incidence and mortality from cancer of the digestive tract and other sites: vegetables were effective in reducing the frequency of digestive tract neoplasms, while fruit reduced the relative risk for cancer of the upper digestive tract, stomach and the urinary tract [93].

However there is no absolute concordance in the field, and two recent meta-analyses point out that some of these associations are quite weak – as the one between gastric cancer and vegetables more than fruit, or the associations detected in cohort studies rather than in case-control studies [94, 95]. For these reasons, within the European Prospective Investigation into Cancer and Nutrition (EPIC) cohort from 10 European countries (including Italy), the relation between the intake of fruit and vegetable and gastric cancer and adenocarcinoma of the esophagus was re-evaluated [96]. Although the sample size of this study is large (521,457 people), and the average follow-up has been 6.5 years, only a possible negative association was detected between gastric cancer of intestinal subtype and vegetable consumption; a nonsignificant association was also found between citrus fruit intake and gastric cancer at the cardias site. As for the adenocarcinoma of the esophagus, non-significant associations of this type of cancer with vegetable intake and with citrus fruit intake were observed. The authors conclude that it is only possible to suggest a protective effect of fruit and vegetables on subtypes or specifically localized gastric cancers as well as on the adenocarcinoma of the esophagus. These findings illustrate the complexity of obtaining clear-cut results in similar studies dealing with nutritional issues, and explaining why there is still no conclusive evidence on such topics and why further cohort studies with more cases are needed. This is also the case for the controversial association between fruit and vegetable consumption and prevention of colorectal cancer, an association in which the high fiber content of these foods is involved. The current opinion, however, is that a diet rich in vegetables and fruits can help prevent colorectal cancer and the precursor adenomatous polyps [97]. The intake of fruit and vegetables is also thought to protect against lung cancer: an Italian, hospital-based, case-control study, has shown a protective effect from lung cancer with a high consumption of carrots and tomatoes, after controlling for several smoking variables [98]. However, a review of the more recent literature demonstrates conflicting results, and, within the EPIC cohort, a protective effect against lung cancer of fruit, but not vegetables, was detected [99]. The same authors concluded that such effect was likely to be small compared to smoking cessation. More recently, fruits and vegetables were studied again in relation with lung cancer and smoking, but in a case-control study [100]. Results were different relatively to the previous study, because in this setting a sporadic consumption of vegetables was associated with a twofold increased risk of lung cancer compared to frequent intake of vegetables. A similar, but less pronounced protective effect was detected for fruit. Nevertheless, also in this study, smoking was the dominant risk factor.

The role of diet and cancer, with special focus on the relation between vegetables and breast cancer, was also analyzed by studying the association of high mammographic breast density (H-MBD) with dietary components in an Italian population [101]. H-MBD is strongly associated with the risk of breast cancer. In this longitudinal study of a Mediterranean population, H-MBD was inversely associated with increasing consumption of vegetables, olive oil, and also with frequent consumption of cheese and high intake of β-carotene, vitamin C, calcium, and potassium. A direct association was, instead, observed with consumption of wine. The observed reduced risk of H-MBD in the presence of high intake of vegetables is consistent with the hypothesis that eating vegetables and, to a lesser extent, fruit might reduce the risk of breast cancer, as suggested mostly from case-control studies [94]. However, other cohort studies have failed to find a significant relation between fruit and vegetable consumption and reduced risk of breast cancer [102, 103]. It is possible that these differences can be attributed to different levels of fruit and vegetable intake, which can make more or less evident the protective effect on breast cancer.

Of course, there is also a strong interest to recognize whether or not there are specific compounds or micronutrients within fruits and vegetables that can be responsible for the potential benefits in cancer prevention. A related matter of discussion is whether bioactive compounds in fruits and vegetables could have the same effects as isolated molecules or, instead, they need the interactions present in the whole food. ß-Carotene, vitamin C and vitamin E showed an inverse relationship with the risk of oral, pharyngeal, esophageal and breast cancer. Furthermore, vitamins C and D, calcium, carotene and riboflavin provided the most consistent protective effects against colorectal cancer [93]. A group of experimental studies suggests that fruits and vegetables could protect against bladder cancer by inhibiting the formation of DNA adducts [104]; flavonoids, a group of antioxidants found in fruits and vegetables, decrease the level of DNA adducts in vivo [105]. High concentration of flavonoids can be found in onions, lettuce and red wine, typical components of the Mediterranean diet.

Another component of vegetarian food that can provide protection from cancer is fiber, which is present mostly in unrefined cereals and, to a lesser extent, in vegetables and fruits. However, the data about the protective effect of fiber against cancer are not fully concordant. For instance, although the stronger evidence of a protective effect of dietary fiber against cancer regards colorectal cancer, the epidemiology of dietary fiber and colorectal cancer is rather inconsistent [106]. Among others, a prospective study in the EPIC cohort, which includes also Italian individuals, showed that in populations with a low-average intake of dietary fibers, increasing the intake of dietary fibers by almost twofold was associated with a reduction of the risk of colorectal cancer by 40% [107]. A variety of mechanisms have been proposed for the protective effects of dietary fiber, among which is noteworthy to recall the decreased transit time of feces and the production of the short chain fatty acid, butyric acid, obtained by degradation of fiber by colonic bacterial microflora. As far as the first mechanism is concerned, a reduced transit time of the fecal content in the intestine reduces also the time of contact of potential carcinogens with the colon epithelium. Butyric acid, instead, has been reported to have antimitotic, differentiating and pro-apoptotic effects on the intestinal epithelial cells [106]. Consistent with a protective role of dietary fibers, an elevated intake of refined grains was associated with an increased risk of cancers of the stomach, colon-rectum, breast, upper digestive tract sites, and thyroid [90].

An additional advantage of the high intake of fruits and vegetables, typical of the Mediterranean diet, relies upon the high content of folate present in fruits, vegetables, but also in legumes and whole grain. In fact, a low intake of folate may increase the risk for breast and colorectal cancers [108, 109], in particular in people who regularly drink alcohol, because alcohol interferes with absorption, metabolism, and storage of folate [110]. A high intake of dietary folate may also contribute to reduce the risk of ovarian cancer, especially among women who consume alcohol regularly [111].

Despite the current uncertainty about the molecular mechanisms that underlie the protective effect of vegetables and fruits, a major hypothesis ascribes such potential to the antioxidant compounds contained in these foods [112]. Reactive oxygen species, formed continuously during metabolic reactions or produced by external sources like radiations, tobacco smoke, and air and food pollutants can produce oxidative damage of all the major molecules of the living cell, including DNA, proteins, and lipids. Damage to the DNA if the mechanisms of repair are overcome, can cause accumulation of genetic mutations, a leading event of carcinogenesis. Plants have evolved an antioxidant-based protection mechanism that makes vegetarian food especially rich in antioxidants, thus providing a significant contribution to the endogenous antioxidant defensive system of animals, including man. Besides the antioxidant activity, other potential anticarcinogenic mechanisms rely upon the induction of detoxification enzymes, inhibition of the formation of nitrosamines, binding and dilution of carcinogens in the digestive tract, and alteration of hormone metabolism. None of these mechanisms, if considered individually, seem to explain the protection of fruits and vegetables on several cancer types; more likely it is the synergy of several mechanisms that can explain the protective effect of fruit and vegetables against the risk of cancer.

In general, vegetables, fruit, dietary fiber, and certain micronutrients appear to protect against cancer, whereas excess of dietary saturated fat [113], calories, and alcohol increases the risk of cancer [88, 114]. This latter factor is linked to an additional built-in protection factor against cancer of the Mediterranean diet: especially in Italy, there is the habit to avoid alcohol consumption other than moderate drinking of wine during the main meals. Wine, which is the most typical alcoholic beverage in Italy, has a small ethanol content compared to most of other alcoholic drinks, and epidemiological studies have associated alcohol intake with increased risk of cancer of the oral cavity, pharynx, larynx, esophagus, and liver; a relationship is also possible between alcohol and cancer of the colon-rectum, pancreas, lung, and breast [88, 115]. On the other hand, wine is rich in polyphenols, like resveratrol, which can exert protective actions as mentioned above. In fact, in one study wine exerted a protective effect against ovarian cancer [116], while in another study the protective effect of wine on ovarian cancer was also observed, but only in the presence of adequate folate intake [117]. It is important to remark that by controlling for alcohol intake, the authors of the latter study were able to exclude that the protective effect of wine was related to its alcohol content. A new area of research is committed to the analysis of possible direct actions of micronutrients on the intracellular signaling pathways controlling cell cycle and cell proliferation, thus affecting tumor progression. There is large experimental evidence, for example, that resveratrol, a polyphenol relatively abundant in red wine, is not only a powerful antioxidant, but is also able to control cell proliferation [118].

As to animal protein-rich foods, most of the evidence indicates an opposite relationship with cancer according to the protein source: multivariate analyses show that the relative risk for the highest tertile of meat intake (≥7 times per week), was 1.7 for stomach, 2.0 for colon, 1.9 for rectal, 1.6 for pancreas, 1.5 for bladder, 1.5 for endometrial, and 1.3 for ovarian cancers, compared with the lowest tertile (≤3 times per week) [90]. Fish consumption appears to reduce risk of cancer of digestive tract, endometrium, ovary and prostate. Because meat is not frequently consumed, while fish is relatively abundant in the Mediterranean diet, once more, it comes out that eating the Mediterranean way confers protection from cancer. It is worth mentioning that in the same study, in which a high intake of red meat was associated with an increased risk of rectal cancer, a similar association was not observed for elevated chicken or fish consumption [119]. Indeed, chicken consumption was negatively, although weakly, associated with colorectal cancer. Consistent, but more detailed results are reported by Larsson et al. [120], who were able to associate red meat consumption with increased risk of colorectal cancer at specific subsites of the large bowel, in particular with distal but not proximal colon or rectum. Also in the EPIC cohort, high consumption of red meat was associated with colorectal cancer risk; in addition, there is some discrepancy in previous results regarding poultry and fish, the former not being associated and the latter being inversely related with the risk of colorectal cancer [121].

As already mentioned, fish is largely represented in the Mediterranean diet, and its consumption in Italy is quite high, especially among sea-coast populations. One of the most relevant compounds of fish, from the dietary point of view, is fish oil. This term refers particularly to omega-3, long-chain, polyunsaturated fatty acids, such as eicosapentaenoic acid and docosahexaenoic acid, which are present at relatively high levels in fish. It has been well documented that the ingestion of these fatty acids improves the lipid profile in man and consequently reduces the cardiovascular risk. In addition, fish oils have been proven to inhibit carcinogenesis in animal and in vitro studies [122]. However, the epidemiological evidence of the benefit of fish intake in the prevention of cancer is not as solid as the experimental data [123]. Intake of fish or fish oil has been considered protective mainly against breast, prostate, and other hormone-related cancers like those of the ovary and endometrium, but this is supported by no more than half of the studies published; the remaining studies did not find any significant relation between the intake of fish or fish oils and the risk of the mentioned forms of cancers [122].

The concept that an excess of dietary sugars can increase the risk of cancer is relatively newer and not generally accepted, although lowering blood glucose, insulin levels, and dietary glycemic index are associated with a reduction of chronic diseases including cancer [124]. In particular breast cancer has been associated with a higher intake of carbohydrates in several, but not all studies. In a recent case-control study Mexican women in the highest quartile of total carbohydrate intake were found to have a relative risk of breast cancer of 2.22 compared to women in the lowest quartile, after adjusting for total energy and other potential confounding variables; this trend was highly statistically significant [125]. Among carbohydrates, sucrose and fructose, but not starch, were associated with the increased risk of breast cancer. This difference is not easy to reconcile with one hypothesis, suggested by the authors, on the biological plausibility of the observed link between carbohydrate intake and cancer: the ingestion of carbohydrates stimulates insulin secretion – which is itself a stimulus for cell growth – and also reduces the plasma and tissue levels of IGF binding proteins 1 and 2, thus increasing the availability of IGF-1. Sucrose, fructose, and starch, instead, increase insulin in the same way and accordingly should have the same carcinogenic potential. A prospective study published very recently did not find any association between dietary carbohydrates, glycemic index, and dietary fiber, and invasive breast cancer in post-menopausal women, but only a modest, subtle association between carbohydrate and fiber intake and low-grade breast cancers [126]. Thus, even if it is advisable to replace high glycemic index foods, such as white bread, with medium-low glycemic index foods, like legumes and pasta, the independent carcinogenic potential of dietary sugars is still a matter of debate more than a proven fact.

In conclusion, there is no doubt that dietary components can influence the risk of several types of cancer in both ways. Although studies on this topic are complicated by the difficulty of acquiring reliable, standardized measurements of food intake, and controversy exists on several issues, the Mediterranean diet can protect from cancer because it is rich in foods that reduce the risk of several types of cancer, such as vegetables, fruit, and fiber, and relatively poor in meat and alcohol. Although further studies are necessary to better analyze the interactions among micronutrients and constituents of vegetables and fruit and other lifestyle risk factors, this healthy diet, typical of Italy, especially along the seacoast, provides an important protecting factor in the complex interaction between genes and environment leading to chronic diseases.

Mediterranean Diet in the Elderly

Several studies have reported nutritional deficiencies in diet of elderly Italians due to insufficient intake of component such as calcium, iron, zinc, thiamin, riboflavin, niacin, beta-carotene and vitamins A, D, and C. The low intake of these elements has been associated with cardiovascular diseases and a variety of cancers (breast, bowel, prostate, lung, stomach, esophagus and pancreas), as well as with other diseases like osteoporosis, diverticula disease, cataract, anemia, decline in the immune system and cognitive functions. A recent study on 847 men and 1,485 women, aged 65 years or older, living in rural areas in northern and southern Italy, demonstrated nutritional deficiency in 50% of the population, with inadequate intake of essential FA, calcium, potassium, and zinc in men, iron in women, and thiamin, riboflavin, niacin, beta- carotene vitamins A, D, E in both sexes [127].

Another study evaluated dietary intake and nutritional status in a random sample of 190 Italians (70–75 years of age) used to a typical Mediterranean diet. Daily energy intake, as assessed by dietary history was 2,208 ± 562 kcal in men and 1,742 ± 527 kcal in women. The general nutritional status of this sample was fairly good, and only few subjects were found at high risk of deficiency with regard to plasma vitamins levels. These data demonstrate that a correct daily intake of energy by Mediterranean diet can prevent vitamin deficiency in the elderly [128].

Moderate red wine drinking mainly during meals is one of the characteristic of Mediterranean diet in Italy, and has possible protective effects on tissue oxidative stress. A study in 26 healthy Italian centenarians, 17 women and 9 men (age range 100–105 years) showed that most of these subjects have been moderate wine consumers (<500 ml/day). Those who had a deterioration of the diet in the last three years of their life, had a significant reduction of total serum antioxidant capacity (TAC), but red wine consumption exerted a protective effect against this trend [129]. Taken together these data indicate that the Mediterranean diet as consumed in Italy, with high intake of olive oil, vegetable, fruit and moderate wine drinking can prevent nutritional deficiencies and may have protective effects against a possible reduction of TAC in old age.

Recent evidence has been published, suggesting a linkage between dietary pattern and human longevity. Many components of the Mediterranean diet, a high ratio of monounsaturated (MUFA) to polyunsaturated fatty acids (PUFA), moderate wine consumption, high consumption of legumes, cereals, vegetables and low consumption of meat can in fact reduce the risk of cancer and cardiovascular diseases [130]. In several studies conducted in Italy and Greece, the Mediterranean dietary pattern was shown to favorably affect life expectancy in the elderly population, especially before age 80. Caution should be exerted in modifying dietary habits in individuals aged >80 years because dietary modification can affect the quality of the last years of life.

Another element of the quality of health and life of aged people that seem to be influenced by the Mediterranean diet is cognitive skill. In the last years the attention of many researchers has focused on the relations between the Mediterranean diet and cognitive impairment – a major component of dementia syndromes and a determinant of disability. In an elderly population of southern Italy with a typical Mediterranean diet, high energy intake of MUFA appeared to be associated with a high level of protection against cognitive decline; in addition, fish and cereal consumption are found to reduce the prevalence of Alzheimer's disease in Europe and North America [131]. Similar studies suggested that consumption of omega-3 PUFA derived from fish is inversely associated with cognitive impairment and cognitive decline at a 3-year follow-up, reduces the risk of heart disease, inhibits carcinogenesis, can reduce blood pressure, and, taken together, improves life expectancy [132].

Some longitudinal studies have focused on the relation between intake of MUFA and all-cause mortality. The higher MUFA intake of the Mediterranean diet was associated with increased survival and appeared to be associated also with a strong protection against age-related cognitive decline (ARCD). A significant reduction of ARCD risk has been found in Italian population samples with high intakes of MUFA from olive oil (>100 g of olive oil per day), although this protective effect may be due not only to the type of FA but also to the presence of concomitant antioxidant compounds (tocopherol and polyphenols). The Mediterranean dietary pattern in Italy, therefore, based on complex carbohydrates, fiber and non-animal fat as olive oil (>100 g/day), might protect against cognitive decline in old age.

Conclusions

Dietary surveys and biochemical analyses performed in Italy and in Northern Europe confirm that dietary habits in the Mediterranean countries maintain to a large extent their traditional characteristics.

There is awareness that cultural differences, including dietary habits, tend to decrease because of the on-going globalization process. Data are already available showing that extreme differences, such as those seen between Scotland or Finland and Italy are progressively decreasing, mainly due to major changes towards healthier dietary habits in Northern Europe. However, a stronger attitude to preserve healthy traditional food habits is also developing in Italy, as compared to the recent past. Institutions, television and daily press frequently recommend to consume more fiber-rich foods like vegetables and legumes, which help control appetite by inducing long lasting satiety. The consumption of fresh fruit is also encouraged for its vitamin content. Fish, lean white meat and MUFA-rich olive oil are also recommended to maintain plasma concentrations of atherogenic lipoproteins, arterial blood pressure and thrombogenic factors as low as possible. These advices are compatible with typical and tasty dishes of the Italian traditional cuisine. Last but not least, the Mediterranean diet should be integrated with regular physical activity in order to prevent the epidemic of obesity, which is impressive in the Mediterranean area. Several features of the dietary habits of Mediterranean populations are now suggested to be helpful for the prevention of cancer.

In general, the dietary habits of Mediterranean populations (especially those living in Italy and Greece) have been found associated with increased life expectancy, and therefore represent a useful reference model, to be incorporated in a healthy lifestyle worldwide.

Acknowledgement

We are grateful to Ms Rosanna Scala for revision of the manuscript and generous assistance during the preparation of the text.

References

1 Fidanza F: The Mediterranean diet in the prevention of coronary heart disease. Diab Nutr Metab 1988;3:169–173.
2 Willet WC, Sacks F, Trichopoulou A, Drescher G, Ferro-Luzzi A, Helsing E, Trichopoulos D: Mediterranean diet pyramid: a cultural model for healthy eating. Am J Clin Nutr 1995;61: 1402S–1406S.
3 Trichopoulou A, Lagiou P: Healthy traditional Mediterranean diet: an expression of culture, history, and lifestyle. Nutr Rev 1997;55:383–389.
4 Keys A: Seven Countries: A Multivariate Analysis of Death and Coronary Artery Disease. Cambridge, Harvard University Press, 1980.
5 Ferro-Luzzi A, Branca F: Mediterranean diet, Italian-style: prototype of a healthy diet. Am J Clin Nutr 1995;61:1338S–1345S.
6 Keys A, Keys M: How to Eat Well and Stay Well, the Mediterranean Way. Garden City, Doubleday, 1975.
7 Fidanza F: The search for the historical roots of the Italian Mediterranean Diet: from antiquity to the first half of the XIX century. Diab Nutr Metab 2002;15:131–135.
8 Fidanza F: Who remembers the true Italian Mediterranean diet? Diab Nutr Metab 2001;14: 119–120.
9 De Lorenzo A, Alberti A, Andreoli A, Iacopino L, Serranò P, Perriello G: Food habits in a southern Italian town (Nicotera) in 1960 and 1966: still a reference Italian Mediterranean diet? Diab Nutr Metab 2001;14:121–125.
10 Fidanza F, Alberti A: The healthy Italian Mediterranean diet temple food guide. Nutr Today 2005;40: 71–78.
11 Alberti-Fidanza A: Mediterranean meal patterns; In Somogyi JC, Koskinen EH, (eds): Nutritional Adaptation to New Life-Styles. Basel, Karger, 1990, vol 45, pp 59–71.
12 Saba A, Turrini A, Mistura G, Cialfa E, Vichi M: Indagine nazionale sui consumi alimentari delle famiglie 1980–1984: alcuni principali risultati. La Rivista della Società Italiana di Scienza dell'Alimentazione 1990;19:53–65.
13 Turrini A, Saba A, Perrone D, Cialfa E, D'Amicis A: Food consumption patterns in Italy: the INN-CA Study 1994–1996. Eur J Clin Nutr 2001;55:571–588.
14 Turrini A, Lombardi-Boccia G: The formulation of the market basket of the Italian total diet 1994–96. Nutr Res 2002;22:1151–1162.
15 Storelli MM, Giacominelli-Stuffler R, Storelli A, D'Addabbo R, Palermo C, Marcotrigliano GO: Survey of total mercury and methylmercury levels in edible fish from the Adriatic Sea. Food Addit Contam 2003;20:1114–1119.
16 Bry GA, Nielsen SJ, Popkin BM: Consumption of high-fructose corn syrup in beverages may play a role in the epidemic of obesity. Am J Clin Nutr 2004;79:537–543.
17 Trevisan M, Krogh V, Freudenheim J, Blake A, Muti P, Panico S, Farinaro E, Mancini M, Menotti A, Ricci G, Council tRGA-RotINR: Consumption of olive oil, butter, and vegetable oils and coronary heart disease risk factors. J Am Med Assoc 1990;263:688–692.
18 Pala V, Sieri S, Masala G, Palli D, Panico S, Vineis P, Sacerdote C, Mattiello A, Galasso R, Salvini S, Ceroti M, Berrino F, Fusconi E, Tumino R, Graziella F, Riboli E, Trichopoulou A, Baibas N, Krogh V: Associations between dietary pattern and lifestyle, anthropometry and other health indicators in the elderly participants of the EPIC-Italy cohort. Nutr Metab Cardiovasc Dis 2006;16: 186–201.

19 Pala V, Berrino F, Vineis P, Palli D, Celentano E, Tumino R, Krogh V: How vegetables are eaten in Italy EPIC centres: still setting a good example? IARC Sci Publ 2002;156:119–121.
20 Hu FB: Dietary pattern analysis: a new direction in nutritional epidemiology. Curr Opin Lipidol 2002;13:3–9.
21 Alberti-Fidanza A, Fidanza F, Chiuchiù MP, Verducci G, Fruttini D: Dietary studies on two rural Italian population groups of the Seven Countries Study. 3. Trend of food and nutrient intake from 1960 to 1991. Eur J Clin Nutr 1999;53:854–860.
22 Alberti-Fidanza A, Fidanza F: Mediterranean Adequacy Index of Italian diets. Publ Health Nutr 2004;7:937–941.
23 Fidanza F, Alberti A, Lanti M, Menotti A: Mediterranean Adequacy Index: correlation with 25-year mortality from coronary heart disease in the Seven Countries Study. Nutr Metab Cardiovasc Dis 2004;14:254–258.
24 Trichopoulou A, Kouris-Blazos A, Wahlqvist ML, Gnardellis C, Lagiou P, Polychronopoulos E: Diet and overall survival in elderly people. Br Med J 1995;311:1457–1460.
25 Trichopoulou A, Bamia C, Trichopoulos D: Mediterranean diet and survival among patients with coronary heart disease in Greece. Arch Intern Med 2005;165:29–35.
26 Trichopoulou A, Orfanos P, Norat T, et al: Modified Mediterranean diet and survival: EPIC-elderly prospective cohort study. Br Med J 2005;330:991.
27 Trichopoulou A, Costacou T, Bamia C, Trichopoulos D: Adherence to a Mediterranean diet and survival in a Greek population. N Engl J Med 2003;348:2599–2608.
28 Huijbregts PP, Feskens E, Rasanen L, Fidanza F, Nissinen A, Menotti A, et al: Dietary pattern and 20 year mortality in elderly men in Finland, Italy and The Netherlands: longitudinal cohort study. Br Med J 1997;315:13–17.
29 Panagiotakos DB, Pitsavos C, Stefanadis C: Dietary patterns: a Mediterranean diet score and its relation to clinical and biological markers of cardiovascular disease risk. Nutr Metab Cardiovasc Dis 2006; in press, available online 9 February 2006.
30 Ciccarone E, Di Castelnuovo A, Salcuni M, Siani A, Giacco A, Donati MB, De Gaetano G, Capani F, Iacoviello L: on behalf of the Gendiabe Investigators: A high-score Mediterranean dietary pattern is associated with a reduced risk of peripheral arterial disease in Italina patients with type 2 diabetes. J Thromb Haemost 2003;1:1744–1752.
31 Barzi F, Woodward M, Marfisi RM, Tavazzi L, Tognoni G, Valagussa F, Marchioloi R: Investigators obotG-P. Mediterranean diet and all-causes mortality after myocardial infarction: results from the GISSI-Prevenzione trial. Eur J Clin Nutr 2003;57:604–611.
32 Knoops KTB, de Groot LC, Fidanza F, Alberti-Fidanza A, Kromhout D, van Staveren WA: Comparison of three different dietary scores in relation to 10-year mortality in elderly European subjects: the HALE project. Eur J Clin Nutr 2006;60:746–755.
33 The Seven Countries Study: The diet and all cause death rate in the Seven Countries Study. Lancet 1981;ii:58–61.
34 Keys A, Menotti A, Karvonen MJ, Aravanis C, Blackburn H, Buzina R, Djordjevic BS, Dontas AS, Fidanza F, Keys MH, Kromhout D, Nedeljkovic S, Punsar S, Seccareccia F, Toshima H: The diet and 15-year death rate in the seven countries study. Am J Epidemiol 1986;124:903–915.
35 Trevisan M, Krogh V, Freudenheim JL, Blake A, Muti P, Panico S, Farinaro E, Mancini M, Menotti A, Ricci G: Diet and coronary heart disease risk factors in a population with varied intake. The Research Group ATS-RF2 of the Italian National Research Council. Prev Med 1990;19:231–241.
36 Rubba P, Iannuzzi A: n–3 to n–6 fatty acids for managing hyperlipidemia, diabetes, hypertension, atherosclerosis: Is there evidence ? Eur J Lipid Sci Technol 2001;103:407–418.
37 Keys A: Dietary survey methods; in Levy R, Rifkind B, Dennis B, Ernst N (eds): Nutrition, Lipids, and Coronary Heart Disease. New York, Raven Press, 1990.
38 Logan RL, Thomson M, Riemersma RA, Oliver MF, Olsson AG, Rossner S, Callmer E, Walldius G, Kaijser L, Carlson LA, Lockerbie L, Luts W: Risk factors for ischemic heart disease in normal men aged 40. Lancet 1978;i:949–955.
39 Riemersma RA, Wood DA, Butler S, Elton RA, Oliver MF, Salo M, Nikkari T, Vartiainen E, Puska P, Gey F, Rubba P, Mancini M, Fidanza F: Linoleic acid content in adipose tissue and coronary heart disease. Br Med J 1986;292:1423–1427.

40 Olsson AG, Holmquist L, Walldius G, Hadell K, Carlson LA, Riccardi G, Rubba P, Pauciullo P, Mancini M: Serum apolipoproteins, lipoproteins and FA in relation to ischemic heart disease in northern and southern European males. Acta Med Scand 1988;223:3–13.

41 Puska P, Nissinen A, Vartiainen E, Dougherty T, Mutanen M, Jacono JM, Korhonen HJ, Pietinen P, Leino U, Moisio S, Huttunen J: Controlled, randomised trial of the effect of dietary fat on blood pressure. Lancet 1983;i:1–5.

42 Fidanza F, Rubba P, Cozzolino G, Mancini M: Food habits of a traditional Mediterranean population from southern Italy. Nutr Metab Cardiovasc Dis 1991;1:71–76.

43 Fulton M, Thomson M, Elton RA, Brown S, Wood DA, Oliver MF: Cigarette smoking, social class and nutrient intake: relevance to coronary heart disease. Eur J Clin Nutr 1988;42:797–803.

44 Rubba P, Mancini M, Fidanza F, Gautiero G, Salo M, Nikkari T, Elton R, Oliver MF: Adipose tissue fatty acids and blood pressure in middle-aged men from southern Italy. Int J Epidemiol 1987;16:528–531.

45 Massaro M, De Caterina R: Vasculoprotective effects of oleic acid: epidemiological background and direct vascular antiatherogenic properties. Nutr Metab Cardiovasc Dis 2002;12:42–51.

46 Howard BV, Van Horn L, Hsia J, et al: Low fat dietary pattern and risk of cardiovascular disease: the women's health initiative randomized controlled dietary modification trial. J Am Med Assoc 2006;295:655–666.

47 Akeson PK, Axelsson IE, Raiha NC, Warm A, Minoli I, Moro G: Fat intake and metabolism in Swedish and Italian infants. Acta Paediatr 2000;89:28–33.

48 Willet W, et al: Reply. Eur J Clin Nutr 2004;58:561.

49 Negri E, La Vecchia C, Pelucchi C, Bertuzzi M, Tavani A: Fiber intake and risk of nonfatal acute myocardial infarction. Eur J Clin Nutr 2003;57:464–470.

50 Strazzullo P, Ferro Luzzi A, Siani A, Scaccini S, Catasta G, Mancini M: Changing the Mediterranean diet: effects on blood pressure. J Hypertens 1986;4:407–412.

51 Vollmer WH, Sacks FM, Ard J, Appel LJ, Bray GA, et al: Effects of diet and sodium intake on blood pressure: subgroup analysis of the DASH sodium trial. Ann Intern Med 2001;135:1019–1028.

52 Rotilio G, Berni Canani R, Barba G, et al: Nutritional recommendations for the prevention of ischemic stroke. Nutr Metab Cardiovasc Dis 2004;14:115–120.

53 Strazzullo P, Scalfi L, Branca F, Cairella G, Garbagnati F, Siani A, Barba G, Rubba P, Mancia G: Nutrition and prevention of ischemic stroke: present knowledge, limitations and future perspectives. Nutr Metab Cardiovasc Dis 2004;14:97–114.

54 Iuliano L, Mauriello A, Sbarigia E, Spagnoli LG, Violi F: Radiolabeled native low-density lipoprotein injected into patients with carotid stenosis accumulates in macrophages of atherosclerotic plaque: effect of vitamin E supplementation. Circulation 2000;101:1249–1254.

55 Wood DA, Oliver MF: Linoleic acid, antioxidant vitamins, and coronary heart disease; in Marmot M, Elliot P (eds): Coronary Heart Disease Epidemiology. London, Oxford University Press, 1992, pp 179–202.

56 Riemersma RA, Oliver M, Elton RA, Alfthan G, Vartiainen E, Salo M, Rubba P, Mancini M, Georgi H, Vuilleumier JP, Gey KF: Plasma antioxidants and coronary heart disease: vitamins C and E, and selenium. Eur J Clin Nutr 1990;44:143–150.

57 Gey KF, Puska P, Jordan P, Moser U, et al: Inverse correlation between plasma vitamin E and mortality from ischemic heart disease in cross-cultural epidemiology. Am J Clin Nutr 1991;53:326s–334s.

58 Parfitt VJ, Rubba P, Bolton C, Marotta G, Hartog M, Mancini M: A comparison of antioxidant status and free radical peroxidation of plasma lipoproteins in healthy young persons from Naples and Bristol. Eur Heart J 1994;15:871–876.

59 Heart Protection Study Collaborative Group: MRC/BHF Heart Protection Study of antioxidant vitamin supplementation in 20,536 high-risk individuals: a randomised placebo-controlled trial. Lancet 2002;360:23–33.

60 Lee IM, Cook NR, Gaziano JM, Gordon D, Ridker PM, Manson JE, Hennekens CH, Buring JE: Vitamin E in the primary prevention of cardiovascular disease and cancer: the Women's Health Study: a randomized controlled trial. J Am Med Assoc 2005;294:56–65.

61 Gruppo Italiano per lo Studio della Sopravvivenza nell' Infarto del Miocardio: Dietary supplementation with n–3 polyunsaturated fatty acids and vitamin E after myocardial infarction: results of the GISSI-Prevenzione trial. Lancet 1999;354:447–455.

62 Salonen JT, Yla-Herttuala S, Yamamoto R, Butler S, Korpela H, Salonen R, Nyyssonen K, Palinski W, Witzum JL: Autoantibody against oxidised LDL and progression of carotid atherosclerosis. Lancet 1992;339:883–887.
63 van de Vijver LPL, Steyger G, van Poppel G, Boer JMA, Kruijssen DACM, Seidell JC, Princen HMG: Autoantibodies against MDA-LDL in subjects with severe and minor atherosclerosis and healthy population control. Atherosclerosis 1996;122:245–253.
64 Kritchevsky SB, Shimokawa T, Tell GS, Dennis B, Carpenter M, Eckfeldt JH, Peacher-Ryan H, Heiss G: Dietary antioxidant and carotid artery wall thickness. The ARIC Study. Circulation 1995;92:2142–2150.
65 Azen SP, Qian D, Mack WJ, Sevanian A, Selzer RH, Liu C, Hodis HN: Effect of supplementary antioxidant vitamin intake on carotid arterial wall intima-media thickness in a controlled clinical trial of cholesterol lowering. Circulation 1996;94:2369–2372.
66 Rubba P, Panico S, Bond MG, Covetti G, Celentano E, Iannuzzi A, Galasso R, Belisario MA, Pastinese A, Sacchetti L, Mancini M, Salvatore F: Site-specific atherosclerotic plaques in the carotid arteries of middle-aged women from southern Italy: associations with traditional risk factors and oxidation markers. Stroke 2001;32:1953–1959.
67 Iannuzzi A, Celentano E, Panico S, Galasso R, Covetti G, Sacchetti L, Zarrilli F, De Michele M, Rubba P: Dietary and circulating antioxidant vitamins in relation to carotid plaques in middle-aged women. Am J Clin Nutr 2002;76:582–587.
68 Violi F, Cangemi R, Sabatino G, Pignatelli P: Vitamin E for the treatment of cardiovascular disease: is there a future? Ann NY Acad Sci 2004;1031:292–304.
69 de Divitiis M, Rubba P: Cholesterol-lowering and vascular reactivity in relation to coronary heart disease. Nutr Metab Cardiovasc Dis 1999;9:133–142.
70 Esposito K, Marfella R, Ciotola M, Di Palo C, Giugliano F, Giugliano G, D'Armiento M, D'Andrea F, Giugliano D: Effect of a Mediterranean-style diet on endothelial dysfunction and markers of vascular inflammation in the metabolic syndrome: a randomized trial. J Am Med Assoc 2004;292:1440–1446.
71 Iuliano L, Micheletta F, Maranghi M, Frati G, Diczfalusy U, Violi F: Bioavailability of vitamin E as function of food intake in healthy subjects: effects on plasma peroxide-scavenging activity and cholesterol-oxidation products. Arterioscler Thromb Vasc Biol 2001;21:E34–E37.
72 Wald DS, Law M, Morris JK: Homocysteine and cardiovascular disease: evidence on causality from a meta-analysis. Br Med J 2002;23:1202.
73 B-Vitamin Treatment Trialists' Collaboration: Homocysteine-lowering trials for prevention of cardiovascular events: a review of the design and power of the large randomized trials. Am Heart J 2006;151:282–287.
74 Toole JF, Malinow MR, Chambless LE, Spence JD, Pettigrew LC, Howard VJ, Sides EG, Wang CH, Stampfer M: Lowering homocysteine in patients with ischemic stroke to prevent recurrent stroke, myocardial infarction, and death: the Vitamin Intervention for Stroke Prevention (VISP) randomized controlled trial. J Am Med Assoc 2004;291:565–575.
75 Bønaa KH, Njølstad I, Ueland PM, Schirmer H, Tverdal A, Steigen T, Wang H, Nordrehaug JE, Arnesen E, Rasmussen K: NORVIT Trial Investigators. Homocysteine lowering and cardiovascular events after acute myocardial infarction. N Engl J Med 2006;354:1578–1588.
76 Cruz JA: Dietary habits and nutritional status in adolescents over Europe: Southern Europe. Eur J Clin Nutr 2000;54:S29–S35.
77 Istituto Auxologico Italiano: Epidemiologia dell'obesità in Italia. 4° rapporto sull'obesità in Italia, 2002.
78 Cacciari E, Milani S, Balsamo A, Dammacco F, De Luca F, Chiarelli F, Pasquino AM, Tonini G, Vanelli M: Italian cross-sectional growth charts for height, weight and BMI (6–20 y). Eur J Clin Nutr 2002;56:171–180.
79 Lobstein T, Frelut ML: Prevalence of overweight among children in Europe. Obes Rev 2003;4:195–200.
80 Notarbartolo A, Barbagallo CM: Eating behaviour, body mass index and lipids of children in a free-living rural Sicilian population. Nutr Metab Cardiovasc Dis 2001;11:60–63.
81 de Ferranti SD, Gauvreau K, Ludwig DS, Neufeld ES, Newburger J, Rifai N: Prevalence of the metabolic syndrome in American adolescents: findings from the Third National Health and Nutrition Examination Survey. Circulation 2004;110:2494–2497.

82 Valerio G, Licenziati MR, Iannuzzi A, Franzese A, Siani P, Riccardi G, Rubba P: Insulin resistance and impaired glucose tolerance in obese children and adolescents from Southern Italy. Nutr Metab Cardiovasc Dis 2006;16:279–284.

83 Iannuzzi A, Licenziati MR, Acampora C, Renis M, Agrusta M, Romano L, Valerio G, Panico S, Trevisan M: Carotid artery stiffness in obese children with the metabolic syndrome. Am J Cardiol 2006;97:528–531.

84 Iannuzzi A, Licenziati MR, Acampora C, Salvatore V, De Marco D, Mayer MC, De Michele M, Russo V: Preclinical changes in the mechanical properties of abdominal aorta in obese children. Metabolism 2004;53:1243–1246.

85 Martinez-Gonzalez MA, Varo JJ, Santos JL, De Irala J, Gibney M, Kearney J, Martinez JA: Prevalence of physical activity during leisure time in the European Union. Med Sci Sports Exerc 2001;1142–1146.

86 Iacobellis G, Ribaudo MC, Zappaterreno A, Iannucci CV, Leonetti F: Prevalence of uncomplicated obesity in an Italian obese population. Obes Res 2005;13:1116–1122.

87 Doll R, Peto R: The causes of cancer: quantitative estimates of avoidable risk of cancer in US today. J Natl Cancer Inst 1981;66:1191–1308.

88 World Cancer Research Fund: Food, Nutrition and the Prevention of Cancer: A Global Perspective. Washington, 1997.

89 World Health Organization: Healthy nutrition. Preventing nutrition-related diseases in Europe; in James WPT (ed): Copenhagen, World Health Organization Regional Office for Europe, 1988, vol 24.

90 La Vecchia C: Mediterranean diet and cancer. Publ Health Nutr 2004;7:965–968.

91 Bosetti C, Gallus S, Trichopoulou A, Talamini R, Franceschi S, Negri E, La Vecchia C: Influence of the Mediterranean diet on the risk of cancers of the upper aerodigestive tract. Cancer Epidemiol Biomarkers Prev 2003;12:1091–1094.

92 Gallus S, Bosetti C, La Vecchia C: Mediterranean diet and cancer risk. Eur J Cancer Prev 2004;13:447–452.

93 La Vecchia C, Altieri A, Tavani A: Vegetable, fruit, antioxidants and cancer: a review of Italian studies. Eur J Nutr 2001;40:261–267.

94 Riboli E, Norat T: Epidemiologic evidence of the protective effect of fruit and vegetables on cancer risk. Am J Clin Nutr 2003;78:S559–S569.

95 IARC: Fruit and vegetables. IARC Handbooks of Cancer Prevention. Lyon, IARC Press, 2003, vol 8.

96 González CA, Pera G, Agudo A, et al: Fruit and vegetable intake and the risk of stomach and oesophagus adenocarcinoma in the European Prospective Investigation into Cancer and Nutrition. Int J Cancer 2005;118:2559–2566.

97 Papas MA, Giovannucci E, Platz EA: Fiber from fruit and colorectal neoplasia. Cancer Epidemiol Biomarkers Prev 2004;13:1267–1270.

98 Fortes C, Forastiere F, Farchi S, Mallone S, Trequattrinni T, Anatra F, Schmid G, Perucci CA: The protective effect of the Mediterranean diet on lung cancer. Nutr Cancer 2003;46:30–37.

99 Miller AB, Altenburg H-P, Bueno-de-Mesquita B, et al: Fruits and vegetables and lung cancer: findings from the European prospective investigation into cancer and nutrition. Int J Cancer 2004;108:269–276.

100 Rylander R, Axelsson G: Lung cancer risk in relation to vegetable and fruit consumption and smoking. Int J Cancer 2006;118:739–743.

101 Masala G, Ambrogetti D, Assedi M, Giorgi D, Del Turco MR, Palli D: Dietary and lifestyle determinants of mammographic breast density: a longitudinal study in a Mediterranean population. Int J Cancer 2006;118:1782–1789.

102 Smith-Warner SA, Spiegelman D, Yuan SS, Adami HO, Beeson WL, van den Brandt PA, Folsom AR, Fraser GE, Freudenheim JL, Goldbhom RA, Graham S, Miller AB, Potter JD, Rohan TE, Speizer FE, Toniolo P, Willet WC, Wolk A, Zeleniuch-Jacquotte A, Hunter DJ: Intake of fruit and vegetables and risk of breast cancer: a pooled analysis of cohort studies. J Am Med Assoc 2001;285:769–776.

103 van Gils CH, Peeters PHM, Bueno-de-Mesquita BH, et al: Consumption of vegetables and fruits and risk of breast cancer. J Am Med Assoc 2005;293:183–193.

104 Peluso M, Airoldi L, Magagnotti C, Fiorini L, Munnia A, Hautefeuille A, Malaveille C, Vineis P: White blood cell DNA adducts and fruit and vegetable consumption in bladder cancer. Carcinogenesis 2000;21:183–187.

105 Cai Q, Rahan RO, Zang R: Dietary flavonoids, quercetin, luteolin and genistein, reduce DNA damage and lipid peroxidation and quench free radicals. Cancer Lett 1997;119:99–108.
106 Zappia V, Della Ragione F, Barbarisi A, Russo GL, Dello Iacovo R: Advances in Nutrition and Cancer. 2. Advances in Experimental Medicine and Biology. New York, Kluwer Academic/Plenum Publisher, 1999, vol. 472.
107 Bingham SA, Day NE, Luben R, et al: Dietary fibre in food and protection against colorectal cancer in the European Prospective Investigation into Cancer and Nutrition (EPIC): an observational study. Lancet 2003;361:1496–1501.
108 La Vecchia C, Negri E, Pelucchi C, Franceschi S: Dietary folate and colorectal cancer. Int J Cancer 2002;102:545–547.
109 Jiang R, Hu FB, Giovannucci EL, Rimm EB, Stampfer MJ, Spiegelman D, et al: Joint association of alcohol and folate intake with risk of major chronic disease in women. Am J Epidemiol 2003;158:760–771.
110 Hillman RS, Steinberg SE: The effects of alcohol on folate metabolism. Ann Rev Med 1982;33: 345–354.
111 Larsson SC, Giovannucci E, Wolk A: Dietary folate intake and incidence of ovarian cancer: the Swedish Mammography Cohort. J Natl Cancer Inst 2004;96:396–402.
112 Visioli F, Grande S, Bogani P, Galli C: The role of antioxidants in the Mediterranean diet: focus on cancer. Eur J Cancer Prev 2004;13:337–343.
113 Linseisen J, Bergstrom E, Gafa L, et al: Consumption of added fats and oils in the European Prospective Investigation into Cancer and Nutrition (EPIC) centres across 10 European countries as assesses by the 24-hour dietary recalls. Publ Health Nutr 2002;5:1227–1242.
114 Steinmetz KA, Potter JD: Vegetables, fruit, and cancer prevention: a review. J Am Diet Assoc 1996;96:1027–1039.
115 International Agency for Research on Cancer: Alcohol drinking; in: Monographs on the Evaluation of the Carcinogenic Risk of Chemicals to Humans, Lyon, 1988, vol 44.
116 Webb PM, Purdie DM, Bain CJ, Green AC: Alcohol, wine, and risk of epithelial ovarian cancer. Cancer Epidemiol Biomarkers Prev 2004;13:592–599.
117 Larsson SC, Wolk A: Wine consumption and epithelial ovarian cancer. Cancer Epidemiol Biomarkers Prev 2004;13:1823–1824.
118 Pervaiz S: Resveratrol: from grapevines to mammalian biology. FASEB J 2003;17:1875–1985.
119 English DR, MacInnis RJ, Hodge AM, Hopper JL, Haydon AM, Giles GG: Red meat, chicken, and fish consumption and risk of colorectal cancer. Cancer Epidemiol Biomarkers Prev 2004;13: 1509–1514.
120 Larsson SC, Rafter J, Holmberg L, Bergkvist L, Wolk A: Red meat consumption and risk of cancers of the proximal colon, distal colon and rectum: the Swedish Mammography Cohort. Int J Cancer 2005;113:829–834.
121 Norat T, Bingham S, Ferrari P, et al: Meat, fish, and colorectal cancer risk: the European Prospective Investigation into Cancer and Nutrition. J Natl Cancer Inst 2005;97:906–916.
122 Larsson SC, Kumlin M, Ingelman-Sundberg M, Wolk A: Dietary long-chain n–3 fatty acids for the prevention of cancer: a review of potential mechanisms. Am J Clin Nutr 2004;79:935–945.
123 Terry PD, Rohan TE, Wolk A: Intakes of fish and marine fatty acids and the risk of cancers of the breast and prostate and of other hormone-related cancers: a review of the epidemiologic evidence. Am J Clin Nutr 2003;77:532–543.
124 Brand-Miller JC: Glycemic load and chronic disease. Nutr Rev 2003;61:S49–S55.
125 Romieu I, Lazcano-Ponce E, Sanchez-Zamorano LM, Willet W, Hernandez-Avila M: Carbohydrates and the risk of breast cancer among Mexican women. Cancer Epidemiol Biomarkers Prev 2004;13: 1283–1289.
126 Giles GG, Simpson JA, English DR, Hodge AM, Gertig DM, MacInnis RJ, Hopper JL: Dietary carbohydrate, fibre, glycaemic index, glycaemic load and the risk of postmenopausal breast cancer. Int J Cancer 2006;118:1843–1847.
127 Correa Leite ML, Nicolosi A, Cristina S, Hauser WA, Pugliese P, Nappi G: Dietary and nutritional patterns in an elderly rural population in Northern and Southern Italy. II: Nutritional profiles associated with food behaviours. Eur J Clin Nutr 2003;57:1522–1529.

128 Inelmen EM, Gimenez GF, Gatto MR, Miotto F, Sergi G, Marccari T, Gonzalez AM, Maggi S, Peruzza S, Pisent C, Enzi G: Dietary intake and nutritional status in Italian elderly subjects. J Nutr Health Aging 2000;4:91–101.
129 Antonini FM, Petruzzi E, Pinzani P, Orlando C, Petruzzi I, Pazzagli M, Masotti G: Effect of diet and red wine consumption on serum total antioxidant capacity (TAC), dehydroepiandrosterone-sulphate (DHEAS) and insulin-like growth factor-1 (IGF-1) in Italian centenarians. Arch Gerontol Geriatr 2005;41:151–157.
130 Lasheras C, Fernandez S, Patterson AM: Mediterranean diet and age with respect to overall survival in institutionalized, nonsmoking elderly people. Am J Clin Nutr 2000;71:987–992.
131 Panza F, Solfrizzi V, Colacicco AM, D'Introno A, Capurso C, Torres F, Del Parigi A, Capurso S, Capurso A: Mediterranean diet and cognitive decline. Publ Health Nutr 2004;7:959–963.
132 Solfrizzi V, Panza F, Capurso A: The role of diet in cognitive decline. J Neural Transm 2003;110: 95–110.

Paolo Rubba, MD
Department of Clinical and Experimental Medicine
Federico II University, Via S. Pansini 5
IT–80131 Napoli (Italy)
Tel. +39 081 746 2300, Fax +39 081 746 2300, E-Mail rubba@unina.it

A Mediterranean Diet Is Not Enough for Health: Physical Fitness Is an Important Additional Contributor to Health for the Adults of Tomorrow

Manuel J. Castillo-Garzón, Jonatan R. Ruiz, Francisco B. Ortega, Angel Gutierrez-Sainz

School of Medicine, University of Granada, Granada and Sotogrande Health Experience, Cadiz, Spain

Is It Only Diet?

Cardiovascular diseases are the major cause of death in Western Societies. Nevertheless, important differences exist among different populations and regions. In Europe, for instance, large differences exist in mortality from coronary heart disease and stroke. These diseases show a clear West-East and South-North gradient with high rates in Eastern and Northern Europe and lower rates in most Mediterranean countries [1]. Interestingly, large regional differences in ischemic heart disease and prevalence of cardiovascular risk factors occur within the same country and even within the same region. These differences are present both in countries with high and low incidence of cardiovascular disease [2].

Classical risk factors for cardiovascular disease include age, sex, hypertension, smoking, diabetes, elevated plasma low-density lipoprotein (LDL)-cholesterol, and low high-density lipoprotein (HDL)-cholesterol, lack of exercise and increased body fat. Nevertheless, the contribution of changes in these factors to trends in coronary event rates can only explain half of the cases [3]. Emerging independent risk factors include abdominal adiposity, high plasma levels of triglycerides, lipoprotein(a), modified LDL-cholesterol particles, homocysteine, several markers of inflammation, and thrombotic risk factors. It is quite possible that even taking all these factors into account, differences in coronary heart disease rates could not be fully explained.

Table 1. Beneficial effects on health of practising regular physical exercise

---

Reduction in the risk of developing ischemic heart disease and other cardiovascular diseases
Reduction in the risk of developing obesity and diabetes
Reduction in the risk of developing (and control of) high blood pressure and dyslipidemia
Reduction in the risk of developing breast and colon cancer
Helps in the control of body weight and improves 'body image'
Improves muscle tone and preserves or increases muscular mass
Strengthens bones and joints
Increases coordination and neuromotor responses; reduces the risk of falls
Improves immune system activity
Reduces depression and anxiety
Promotes wellbeing and social integration

Growing evidence demonstrates that the Mediterranean life-style is beneficial to health. The evidence is stronger for coronary heart disease, but it also applies to stroke and some forms of cancer [4–6]. Diet is one outstanding component of the Mediterranean life-style. Large life-style and dietary variations occur in different regions and countries. In many of them, a progressive departure from the traditional Mediterranean life-style and diet is being observed [7]. In this departure, more affluent economies and younger subjects are, probably, more easily influenced.

In addition to diet, a sedentary life-style is a major risk factor for noncommunicable diseases (e.g. coronary heart disease, stroke, obesity, hypertension, type 2 diabetes, allergies and several types of cancers) and is close to overtaking tobacco as the leading cause of preventable death [8]. The protective effect of regular physical activity on the above mentioned diseases has been widely reported in young people, in adults and in the elderly. It is now well known that regular participation in moderate and vigorous levels of exercise can lead to many health benefits (table 1).

The Spanish-Mediterranean Life-Style (and Diet)

The Spanish-Mediterranean life-style (and diet) is that usually followed by the inhabitants of Spain. Nevertheless, geographical, economic and social differences result in many different dietary practices and physical activity patterns. This, obviously, precludes a single definition of the Spanish-Mediterranean life-style. Nonetheless, regarding diet, there is a dietary pattern that is common in the different diets in the country. This traditional dietary pattern is composed of a cluster of basic foods that have been easily available in the region during centuries. This determines a diet that is high in fruits, green and root vegetables, bread, other forms of cereals, beans, nuts and seeds of different types. A common and outstanding characteristic of the Spanish Mediterranean diet is the use of olive oil which represents the more important source of fat in the diet. Animal products intake includes eggs, dairy products and poultry. There are significant variations in the intakes of fish, red meat (pork, beef, lamb) and meat derived products. Red wine and beer have been traditionally consumed. A main difference between the Spanish-Mediterranean diet and other Mediterranean diets is the lower intake of pasta and potatoes, and the higher intake of bread, legumes and fish [9, 10]. Many of these components may have an effect on cardiovascular risk factors, particularly by influencing the plasma lipid profile.

One specific characteristic of the traditional Spanish-Mediterranean lifestyle is the time spent outdoor which is favored by the favorable weather conditions. This may determine higher levels of physical activity. In Spain, the timetable for meals is different from other countries. The main meal of the day is usually taken in early afternoon (around 2–3 p.m.) and the dinner is late in the evening (around 10 p.m.) and rather light. There is a widely spread culture of eating outside the home in an informal way and usually standing up. It is the typical 'tapas' eating. These 'tapas' are taken between meals and occasionally represent an alternative to a more formal meal.

Diet and Physical Activity Interaction

Diet and physical activity interact in the development and prevention of ischemic heart disease and several other health conditions. Both factors affect the plasma lipid profile and body composition, and probably influence other risk factors. In fact, a physiological means of influencing diet-induced modifications of the plasma lipid profile and body fat content is physical activity [11]. Physical activity favorably influences all three components of the atherogenic lipoprotein phenotype: the HDL-cholesterol concentration may increase, LDL-cholesterol may decrease, and serum triglycerides can also be reduced [12, 13]. In addition, physical activity precludes body fat accumulation. Complex interactions between diet, physical activity, life-style, lipoprotein metabolism and other factors determine the development of atherosclerosis and its complications. These interactions may start early in life. In this way, adolescence is a critical period because it is at that time when the individual takes control of his/her own life-style and diet.

We have studied a representative sample of Spanish adolescents aged 13–18.5 years participating in the 'Alimentación y Valoración del Estado Nutricional de los Adolescentes' (AVENA) study (www.estudioavena.com). The

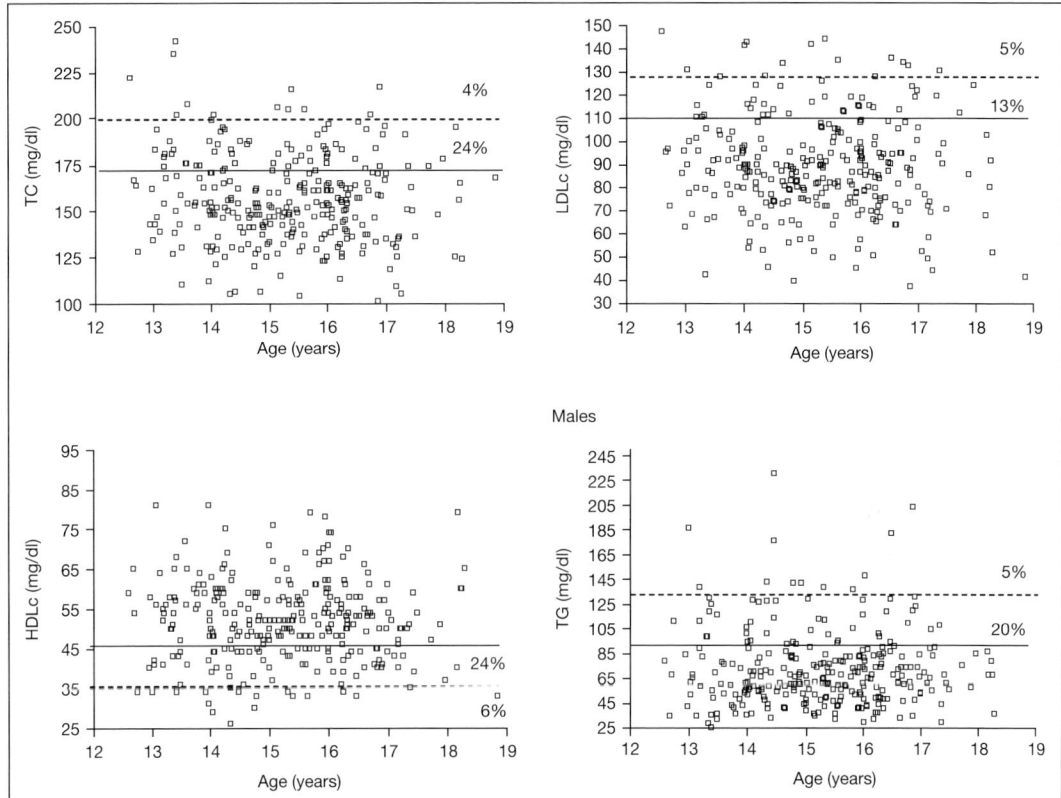

Fig. 1. Serum levels of total cholesterol (TC), low-density lipoprotein cholesterol (LDLc), high-density lipoprotein cholesterol (HDLc) and triglycerides (TG) in male Spanish adolescents. Solid lines represent the limit level considered as healthy. Broken lines represent the limit level considered as unhealthy. Subjects between both lines can be considered as borderline. [Ruiz et al., unpubl. data].

AVENA study is a population-based cross-sectional survey conducted in five different geographic areas of Spain (Madrid, Murcia, Granada, Santander and Zaragoza), addressing genetic and environmental factors in relation to metabolic traits during adolescence [14]. Some interesting data regarding cardiovascular risk factors are being obtained from this study. Interestingly, we have observed a high prevalence of an unfavorable plasma lipid profile, both in boys (fig. 1) and girls (fig. 2) [15]. Similarly, it is well known the high prevalence of obesity in Mediterranean children and adolescents (fig. 3) [16]. These results underline the importance of implementing effective measures for preventing the deleterious consequences that these conditions are going to have in the health of tomorrow's

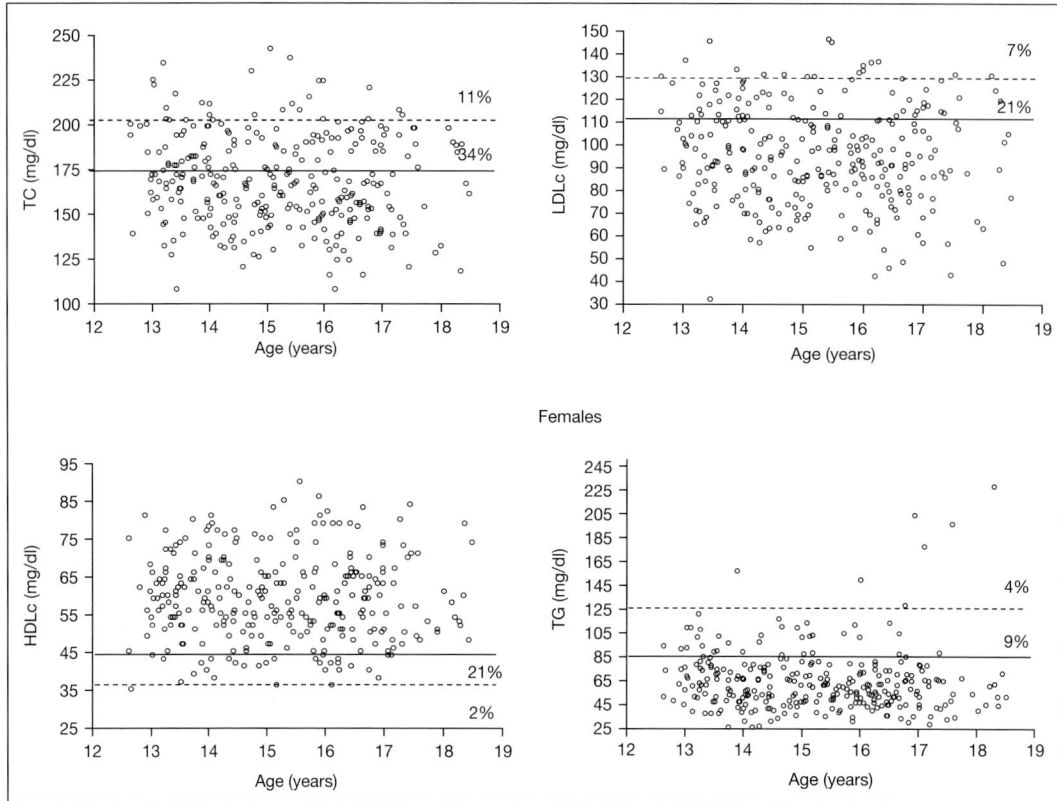

Fig. 2. Serum levels of total cholesterol (TC), low-density lipoprotein cholesterol (LDLc), high-density lipoprotein cholesterol (HDLc) and triglycerides (TG) in female Spanish adolescents. Solid lines represent the limit level considered as healthy. Broken lines represent the limit levels considered as unhealthy. Subjects between both lines can be considered as borderline. [Ruiz et al., unpubl. data].

adults. One positive measure is the return to the traditional Spanish-Mediterranean diet; the other is to increase the levels of physical activity. In other words, the return to the traditional Spanish-Mediterranean life-style.

Physical Activity, Physical Exercise and Physical Fitness

Regular physical activity stimulates functional adaptation of all tissues and organs in the body, thereby also making them less vulnerable to lifestyle-related degenerative and chronic diseases. Physical activity refers to any body movement produced by muscle action that increases energy expenditure. Physical exercise refers to planned, structured, repetitive and purposeful physical activity.

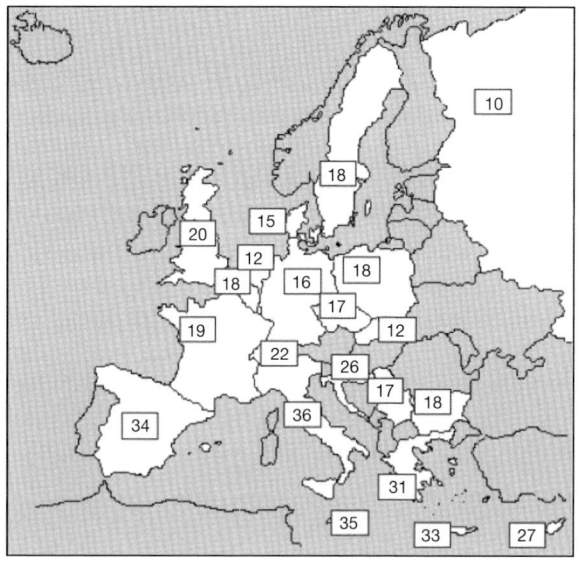

Fig. 3. Prevalence (%) of children (7–10 years old) with overweight in Europe [16].

Physical fitness is the capacity to perform physical exercise. Physical fitness makes reference to the full range of physical qualities, e.g. aerobic capacity, muscle strength, speed, agility, coordination and flexibility. It can be understood as an integrated measurement of most, if not all, the body structures and functions (skeletomuscular, cardiorespiratory, hematocirculatory, psychoneurological and endocrine-metabolic) involved in the performance of physical activity and/or physical exercise [17]. Thus, being physically fit implies that the response of these functions and structures will be adequate. A person cannot be more physically fit than that allowed by the function or structure in lowest condition. Health-oriented physical fitness includes those components of physical fitness more associated with aspects of good health and/or disease prevention [17].

Physical Fitness as a Health Determinant

Aerobic capacity or cardiorespiratory fitness is one of the key components of physical fitness. Maximum aerobic capacity is expressed in terms of maximum oxygen consumption (VO_{2max}). The VO_{2max} can be expressed with respect to subject weight (ml/kg/min), in absolute terms (l/min) or in metabolic equivalents (METs). One MET is the energy expenditure at rest ($\sim$3.5 ml/kg/min). Thus, if a subject has a VO_{2max} of 42 ml/kg/min, he/she also has an energy expenditure of 12 METS (i.e. he/she is able to increase his/her resting energy expenditure 12-fold).

A number of important prospective studies have shown that VO_{2max} is the most important predictor of all-cause mortality, and in particular of cardiovascular death. This is true for both healthy persons and for people with cardiovascular disease [18], and for both men [19–21] and women [22, 23] of different ages [24]. An almost linear reduction in mortality is seen as the cardiorespiratory fitness increases [23, 24]. For each increase of 1 MET, there is a 12% increase in the life expectancy of men [24] and a 17% increase in women [22]. This is even more evident if cardiovascular mortality is considered alone, and again is true for both men [18, 21] and women [22, 23]. An inverse relationship has also been found between cardiorespiratory fitness and mortality due to cancer independently of age, alcohol intake, diabetes mellitus and tobacco [25–28]. Similarly, it has been shown that VO_{2max} is associated with insulin sensitivity [29]; low VO_{2max} levels are also associated with metabolic syndrome (abdominal obesity, glucose intolerance, type II diabetes, hypertension, hyperlipidemia and insulin resistance) [30, 31]. High levels of cardiorespiratory fitness reduce the neuronal losses associated with aging [32] and protects against cognitive dysfunction [33].

Handgrip strength, assessed by the manual dynamometer test, is currently considered to be a reliable marker of health and well-being and a potent predictor of mortality and the expectancy of being able to live independently [34, 35]. Efforts are made to reduce the errors associated with its measurement in adolescents [36] and adults [37].

Physical Fitness and Cardiovascular Risk Factors in Mediterranean Adolescents

Cardiorespiratory Fitness and Traditional Cardiovascular Risk Factors

Cardiorespiratory fitness is a direct marker of physiological status and reflects the overall capacity of the cardiovascular and respiratory systems. Results from several cross-sectional studies have clearly shown strong negative associations between cardiorespiratory fitness and cardiovascular risk factors not only in adults but also in children and adolescents (table 2). In addition, results from prospective studies suggest that high cardiorespiratory fitness during childhood seems to provide more health protection in adulthood.

Associations between increased cardiorespiratory fitness and several cardiovascular risk factors have been repeatedly found. As it is known, elevated levels of triglycerides are strongly associated with an increased risk of coronary artery disease. In Spanish adolescents (aged 13–18.5 years) it was found a negative correlation between cardiorespiratory fitness and triglycerides, especially in males (fig. 4). In females, a trend toward lower levels of triglycerides with increasing fitness was also observed. These findings concur with the results obtained in children and adolescents from other European countries (table 2). Indeed, a negative correlation between cardiorespiratory fitness and triglycerides has been found in Danish, Swedish and Estonian children from the European Youth Heart Study, which is also in agreement with findings from their American peers (table 2).

Similar associations were also observed between cardiorespiratory fitness and LDL-cholesterol. There was a trend indicating lower levels of LDL-cholesterol with higher levels of fitness in both males and females (fig. 5). These findings are noteworthy since it is known that LDL-cholesterol and their oxidized derivatives initiate and promote the atherosclerotic process, leading to the development of coronary artery disease.

Plasma HDL-cholesterol has anti-atherogenic proprieties with its concentration inversely related to risk of coronary artery disease. It is estimated that for every 1 mg/dl (0.026 mmol/l) increase in HDL-cholesterol, the risk for a coronary heart disease event is reduced by 2% in men and at least 3% in women. Cardiorespiratory fitness has been shown to be negatively correlated with HDL-cholesterol in children, adolescents and adult population. Figure 6 clearly shows the associations between fitness and HDL-cholesterol. This is also the case for fitness and apolipoprotein (apo) A-1 (fig. 7). Apo A-1 is the most abundant protein of HDL-cholesterol. An increase in the apo A-1 can lead to an increase of HDL-particles. Alternatively, increased catabolism or removal of apo A-1 will lead to a reduction in plasma HDL-cholesterol levels.

A more favorable metabolic profile (computed with age and gender specific standardized values of triglycerides, LDL-cholesterol, HDL-cholesterol and fasting glycemia) with increased levels of cardiorespiratory fitness has also been shown in Spanish adolescents [13]. Figure 8 shows the association of cardiorespiratory fitness and metabolic profile in non-overweight and overweight adolescents. These results suggest that both fitness and weight management are necessary for the prevention of lipid-related cardiovascular risk in adolescents. In fact, the odds ratio for having an unfavorable lipid profile is increased in subjects with low cardiorespiratory fitness even after adjusting for age and waist circumference (fig. 9).

Cardiorespiratory Fitness and Emerging Cardiovascular Risk Factors

Cardiorespiratory fitness has also been associated with recently recognized cardiovascular risk factors such as low grade inflammation markers (e.g. C-reactive protein, fibrinogen, ceruloplasmin, complement factor C3 and C4) and homocysteine. Findings from the AVENA study suggest that cardiorespiratory

Table 2. Summary of recent studies examining the associations between cardiorespiratory fitness and health-related variables in children and adolescents

Study	Type of study	Subjects	Age	Outcome
Gutin et al. [38]	cross-sectional	boys = 116 girls = 166	14–18 years	boys and girls CRF was inversely associated with insulin concentrations, and the adverse impact of low CRF was greater in boys than in girls
Brage et al. [39]	cross-sectional	boys = 279 girls = 380	8–10 years	boys and girls CRF was inversely associated with insulin, TG, systolic BP, and skinfold thicknesses ($p \leq 0.033$). CRF was inversely associated with metabolic syndrome Z score ($p \leq 0.031$). CRF was positively associated with HDLc ($p = 0.002$)
Reed et al. [40]	cross-sectional	boys = 55 girls = 44	9–11 years	boys and girls CRF accounted for 37% of the variance in large artery compliance. Highest CRF quartile had greater compliance than children in the two lowest CRF quartiles, by as much as 34%
Eisenmann et al. [41]	cross-sectional	Boys = 416 Girls = 345	9–18 years	CRF and BMI showed an independent association with cardiovascular risk factors
Gutin et al. [42]	cross-sectional	boys = 187 girls = 211	14–18 years	higher CRF and lower fatness were associated with favorable lipid profile; for most of the variables, fatness was slightly greater than the influence of CRF

Ruiz et al. [43]	cross-sectional	boys = 429 girls = 444	9–10 years	boys and girls CRF was inversely associated with insulin resistance, and skinfold thicknesses (p < 0.001). CRF was inversely associated with metabolic syndrome Z score (p ≤ 0.02) CRF was negatively associated with TG in girls (p = 0.026)
Andersen et al. [44]	prospective	boys = 133 girls = 172	16–19 years to 24–27 years	boys and girls CRF was associated with cardiovascular disease risk factors; the probability for 'a case' at the first examination to be 'a case' at the second was 6.0
Boreham et al. [45]	prospective	boys = 251 girls = 203	12–15 – 20–25 years	boys and girls CRF was inversely associated with arterial stiffness
Eisenmann et al. [46]	prospective	boys = 36 girls = 12	15.9–27.2 years	boys and girls adolescent CRF is related only to adult BMI, WC and %BF (p < 0.05).
Ferreira et al. [47]	prospective	boys = 175 girls = 189	13–36 years	boys and girls CRF changes were inversely associated with prevalence of metabolic syndrome

%BF = Percentage of body fat; BMI = body mass index; BP = blood pressure; CRF = cardiorespiratory fitness; HDLc = high-density lipoprotein cholesterol; TG = triglycerides; WC = waist circumference.

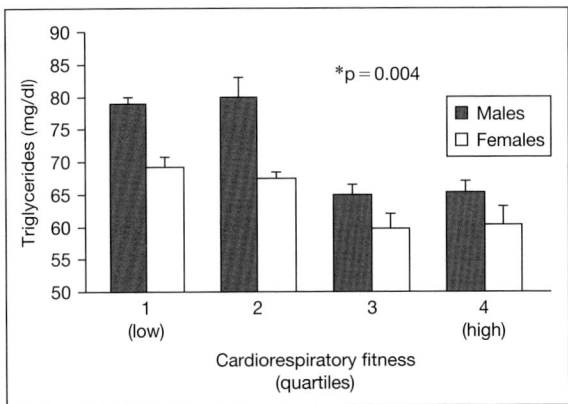

Fig. 4. Associations between triglycerides levels and cardiorespiratory fitness quartiles in male and female Spanish adolescents. Data shown as mean and SEM. * p for trend for males [13].

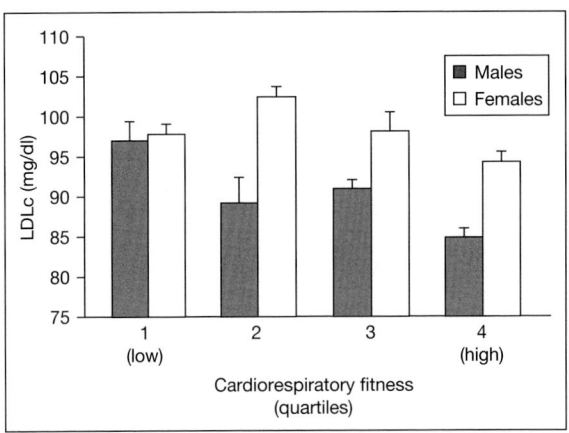

Fig. 5. Associations between low-density lipoprotein cholesterol (LDLc) levels and cardiorespiratory fitness quartiles in male and female Spanish adolescents. Data shown as mean and SEM [13].

fitness is negatively associated with homocysteine levels in female adolescents after controlling for age, puberty, birth weight, smoking, socioeconomic status, sum of six skinfolds and methylenetetrahydrofolate reductase 677C>T genotype [48]. These findings support a previous study examining the relationship between homocysteine and cardiorespiratory fitness in adults [49]. Kuo et al.

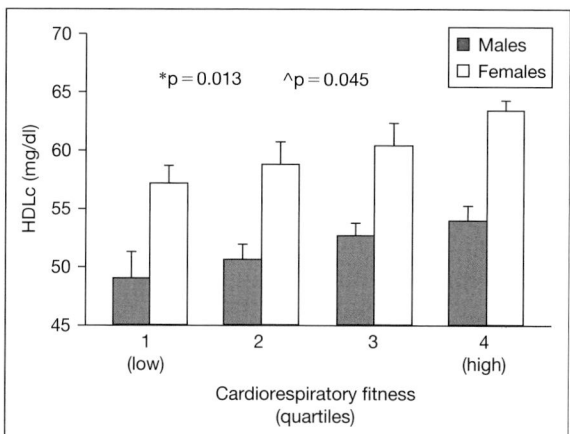

Fig. 6. Associations between high-density lipoprotein cholesterol (HDLc) levels and cardiorespiratory fitness quartiles in male and female Spanish adolescents aged. Data shown as mean and SEM. * p for trend for males; ^ p for trend for females [13].

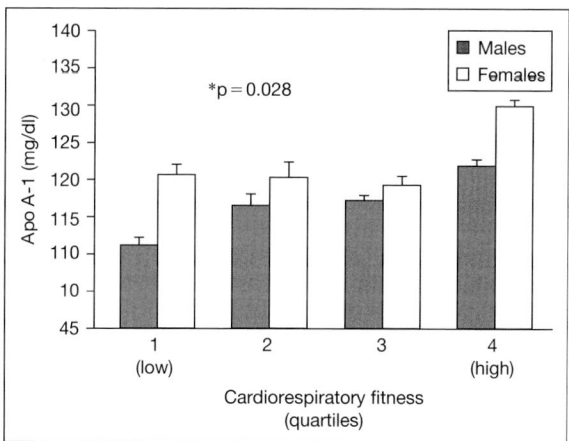

Fig. 7. Associations between apolipoprotein (apo) A-1 levels and cardiorespiratory fitness quartiles in male and female Spanish adolescents aged 13–18.5 years. Data shown as mean and SEM. * p for trend for males [13].

[49] showed that high homocysteine levels were negatively associated with estimated cardiorespiratory fitness in adult women. Moreover, one longitudinal study followed 499 independent community-dwelling elderly for 3 years and found that people with elevated homocysteine levels were at an increased risk of decline in physical function [50]. However, cardiorespiratory fitness data

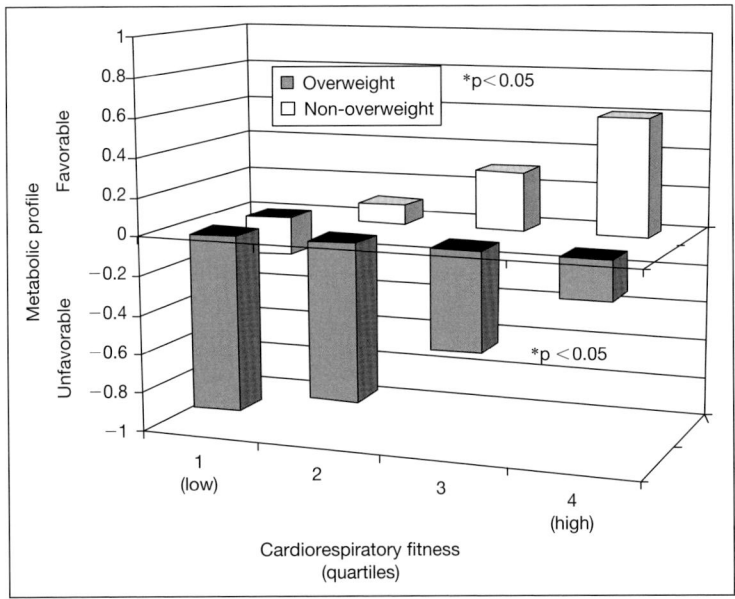

Fig. 8. Association between metabolic profile (computed with age- and gender-specific standardized values of triglycerides, low density lipoprotein cholesterol, high density lipoprotein cholesterol and fasting glycemia) and cardiorespiratory fitness quartiles in non-overweight and overweight Spanish adolescents. The higher is the metabolic profile the healthier. Weight categories were constructed following the International Obesity Task Force-proposed gender- and age-adjusted BMI cutoff points. Data shown as mean and SEM. *p for trend in both overweight and non-overweight categories [13].

were not provided and a gender comparison was not performed. These results should stimulate a debate on whether the metabolism of homocysteine could be one way in which the benefits of high cardiorespiratory fitness are exerted.

Cardiorespiratory fitness has also been shown to be associated with C-reactive protein and C3 in Spanish adolescents [51]. Similarly, Halle et al. [52] showed that cardiorespiratory fitness was negatively associated with low-grade inflammation in normal weight and overweight children aged 12 years. They reported that interleukin 6 levels were as low for obese and fit as for lean and unfit children, while the higher interleukin 6 levels were found in the obese and unfit group. In contrast, they also showed that tumor-necrosis factor-α seemed to be primarily dependent on cardiorespiratory fitness but not obesity since similar levels were found for non-obese as well as for obese children with low cardiorespiratory fitness.

Despite the evidence on the association between cardiorespiratory fitness and emerging and traditional cardiovascular risk factors in young and adult

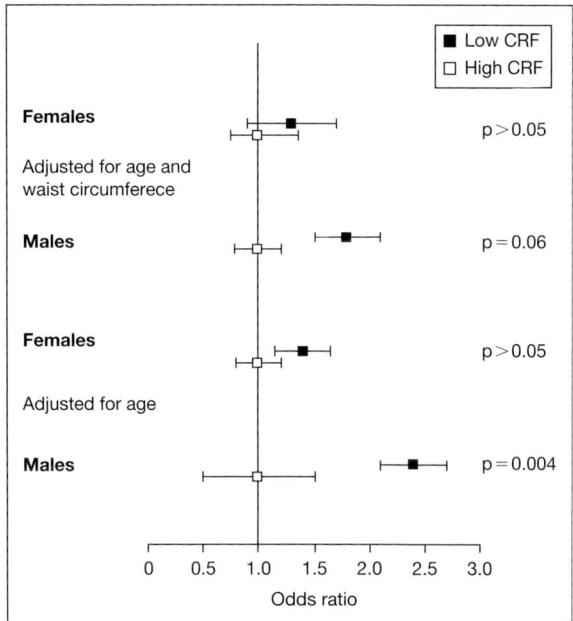

Fig. 9. Odds ratio for having an unfavorable lipid profile (triglycerides, high-density lipoprotein cholesterol, apolipoprotein A-1, apolipoprotein B-100, total cholesterol and high-density lipoprotein cholesterol ratio) in male and female Spanish adolescents.

populations, it is still uncertain whether health criterion values for cardiorespiratory fitness can be identified and the implications of these from the public health perspective. In this respect, several health-related threshold values of cardiorespiratory fitness have been suggested by world-wide recognized organizations [53, 54]. Based on expert judgment, the European Group of Pediatric Work Physiology considered a VO_{2max} of $\geq$35 ml/kg/min for girls and $\geq$40 ml/kg/min for boys as a 'Health Indicator' [53]. The Cooper Institute for Aerobics Research suggested $\geq$38 and $\geq$42 ml/kg/min for girls and boys respectively as a criterion standard for the 'Healthy Fitness Zone' [54]. The cutoff points proposed by the Cooper Institute for adolescents were extrapolated from the adults established thresholds.

Muscle Strength and Cardiovascular Risk Factors

Muscle strength refers to a balanced, healthy functioning of the musculoskeletal system and requires that a specific muscle or muscle group be able to generate force or torque. Muscle strength can also be a surrogate measure of both muscular endurance (that is the capacity to resist repeated contractions

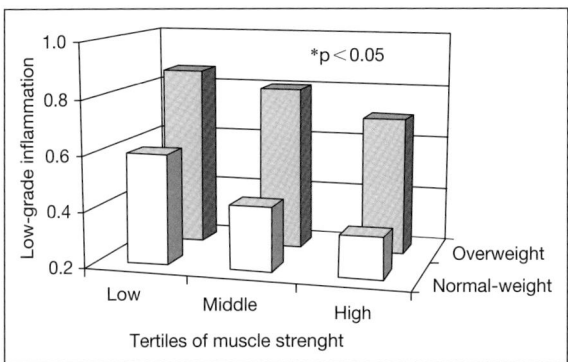

Fig. 10. Associations between tertiles of muscle strength and low-grade inflammation (estimated as a compound index of C-reactive protein and C3). These results are presented according to weight categories in Spanish adolescents. Weight categories were constructed following the International Obesity Task Force-proposed gender- and age-adjusted body mass index cut-off points. *p value from the regression analyses for the overweight category. [Ruiz et al., unpubl. data].

over time or maintain a maximal voluntary contraction for a prolonged period of time), and explosive strength (that is the capacity to carry out a maximal, dynamic contraction of a muscle or muscle group).

The importance of resistance exercise in promoting health and preventing disease has become increasingly recognized. Resistance exercise improves skeletal muscle strength and power, but also contributes to the prevention and management of atherosclerotic coronary heart disease, hypertension, diabetes, and overweight and obesity in adults. Muscle strength has been suggested to be inversely associated with all-cause mortality in men and women, independent of cardiorespiratory fitness levels [55]. However, little is known whether the health benefits of resistance exercise are independent of, or additive to, those already established for large muscle dynamic aerobic activity. Results from the AVENA study revealed significant associations between muscle strength and low-grade inflammation. It is known that low-grade inflammation seems to play a role in the pathogenesis of atherosclerosis from early ages, suggesting that preventive measures should start early in life. Figure 10 shows the associations between muscle strength and a compound index of low-grade inflammation integrated by C-reactive protein and C3, according to weight categories. Regression analysis was performed on muscle strength and the logarithmic of this index as continuous variables separately for non-overweight and overweight; however, in figure 10 they are broken into tertiles to illustrate the nature of the association. C-reactive protein has been recognized as cardiovascular risk factors, and nowadays there is increasing evidence about the link between C3 and cardiovascular disease.

Taken together, these findings support the concept that cardiorespiratory fitness and muscle strength may exert a protective effect on the cardiovascular system from an early age [56]. In fact, it is biologically plausible that a high fitness level provides more health protection than low fitness, even in healthy adolescents as has been found in adults. Prospective studies are needed to examine the independent and joint effects of cardiorespiratory fitness and muscle strength in preventing the development of cardiovascular risk factors among young people and adults. For public health strategies and preventive purposes it is of interest to understand the associations between diet, cardiorespiratory fitness, muscle fitness and cardiovascular risk factors from early ages on.

Body Composition and Cardiovascular Risk Factors in Mediterranean Adolescence

Childhood overweight or obesity is associated with a variety of adverse consequences both at that early age and later in life. Since childhood obesity is now recognized as a worldwide epidemic [16] it seems relevant to study, in children and adolescents, the association between total body fatness and physical activity and physical fitness, particularly in regions which have been traditionally protected given their favorable diet and life-style. It is known that the amount of fatness is associated with a poor health status, but it is also important how the fat depots are distributed in the body. In fact, central body fatness is associated with coronary heart disease morbidity and mortality and coronary heart disease risk factors including dyslipidemia, insulin resistance and hypertension [57]. Most disturbances related to abdominal obesity have been established to show their onset during childhood [58]. Therefore, in this section both total and central/abdominal adiposity and their relationships with physical activity and cardiorespiratory fitness in children and adolescents are presented.

Physical Activity, Fitness and Total Body Fat
Total Body Fat in Young Populations
Defining obesity or overweight for children and adolescents is difficult, and there is no generally accepted definition of overweight or obesity for youths. However, body mass index (BMI) is a widely used tool to identify overweight and obese children and adolescents [59]. Indeed, we have observed elevated overweight and obesity prevalence in Spanish adolescents [60], similar to those observed in other European countries (including Mediterranean diet's countries) (fig. 3). Factors, such as socioeconomic status, seem to be inversely related to the overweight + obesity prevalence. Of note is that the rate of change in overweight prevalence in Spanish adolescents seems to be

increasing [60]. Particularly in Mediterranean countries, there is an urge to establish preventive measures to fight against this alarming increasing in the childhood obesity epidemic. Measures to improve fitness could play a key role not only in obesity prevention but also in improving the health of the adults of tomorrow.

Although the BMI criterion is the most frequently used, an important number of adolescents classified as overweight or obese do not have really high adiposity (32.1% of females and 42% of males) [61]. Therefore, whenever possible, the anthropometric assessment of body composition should include a body fat estimation (i.e. from skinfold thickness). In this context, body fat reference data from Spanish adolescents have been recently reported, helping us to classify adolescents in comparison with a well-established reference population, and to estimate the proportion of adolescents with high or low adiposity amounts [62].

Associations of Total Body Fat with Physical Activity and Fitness

A sedentary lifestyle and a significant reduction in daily physical activity are one of the key factors of the obesity epidemic in children and adolescents. By contrast, high cardiorespiratory fitness during childhood and adolescence has been associated not only with a healthier cardiovascular profile during these years but also later in life (table 2). For preventive purposes, it is of interest to understand the relative importance of the amount and intensity of physical activity not only on total body fat but also in cardiorespiratory fitness levels. New data have shown positive associations between physical activity, especially vigorous physical activity (>6 METs) and cardiorespiratory fitness (fig. 11) [63], as well as negative associations between vigorous physical activity and fatness in children and adolescents (fig. 12) [63, 64]. These results suggest that a certain level of physical activity needs to be achieved in order to improve the fitness and fatness status. Vigorous physical activity seems to be more relevant in increasing fitness and reducing body fat in young people. From a public health perspective these findings are particularly relevant.

Physical Activity, Fitness and Body Fat Distribution
Body Fat Distribution in Young Populations

The study of fat distribution among children and adolescents is complex because there are marked changes in circumferences and skinfold thickness during growth and development [65]. The two types of fat depots are abdominal and truncal fat. In population studies, the best anthropometric marker of abdominal obesity is waist circumference. Waist circumference correlates well with intra-abdominal and subcutaneous fat measured by magnetic resonance

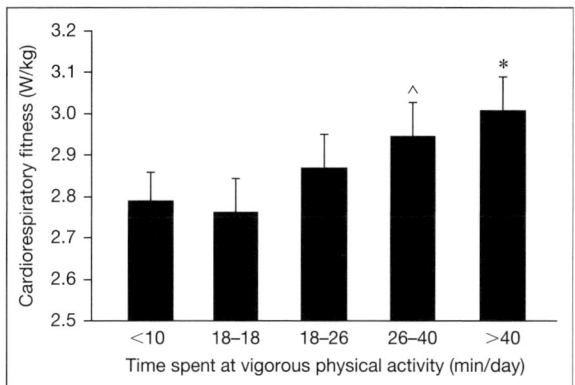

Fig. 11. Mean cardiorespiratory fitness stratified by time spent at vigorous physical activity in Swedish and Estonian children. Error bars represent 95% CIs. * A significant difference was observed between those who accumulated >40 min/day of vigorous physical activity and those who accumulated <18 min/day at this intensity level. ^ A significant difference was also observed between children who accumulated 26–40 min/day of vigorous physical activity compared to those who accumulated 10–18 min/day at this level of intensity [63].

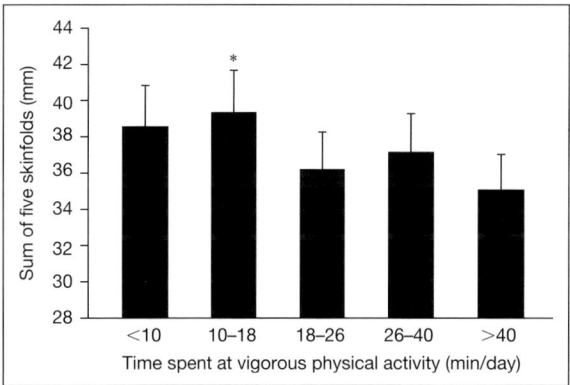

Fig. 12. Mean sum of five skinfolds (body fat) stratified by time spent at vigorous physical activity in Swedish and Estonian children. Errors bars represent 95% CIs. * A significant difference was observed between those who accumulated >40 min/day of vigorous physical activity and those who accumulated 10–18 min/day at this intensity level [63].

imaging in children and adolescents [66]. Waist circumference is a good tool for the screening of total body fat and the metabolic syndrome. That is why waist circumference is also a central feature of the metabolic syndrome and several diagnostic criteria of the condition include this marker in the definition

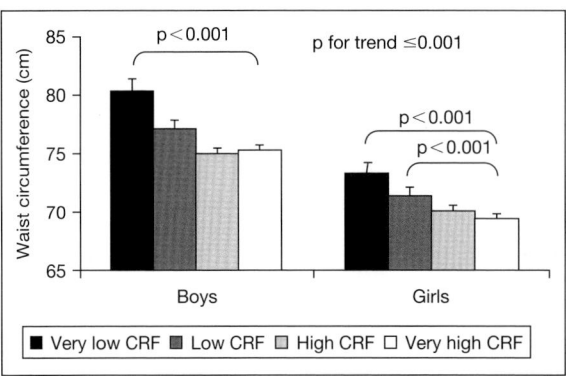

Fig. 13. Waist circumference (means ± standard error of the mean) according to cardiorespiratory fitness (CRF) quartiles in Spanish adolescents [70].

[67]. In the absence of a recognized definition of increased central adiposity in young people, the terms 'overweight' and 'obesity' referred to central adiposity are currently being arbitrarily defined. Therefore, they have been recently reported reference data for waist circumference and other fat patterning indices from a large sample of Spanish adolescents [Moreno et al., unpubl. data]. These data, together with data from other countries, will help to establish international central obesity criteria for adolescents, giving the possibility to estimate the proportion of adolescents with high or low regional adiposity.

Associations of Body Fat Distribution with Physical Activity and Fitness

It has been reported that, even within a given BMI category, children and adolescents with a large waist circumference are more likely to have abnormal cardiovascular disease risk factors compared to those with a small waist circumference [68]. Consequently, waist circumference could be a useful tool for studying obesity in adolescents. In adults, several studies have reported that individuals with better cardiorespiratory fitness have less abdominal fat and/or smaller waist circumferences for a given BMI [69]. However, the results obtained so far on the relationship between physical activity and central obesity in children and adolescents are also inconsistent.

Recent results from Spanish adolescents [70] suggest that moderate to high levels of cardiorespiratory fitness, but not self-reported physical activity, are associated with lower abdominal adiposity, as measured by waist circumference (fig. 13). However, given that the questionnaire used in that study does not provide either the intensity level of physical activity or the frequency of

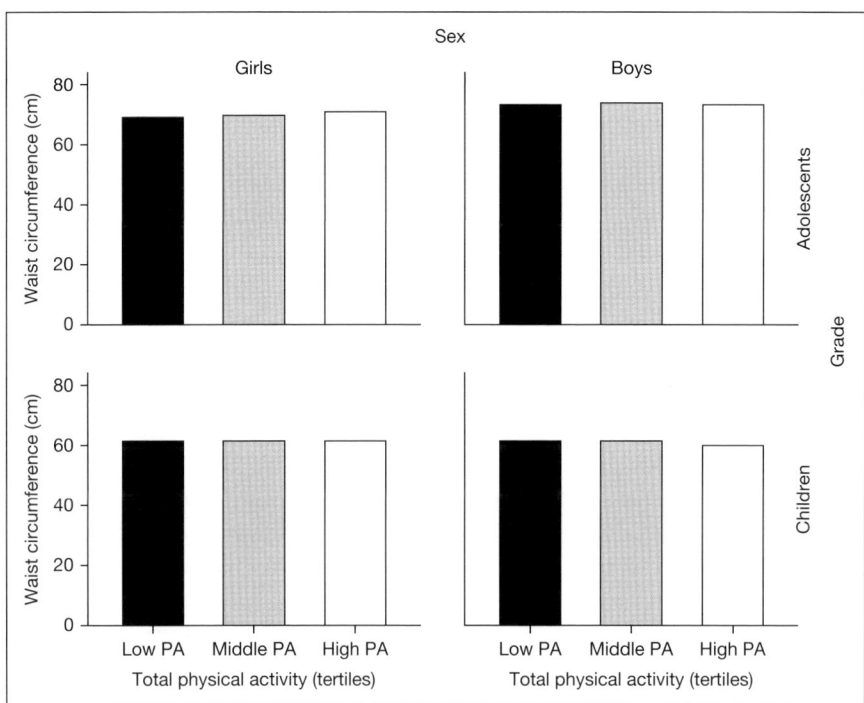

Fig. 14. Waist circumference (means) according to total physical activity (PA) in Swedish children and adolescents. Data were adjusted for age group and height. Total PA was not associated with waist circumference. No relationship was found between the PA intensities levels (moderate, vigorous, or moderate plus vigorous) and waist circumference. [Ortega et al., unpubl. data].

physical activity, it is necessary to be cautious with the physical activity-related conclusions from that study. Research with objective methods for measuring physical activity, such as accelerometry, will provide accurate information about physical activity patterns (intensity, frequency and duration), helping to clarify this issue. In this context, data obtained from the Swedish part of the European Youth Heart Study using physical activity objectively measured, has recently obtained the same conclusion [Ortega et al., unpubl data]. Both in children and adolescents, physical activity (either total, moderate or vigorous) is not associated with abdominal adiposity, as measured by waist circumference (fig. 14). This is not the case with cardiorespiratory fitness. These results suggest that the beneficial effects of physical activity on abdominal adiposity may be explained by its association with cardiorespiratory fitness in children and adolescents.

Conclusion

Growing evidence demonstrates that the Mediterranean life-style is beneficial to health, especially for coronary heart disease, stroke and some forms of cancer. Diet is one outstanding component of the Mediterranean life-style. But it is not only diet – physical activity is another critical component. Diet and physical activity interact in the development (or prevention) of coronary heart disease and several other health conditions. These interactions may start early in life. In this way, adolescence is a critical period because it is at that time when the individual takes control of his/her own life-style and diet. Large life-style and dietary variations occur in different regions and countries. In many of them, a progressive departure from the traditional Mediterranean life-style and diet is being observed. In Spain, a high prevalence of an unfavorable plasma lipid profile has been observed both in boys and girls. Similarly, the high prevalence of obesity in Mediterranean children and adolescents is well known. But it is not only physical activity. Physical fitness (especially cardiorespiratory fitness and muscle strength) is strongly associated with cardiovascular risk factors. For public health strategies and preventive purposes it is of interest to understand the associations of diet, physical activity and fitness on cardiovascular risk factors from early ages on. It is important to implement measures for preventing the deleterious consequences that these conditions are going to have in the health of tomorrow's adults [71]. One positive measure is the return to the traditional Mediterranean diet; the other is to increase the levels of physical activity in order to improve physical fitness. Measures to improve fitness could play a key role in improving the health of the adults of tomorrow.

Acknowledgements

This paper reviews, among others, data (published or yet unpublished) derived from the AVENA Study (www.estudioavena.com) and the European Youth Heart Study. We thank Prof. Michael Sjöström, from the Unit for Preventive Nutrition, Karolinska Institutet, for fruitful discussion and the opportunity to use data from the European Youth Heart Study. We thank our colleagues from the AVENA Study Group for their contribution in data collection and results discussion.

References

1 Kromhout D: Epidemiology of cardiovascular diseases in Europe. Publ Health Nutr 2001;4:441–457.
2 Lopez AD, Mathers CD, Ezzati M, Jamison DT, Murray CJ: Global and regional burden of disease and risk factors, 2001: systematic analysis of population health data. Lancet 2006;367:1747–1757.

3   Kuulasmaa K, Tunstall-Pedoe H, Dobson A, Fortmann S, Sans S, Tolonen H, Evans A, Ferrario M, Tuomilehto J: Estimation of contribution of changes in classic risk factors to trends in coronary-event rates across the WHO MONICA Project populations. Lancet 2000;355:675–687.
4   Simopoulos AP, Visioli F: Mediterranean Diets. World Rev Nutr Diet. Basel, Karger, 2000, vol 87, pp 1–184.
5   Kok FJ, Kromhout D: Atherosclerosis. Epidemiological studies on the health effects of a Mediterranean diet. Eur J Nutr 2004;43:I/2–I/5.
6   Trichopoulou A: Traditional Mediterranean diet and longevity in the elderly: a review. Publ Health Nutr 2004;7:943–947.
7   Tur JA, Romaguera D, Pons A: Food consumption patterns in a Mediterranean region: does the Mediterranean diet still exist? Ann Nutr Metab 2004;48:193–201.
8   Mokdad AH, Marks JS, Stroup DF, Gerberding JL: Actual causes of death in the United States, 2000. JAMA 2004;291:1238–1245.
9   Moreiras-Varela O: The Mediterranean diet in Spain. Eur J Clin Nutr 1989;43:83–87.
10 Castillo-Garzon MJ: Changing the Spanish Mediterranean diet: effects on plasma lipids; in Watson R (ed): Wild-Type Diet. New York, Humana Press, in press.
11 Delgado M, Gonzalez-Gross M, Cano MD, Gutierrez A, Castillo M: Physical exercise reverses diet-induced increases in LDL-cholesterol and apo B levels in healthy ovo-lactovegetarian subjects. Nutr Res 2000;20:1707–1714.
12 Ruiz JR, Mesa JL, Mingorance I, Rodriguez-Cuartero A, Castillo MJ: Sports requiring stressful physical exertion cause abnormalities in plasma lipid profile. Rev Esp Cardiol 2004;57:499–506.
13 Mesa JL, Ruiz J, Ortega FB, Warnberg J, Gonzalez-Lamuno D, Moreno LA, Gutierrez A, Castillo MJ: Aerobic physical fitness in relation to blood lipids and fasting glycaemia in adolescents: influence of weight status. Nutr Metab Cardiovasc Dis 2006;285–293.
14 Gonzalez-Gross M, Castillo MJ, Moreno L, Moreno L, Nova E, Gonzalez-Lamuno D, Perez-Llamas F, Gutierrez A, Garaulet M, Joyanes M, Leiva A, Marcos A: Feeding and assessment of nutritional status of spanish adolescents (AVENA study). Evaluation of risks and interventional proposal. I. Methodology. Nutr Hosp 2003;18:15–28.
15 Ruiz JR, Ortega FB, Moreno LA, Wärnberg J, Gonzalez-Gross M, Cano MD, Gutierrez A, Castillo MJ, the AVENA Study Group: Serum lipid and lipoprotein reference values of Spanish adolescents; The AVENA study. Soz Praventiv Med 2006;51:99–109.
16 Flodmark CE, Lissau I, Moreno LA, Pietrobelli A, Widhalm K: New insights into the field of children and adolescents' obesity: the European perspective. Int J Obes 2004;28:1189–1196.
17 Castillo MJ, Ruiz JR, Ortega FB, Gutierrez A: Anti-aging therapy through fitness enhancement. Clin Intervent Aging 2006;1:213–220.
18 Carnethon MR, Gidding SS, Nehgme R, Sidney S, Jacobs DR Jr, Liu K: Cardiorespiratory fitness in young adulthood and the development of cardiovascular disease risk factors. JAMA 2003;290:3092–3100.
19 Laukkanen JA, Lakka TA, Rauramaa R, Kuhanen R, Venalainen JM, Salonen R, Salonen JT: Cardiovascular fitness as a predictor of mortality in men. Arch Intern Med 2001;161:825–831.
20 Balady GJ: Survival of the fittest: more evidence. N Engl J Med 2002;346:852–854.
21 Kurl S, Laukkanen JA, Rauramaa R, Lakka TA, Sivenius J, Salonen JT: Cardiorespiratory fitness and the risk for stroke in men. Arch Intern Med 2003;163:1682–1688.
22 Gulati M, Pandey DK, Arnsdorf MF, Lauderdale DS, Thisted RA, Wicklund RH, Al-Hani AJ, Black HR: Exercise capacity and the risk of death in women: the St James Women Take Heart Project. Circulation 2003;108:1554–1559.
23 Mora S, Redberg RF, Cui Y, Whiteman MK, Flaws JA, Sharrett AR, Blumenthal RS: Ability of exercise testing to predict cardiovascular and all-cause death in asymptomatic women: a 20-year follow-up of the lipid research clinics prevalence study. JAMA 2003;290:1600–1607.
24 Myers J, Prakash M, Froelicher V, Do D, Partington S, Atwood JE: Exercise capacity and mortality among men referred for exercise testing. N Engl J Med 2002;346:793–801.
25 Lee CD, Blair SN: Cardiorespiratory fitness and smoking-related and total cancer mortality in men. Med Sci Sports Exerc 2002;34:735–739.

26 Evenson KR, Stevens J, Cai J, Thomas R, Thomas O: The effect of cardiorespiratory fitness and obesity on cancer mortality in women and men. Med Sci Sports Exerc 2003;35: 270–277.
27 Lee CD, Folsom AR, Blair SN: Physical activity and stroke risk. Stroke 2003;34:2475–2481.
28 Sawada SS, Muto T, Tanaka H, Lee IM, Paffenbarger RS Jr, Shindo M, Blair SN: Cardiorespiratory fitness and cancer mortality in Japanese men: a prospective study. Med Sci Sports Exerc 2003;35:1546–1550.
29 Seibaek M, Vestergaard H, Burchardt H, Sloth C, Torp-Pedersen C, Nielsen SL, Hildebrandt P, Pedersen O: Insulin resistance and maximal oxygen uptake. Clin Cardiol 2003;26:515–520.
30 Bertoli A, Di Daniele N, Ceccobelli M, Ficara A, Girasoli C, De Lorenzo A: Lipid profile, BMI, body fat distribution, and aerobic fitness in men with metabolic syndrome. Acta Diabetol 2003;40: 130S–133S.
31 Lakka TA, Laaksonen DE, Lakka HM, Mannikko N, Niskanen LK, Rauramaa R, Salonen JT: Sedentary lifestyle, poor cardiorespiratory fitness, and the metabolic syndrome. Med Sci Sports Exerc 2003;35:1279–1286.
32 Colcombe SJ, Erickson KI, Raz N, Webb AG, Cohen NJ, McAuley E, Kramer AF: Aerobic fitness reduces brain tissue loss in ageing humans. J Gerontol [A] 2003;58:176–180.
33 Barnes DE, Yaffe K, Satariano WA, Tager IB: A longitudinal study of cardiorespiratory fitness and cognitive function in healthy older adults. J Am Geriatr Soc 2003;51:459–465.
34 Metter EJ, Talbot LA, Schrager M, Conwit R: Skeletal muscle strength as a predictor of all-cause mortality in healthy men. J Gerontol [A] 2002;57:B359–B365.
35 Seguin R, Nelson ME: The benefits of strength training for older adults. Am J Prev Med 2003;25:S141–S149.
36 Ruiz JR, España-Romero V, Ortega FB, Sjostrom M, Castillo MJ, Gutierrez A: Hand span influences optimal grip span in male and female teenagers. J Hand Surg Am. 2006;31:1367–1372.
37 Ruiz JR, Mesa JL, Castillo MJ, Gutierrez A: Hand size influences optimal grip span in women but not in men. J Hand Surg 2002;27:897–901.
38 Gutin B, Yin Z, Humphries MC, Hoffman WH, Gower B, Barbeau P: Relations of fatness and fitness to fasting insulin in black and white adolescents. J Pediatr 2004;145:737–743.
39 Brage S, Wedderkopp N, Ekelund U, Franks PW, Wareham NJ, Andersen LB, Froberg K: European Youth Heart Study (EYHS): Features of the metabolic syndrome are associated with objectively measured physical activity and fitness in Danish children: the European Youth Heart Study (EYHS). Diabetes Care 2004;27:2141–2148.
40 Reed KE, Warburton DE, Lewanczuk RZ, Haykowsky MJ, Scott JM, Whitney CL, McGavock JM, McKay HA: Arterial compliance in young children: the role of aerobic fitness. Eur J Cardiovasc Prev Rehabil 2005;12:492–497.
41 Eisenmann JC, Katzmarzyk PT, Perusse L, Tremblay A, Despres JP, Bouchard C: Aerobic fitness, body mass index, and CVD risk factors among adolescents: the Quebec family study. Int J Obes Relat Metab Disord 2005;29:1077–1083.
42 Gutin B, Yin Z, Humphries MC, Bassali R, Le NA, Daniels S, Barbeau P: Relations of body fatness and cardiovascular fitness to lipid profile in black and white adolescents. Pediatr Res 2005;58:78–82.
43 Ruiz JR, Ortega FB, Meusel D, Harro M, Oja P, Sjöström M: Cardiorespiratory fitness is associated with features of metabolic risk factors in children. Should cardiorespiratory fitness be assessed in a European health monitoring system? The European Youth Heart Study. J Publ Health 2006;14:94–102.
44 Andersen LB, Hasselstrøm H, Grønfeldt V, Hansen SE, Froberg K: The relationship between physical fitness and clustered risk, and tracking of clustered risk from adolescence to young adulthood: eight years follow-up in the Danish Youth and Sport Study. Int J Behav Nutr Phys Fitness 2004;1:6.
45 Boreham CA, Ferreira I, Twisk JW, Gallagher AM, Savage MJ, Murray LJ: Cardiorespiratory fitness, physical activity, and arterial stiffness: The Northern Ireland Young Hearts Project. Hypertension 2004;44:721–726.
46 Eisenmann JC, Wickel EE, Welk GJ, Blair SN: Relationship between adolescent fitness and fatness and cardiovascular disease risk factors in adulthood: the Aerobics Center Longitudinal Study (ACLS). Am Heart J 2005;149:46–53.

47 Ferreira I, Henry RM, Twisk JW, van Mechelen W, Kemper HC, Stehouwer CD: The metabolic syndrome, cardiopulmonary fitness, and subcutaneous trunk fat as independent determinants of arterial stiffness: the Amsterdam Growth and Health Longitudinal Study. Arch Intern Med 2005;165:875–882.
48 Ruiz JR, Sola R, Gonzalez-Gross M, Ortega FB, Vicente-Rodriguez G, Garcia-Fuentes M, Gutierrez A, Sjöström M, Pietrzik K, Castillo MJ: Cardiovascular fitness is negatively associated with homocysteine levels in female adolescents. Arch Pediatr Adolesc Med. In press.
49 Kuo HK, Yen CJ, Bean JF: Levels of homocysteine are inversely associated with cardiovascular fitness in women, but not in men: data from the National Health and Nutrition Examination Survey 1999–2002. J Intern Med 2005;258:328–335.
50 Kado DM, Bucur A, Selhub J, Rowe JW, Seeman T: Homocysteine levels and decline in physical function. Studies of successful aging. Am J Med 2002;113:537–542.
51 Wärnberg J: Inflammatory Status in Adolescents; the Impact of Health Determinants Such As Overweight and Fitness. Thesis, Karolinska University Press, Stockholm, 2006.
52 Halle M, Berg A, Northoff H, Keul J: Importance of TNF-alpha and leptin in obesity and insulin resistance: a hypothesis on the impact of physical exercise. Exerc Immunol Rev 1998;4: 77–94.
53 Bell RD, Macek M, Rutenfranz J, Saris WHM: Health indicators and risk factors of cardiovascular diseases during childhood and adolescence; in Rutenfranz J, Mocelin R, Klimt F (eds): Children and Exercise. Part XII. Champaign, Human Kinetics, 1986, pp 19–27.
54 Cooper Institute for Aerobics Research: FITNESSGRAM Test Administration Manual. Champaign, Human Kinetics, 1999.
55 Jurca R, Lamonte MJ, Barlow CE, Kampert JB, Church TS, Blair SN: Association of muscular strength with incidence of metabolic syndrome in men. Med Sci Sports Exerc 2005;37: 1849–1855.
56 Ruiz JR, Ortega FB, Gutierrez A, Meusel D, Sjöström M, Castillo MJ, on behalf of the HELENA Study Group: Health-related fitness assessment in childhood and adolescence: a European approach based on the AVENA, EYHS and HELENA studies. J Publ Health 2006;14:269–277.
57 Rexrode KM, Carey VJ, Hennekens CH, Walters EE, Colditz GA, Stampfer MJ, Willett WC, Manson JE: Abdominal adiposity and coronary heart disease in women. JAMA 1998;280: 1843–1848.
58 Freedman DS, Serdula MK, Srinivasan SR, Berenson GS: Relation of circumferences and skinfold thicknesses to lipid and insulin concentrations in children and adolescents: the Bogalusa Heart Study. Am J Clin Nutr 1999;69:308–317.
59 Cole TJ, Bellizzi MC, Flegal KM, Dietz WH: Establishing a standard definition for child overweight and obesity worldwide: international survey. BMJ 2000;320:1240–1243.
60 Moreno LA, Mesana MI, Fleta J, Ruiz JR, Gonzalez-Gross M, Sarria A, Marcos A, Bueno M, Group AS: Overweight, obesity and body fat composition in spanish adolescents. The AVENA Study. Ann Nutr Metab 2005;49:71–76.
61 Rodriguez G, Moreno LA, Blay MG, Blay VA, Garagorri JM, Sarria A, Bueno M: Body composition in adolescents: measurements and metabolic aspects. Int J Obes 2004;3:S54–S58.
62 Moreno LA, Mesana MI, Gonzalez-Gross M, Gil CM, Fleta J, Warnberg J, Ruiz JR, Sarria A, Marcos A, Bueno M: Anthropometric body fat composition reference values in Spanish adolescents. The AVENA Study. Eur J Clin Nutr 2006;60:191–196.
63 Ruiz JR, Rizzo NS, Hurtig-Wennlöf A, Ortega FB, Warnberg J, Sjöström M: Relations of total physical activity and intensity to fitness and fatness in children: The European Youth Heart Study. Am J Clin Nutr 2006;84:298–302.
64 Gutin B, Yin Z, Humphries MC, Barbeau P: Relations of moderate and vigorous physical activity to fitness and fatness in adolescents. Am J Clin Nutr 2005;81:746–750.
65 Ruiz JR, Ortega FB, Moreno LA, Wärnberg J, Mesa JL, Gonzalez-Gross M, Tresaco B, Cano MD, Marcos A, Gutierrez A, Castillo MJ, the AVENA Study Group: Serum lipid and lipoprotein profile during pubertal development in Spanish adolescents aged 13–18.5 years. The AVENA Study. Horm Metabol Res. In press.
66 Brambilla P, Bedogni G, Moreno LA, Goran MI, Gutin B, Fox KR, Peters DM, Barbeau P, De Simone M, Pietrobelli A: Crossvalidation of anthropometry against magnetic resonance imaging

for the assessment of visceral and subcutaneous adipose tissue in children. Int J Obes 2006;30: 23–30.
67 Bueno G, Bueno O, Moreno LA, García R, Tresaco B, Garagorri JM: Diversity of metabolic syndrome risk factors in obese children and adolescents. J Physiol Biochem. In press.
68 Janssen I, Katzmarzyk PT, Srinivasan SR, Chen W, Malina RM, Bouchard C, Berenson GS: Combined influence of body mass index and waist circumference on coronary artery disease risk factors among children and adolescents. Pediatrics 2005;115:1623–1630.
69 Janssen I, Katzmarzyk PT, Ross R: Waist circumference and not body mass index explains obesity-related health risk. Am J Clin Nutr 2004;79:379–384.
70 Ortega FB, Tresaco B, Ruiz JR, Moreno LA, Martin-Matillas M, Mesa JL, Warnberg J, Bueno M, Tercedor P, Gutiérrez A, Castillo MJ: Cardiorespiratory fitness is associated with favorable abdominal adiposity in adolescents. Obes Res. In press.
71 Castillo Garzon MJ, Ortega Porcel FB, Ruiz J: [Improvement of physical fitness as anti-aging intervention]. Med Clin 2005;124:146–155.

Prof. Manuel J. Castillo-Garzón
Department of Physiology, School of Medicine
University of Granada
ES–18071 Granada (Spain)
Tel. +34 958 243540, Fax +34 958 249015, E-Mail mcgarzon@ugr.es

Mediterranean Diet in the Maghreb: An Update

Sabrina Zeghichi-Hamri[a], *Stamatina Kallithraka*[b]

[a]Laboratoire Nutrition, Vieillissement et Maladies Cardiovasculaires, UFR de Médecine et de Pharmacie, Domaine de la Merci, La Tronche, France;
[b]Wine Institute of Athens/NAGREF, Likovrisi, Athens, Greece

The health of the individual and the population in general is the result of interactions between genetics and a number of environmental factors. Nutrition is an environmental factor of major importance [1, 2]. The nutritional regulation occurs both by macro- and micronutrients [3]. Both micro- and macronutrients control gene expression leading to changes in cell growth, differentiation, or metabolism. Defining the molecular basis for nutrient control of gene expression provides insight into the diverse actions of nutrients in both normal and pathophysiological states and may provide novel approaches for the control of chronic diseases such as coronary artery disease, hypertension, insulin resistance, obesity and cancer [4, 5].

The Mediterranean diet has gained enormous popularity lately, mainly because it has been associated with lower death rates from coronary heart disease [6] and certain types of cancer [7], such as breast, colon, and gastric cancer. It has been suggested that certain characteristics of this diet, such as a relatively high consumption of fish, olive oil, vegetables and fruits, and low consumption of meat and animal fat were connected with the low prevalence of the above diseases [8]. Moreover, a majority of published studies refer to the fact that the incidence of some other diseases such as osteoporosis, obesity and dental caries is lower in the Mediterranean region in comparison with the western and Nordic countries [9].

However, more recent data [9–11] indicate that in the last 35 years the food pattern of the Mediterranean populations has been subjected to substantial changes. Significant changes have occurred in consumption of some, but not all, foods in both positive and negative directions with respect to dietary recommendations. Furthermore, the term 'Mediterranean diet' is very loose since geographical, political and religious differences prevent a uniform dietary pattern across the Mediterranean countries and directly influence the dietary customs and habits. Thus, defining the Mediterranean diet at a regional level may provide more information than describing a common Mediterranean food pattern. Under these constraints, we will discuss the current Mediterranean diet in the region of northwestern Africa (which is also called the Maghreb). The Maghreb consists of four countries: Algeria, Libya, Morocco and Tunisia. We will compare it with the dietary patterns of the 1970s.

Generally speaking, the northern part of the Maghreb region is green and fertile with a temperate climate but soon after leaving the coastal area, the Sahara desert starts with an arid and extremely dry climate.

The native population of the Maghreb is mostly Arabs and Berbers who belong mainly to the Islamic religion. During the last 60 years, important changes have occurred in this region as a result of the termination of colonial rule. Since independence, the Maghreb countries have experienced decisive social, economic, and political changes leading to their present situation.

Recent Dietary Trends in Algeria, Libya, Morocco and Tunisia

While discussing the food consumption pattern of the populations in the Maghreb, it should be understood that we are not talking about a uniform dietary pattern of the four countries, but rather about relatively specific diets.

The composition of the diets of the four Maghreb countries, in terms of absolute quantities per consumption unit per year, is shown in figure 1. The source of the food consumption data are mostly generated nationally, but collected, analyzed and published in a standardized manner by the FAO. Although there are serious limitations to this data source, it presents practically the only standardized and consistent database available for cross-country comparison [10].

As shown in figure 1, there are differences in the consumption of specific food items among the Maghreb countries for the period 2000–2003, regarding the absolute quantities consumed. More specifically, Algeria is the country with the lowest consumption of fruits and vegetables, in comparison with the rest of the Maghreb countries. Regarding animal products (meat and eggs), Algerians consume fewer quantities than their neighbors do, but they are first in milk consumption. Regarding fish and seafood, Moroccans and Tunisians consume the highest per capita quantities whereas Algerians the lowest. Libya is the country with the lowest cereal and cereal product consumption in comparison with the rest of the Maghreb countries. Additionally, Libyans consume more vegetable oils and animal fats as well as animal products (meat and eggs), and vegetables than their neighbors do. Morocco has the highest intake of cereals and sweeteners and the

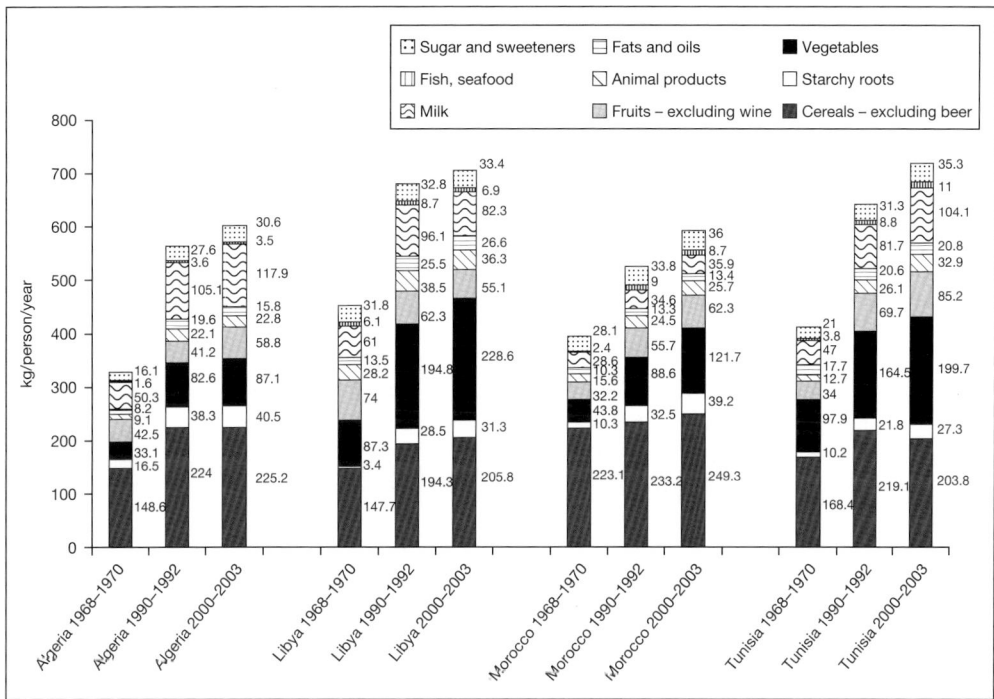

Fig. 1. Average per capita consumption (kg/person/year) of various food groups for Algeria, Libya, Morocco and Tunisia for the years 1968–1970, 1990–1992 and 2000–2003. Values are shown on the right of each food category (FAO, statistics division).

lowest of milk, fats, and oils among the Maghreb countries. Finally, Tunisians consume the highest amounts of fish and seafood as well as fruits in comparison with their neighbors.

On this basis, we could describe the diet of the Maghreb as relatively low in total fat, high in consumption of cereals and vegetable products, and low in animal products. Alcohol and wine consumption (not shown here) is very low mainly due to religious restriction.

Although it might appear self-evident that the Maghreb countries are Mediterranean, since they border the Mediterranean Sea, the food patterns of the Maghreb population are quiet different compared to those of some European Mediterranean populations. For example, cereal per capita consumption in Spain, France, Italy and Greece in 2000–2003 is remarkably lower than in the Maghreb countries (fig. 2). Furthermore, the Maghreb diet contains much less animal products (milk, meat and eggs) than Spain, France, Italy and Greece. The same applies for the USA and UK (non-Mediterranean European countries).

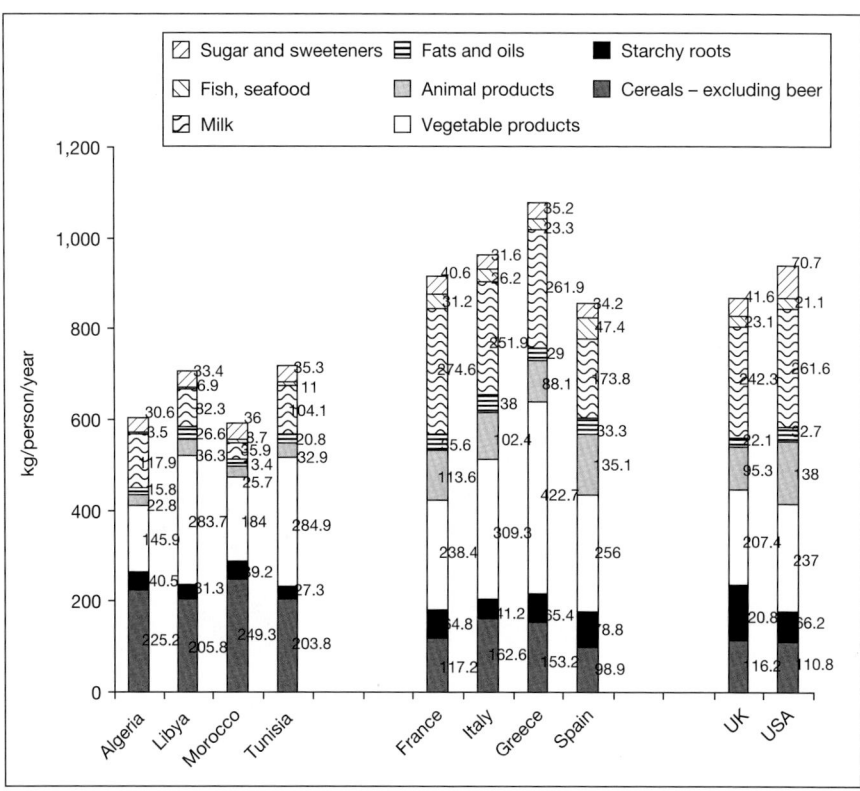

Fig. 2. Average per capita consumption (kg/person/year) of various food groups for the Maghreb countries (Algeria, Libya, Morocco and Tunisia), some Mediterranean European countries, the United Kingdom and the USA for the years 2002–2003. Values are shown on the right of each food category (FAO, statistics division).

Quite unexpectedly, the Maghreb diet is lower in vegetable product consumption except for Libyans and Tunisians who consume higher amounts of vegetables than the French, Italian and Spaniards. Fat and oil consumption also provides an unexpected picture since the Maghreb diet is much lower in fats and oils than the diet in Spain, France, Italy, Greece, UK and USA. Another large variation among the food habits of some European Mediterranean countries and the Maghreb is that of fish consumption. Spain, Italy, France and Greece consume almost three times more fish than the Maghreb countries. We should underline at this point that fish is not easily available in the Maghreb due to difficulties in its preservation and transportation. This problem is even more difficult in the southern part of these countries. Finally, the consumption of sweeteners is almost the same in the Maghreb and the four European Mediterranean countries.

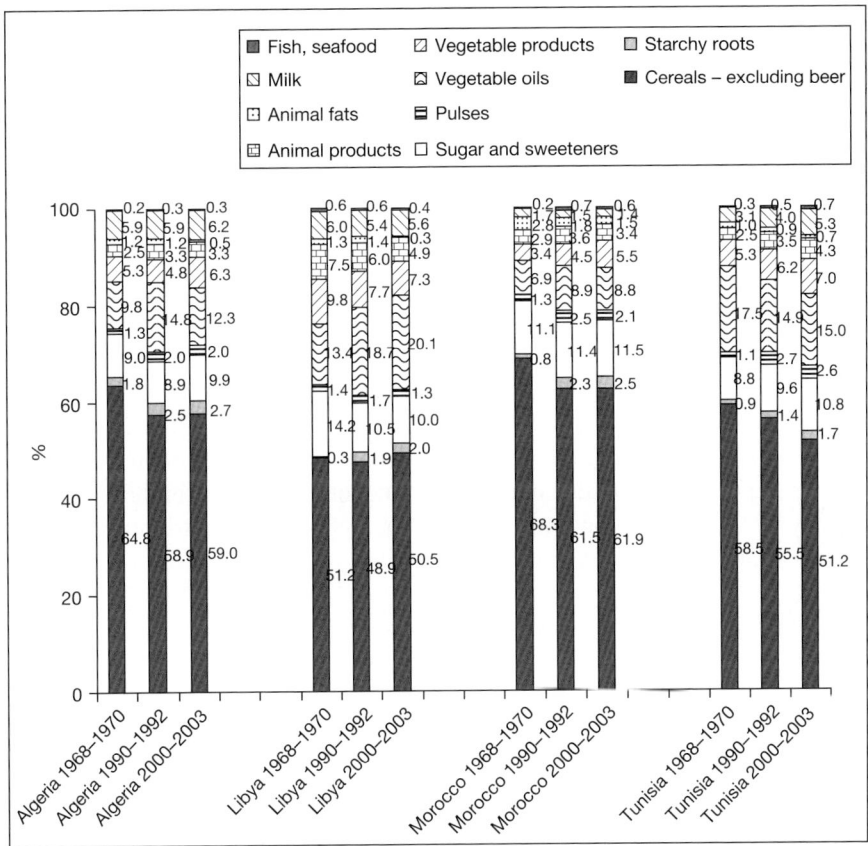

Fig. 3. Percent contribution of various food groups to total dietary energy intake (calories/person/day) in Algeria, Libya, Morocco and Tunisia for the years 1968–1970, 1990–1992 and 2000–2003. Values are shown on the right of each food category (FAO, statistics division).

Taking into account the above-mentioned differences, it is quite clear that the Mediterranean diet is not a homogenous nutritional model. There are several Mediterranean nations with varied cultures, traditions, incomes and dietary habits resulting in a wide variation of the dietary patterns within the Mediterranean region.

To better illustrate the differences among the Maghreb countries, the contribution of the various food groups to total energy supply, for the years 2000–2003, has been calculated and it is presented in figure 3. This provides a visual representation of the differences, but the absolute values should be kept in mind, in order not to lose the overall perspective. The picture remains essentially the same and confirms that the countries of the Maghreb consume relatively high amounts of cereals, sugars, and vegetable oils and less products of animal origin. Since fruits and vegetables have a low contribution to total energy intake, absolute values will be used in order to draw conclusions concerning their consumption.

The most striking feature is the large consumption of cereals (particularly wheat and barley). Their contribution to total energy supply ranges from about 50.5% in Libya to 61.9% in Morocco (fig. 3). In addition, cereals are the richest fiber sources. It has been suggested that diets high in fiber are associated with reduced risk for coronary heart disease [12]. Some evidence from epidemiological studies also suggests that an overall increase in the intake of foods high in fiber might decrease the risk for diabetes mellitus, colon cancer, hemorrhoids and constipation [12, 13]. Furthermore, cereals are the major protein source for these countries since they provide more than 45% of the dietary proteins (the calculations were based on the amount of cereal protein, in grams, consumed per person per day in relation to the total amount of protein received per day by the various food groups). In more detail, their contribution to total protein intake is 62% in Algeria, 46% in Libya, 67% in Morocco and 56% in Tunisia.

Vegetable oils are the second highest energy source for the Maghreb population (contributing to total energy intake from 12.3% in Algeria to 20.1% in Libya) followed by sweeteners (with a contribution to total energy from about 10% in Algeria to 11.5% in Morocco). Energy provided by milk contributes to total energy supply from 1.4% in Morocco to 6.2% in Algeria. Animal products are a low energy source for the Maghreb population since they provide only 3.3% (in Algeria), 3.4% in Morocco, 4.3% in (Tunisia) and 4.9% (in Libya) of the total energy intake. Fish has a remarkably low contribution to energy intake ranging from 0.3 and 0.4% (in Algeria and Libya, respectively) to 0.6 and 0.7% (in Morocco and Tunisia, respectively).

Time Trends

The data reviewed so far refer to recent food habits in the Maghreb region. In order to examine the evolution of the food consumption patterns with time, data from the periods 1968–1970 and 1990–1992 have also been included in figures 1 and 3 as separate columns. Since we did not notice large differences in food intake between the periods 2000–2003 and 1990–1992, this later period will not be discussed in this paper. From figure 1, one notices an increase in the consumption (kg/person/year) of all individual food groups in all countries. Consequently, the total consumption (kg/person/year) of food has increased considerably the last 33 years. More specifically, during the period 2000–2003

Moroccans consumed about 198 kg of food (per person per year) more than the amount they consumed in 1968–1970. The same trend has been observed for the rest of the Maghreb countries with Libyans consuming 253 kg, Algerians 276 kg and Tunisians 307 kg more food (per person per year) compared with the quantities they were consuming 33 years ago. Further evidence is provided by the observed increase in the total energy intake of the Maghreb population for the years 2000–2003. Moroccans, Tunisians, Libyans and Algerians were supplied with 614 (20% increase), 888 (28% increase), 937 (20% increase) and 1,200 (41% increase) more cal/day, respectively, than 33 years ago.

Some beneficial changes are the rise in cereals, vegetable products and fish consumption. However, during the same period, animal products and fat and oil consumption also rose.

Since the consumption of all food categories has increased with time, it is difficult to draw any conclusions concerning the changes in food patterns by referring only to the above figures. Therefore, the comparison of the contribution of the various food groups to total energy supply in 1968–1970 with that in 2000–2003 could provide more useful information. More specifically, figure 3 shows a decrease in cereal consumption, in relation to the consumption of other food groups, in all four countries. The most considerable difference, however, is the observed increase in the contribution of vegetable oils to total energy intake in Algeria, Morocco and Libya. In 1968–1970 the vegetable oil contribution to total energy was 9.2, 6.9 and 13.4%, whereas in 2000–2003 it increased to 12.3, 8.8 and 20.1, respectively. The exception is Tunisia, where the contribution of vegetable oils to total energy intake decreased from 17.5% in 1968–1970 to 15% in 2000–2003. Animal product contribution to total energy increased in Algeria, Morocco and Tunisia from 2.5, 2.5 and 2.9% in 1968–1970 to 3.3, 3.4 and 4.3 in 2000–2003, whereas one notices a considerable decrease of animal product contribution to total energy in Libya (from 7.5 to 4.9%) during the same periods. The contribution of sweeteners to total energy in 2000–2003 is almost the same with that in 1968–1970 with the exception of Libya where a decrease from 14.2 to 10% was observed. Fish consumption has increased almost two times in Algeria, three times in Tunisia and four times in Morocco, whereas it remains almost the same in Libya compared with the quantities consumed during 1968–1970. Animal fat, which has a low contribution to total energy at both periods examined, contributes considerably less to total energy intake in 2000–2003. Milk contribution has remained basically the same in Algeria, Libya and Morocco whereas in Tunisia it has increased almost 2.2%.

To further refine the picture regarding diet in the Maghreb, the consumption of fruits and vegetables, animal products and of fats and oils will be discussed separately, in more detail.

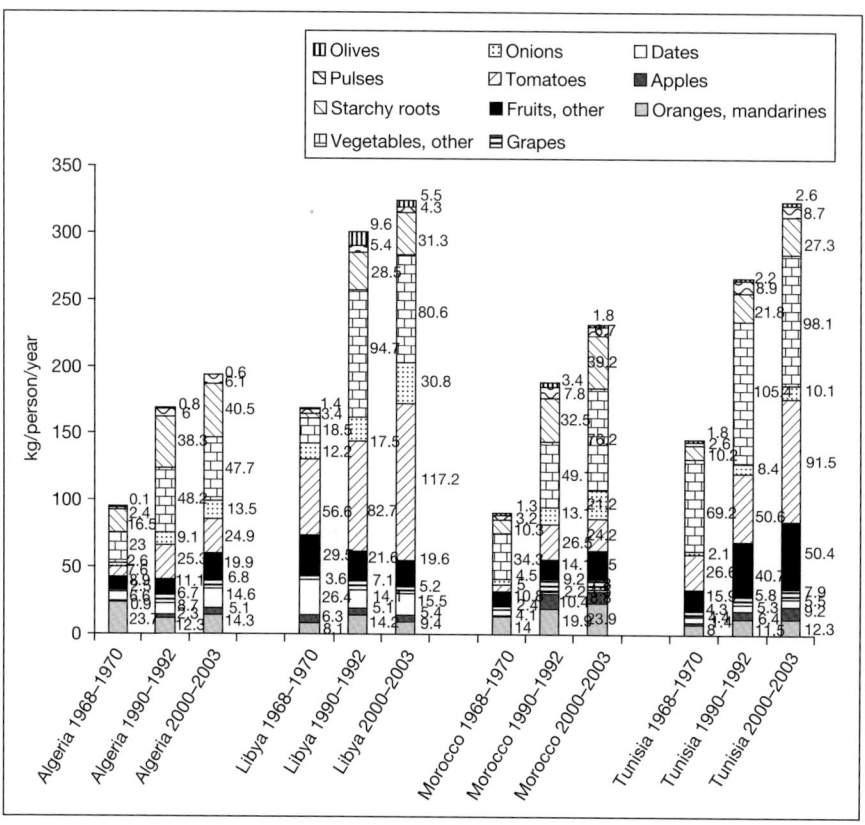

Fig. 4. Average per capita consumption (kg/person/year) of fruits, vegetables, pulses and starchy roots for Algeria, Libya, Morocco and Tunisia for the years 1968–1970, 1990–1992 and 2000–2003. Values are shown on the right of each food category (FAO, statistics division).

Fruits and Vegetables

A closer look at the fruit and vegetable group provides some interesting information (fig. 4). The consumption is expressed in kg/person/year rather than in % energy, because the contribution of these foods to total energy intake is very small due to their low energy density.

The highest consumption of total amount of fruits, vegetables (tomatoes, onion, carrots, spinach, cabbage, lettuce, peppers, etc.), starchy roots (potatoes) and pulses, for the years 2000–2003, is observed in Libya (total 325 kg) and Tunisia (324 kg). Moroccans and Algerians consume less vegetable products than their neighbors (233 and 194 kg, respectively). The quantities of fruits, vegetables, starchy roots and pulses consumed at this period in Libya, Tunisia,

Morocco and Algeria are almost twice more than the amount consumed in 1968–1970 (169, 147, 91 and 95 kg, respectively).

The patterns of fruits and vegetable consumption for the Maghreb countries can be seen in figure 4. In 2000–2003, fruit consumption was quite high in all countries especially of oranges and mandarins, apples, grapes and dates. Regarding olives, Tunisia and Libya consume the highest amount (2.6 and 6.6 kg, respectively) comparing to Morocco and Algeria (0.6 and 1.8 kg, respectively). The vegetables consumed are mainly tomatoes. Tunisia and Libya have the highest tomato intake (117 and 92.5 kg, respectively). Concerning starchy roots, potatoes are almost the only source; Algeria and Morocco show the highest potato intake (40.5 and 39.2 kg). Finally, the highest consumption of pulses is observed in Tunisia (about 9 kg) and the lowest in Libya (4.3 kg).

Per capita fruit consumption in the Maghreb (65.4 kg) is much lower in comparison with some European Mediterranean countries (France, Spain, Italy and Greece where fruit consumption is 95.5, 112.7, 131 and 147 kg, respectively). Concerning vegetable consumption the average value in the Maghreb (159.3 kg) is higher than in France and Spain (143 and 143.3 kg, respectively) whereas Italy and Greece have the highest vegetable intake (178 and 275.7 kg, respectively). This average value becomes considerably higher if we compare it with the vegetable consumption in the UK and the USA (91.5 and 123 kg, respectively). The consumption of starchy food is higher in France, Italy, Greece and Spain (64.8, 41.2, 65.4 and 78.8 kg, respectively) compared with the Maghreb countries (average 34.5 kg). However, the consumption of pulses is higher in the Maghreb countries (average 6.5 kg) than in France (2.1 kg) and Greece (4.8 kg) and almost the same in Italy and Spain (5.6 and 5.7 kg).

Nutritional Aspects

Consumption of fruits and vegetables has been associated with protection against various diseases, including cardiovascular, cerebrovascular disease and cancer [14–16]. It is not known for certain which active dietary constituents contribute to the beneficial effects, but it is often assumed that antioxidant nutrients contribute to this defense. Results from intervention trials on the protective effect of the supplementation with antioxidants such as β-carotene and vitamin E are not conclusive [17–20]. Therefore, the beneficial effect of a high intake of fruits and vegetables on the risk of cardiovascular disease and cancer may rely not on the effect of the well-characterized antioxidants, such as vitamins E, C and β-carotene, but rather on some other antioxidants or non-antioxidant phytochemicals or by an additive action of different compounds present in foods such as alpha-linolenic acid, various phenolic compounds and fiber [21].

In the last two decades, emphasis has been given to natural antioxidants because of a trend toward natural ingredients in foods. Antioxidants quench free radicals in the human body, which may lead to the protection from chronic diseases [26]. Free radicals are believed to play a role in more than 60 different health conditions, including the aging process, cancer and atherosclerosis. Reducing exposure to free radicals and increasing intake of antioxidant nutrients may reduce the risk of free radical-related health problems [22, 23].

A variety of antioxidant enzymes (such as superoxide dismutase, catalase and glutathione peroxidase), and antioxidants (vitamin C, vitamin E, β-carotene, lutein, lycopene, vitamin B_3 and vitamin B_6) may be the best way to provide the body with the most complete protection against free radical damage [22]. However, the consequences of dietary intake of these antioxidants are difficult to separate by epidemiological studies from other important phytochemicals such as flavonoids [24, 25].

Phytochemicals are bioactive non-nutrient substances that plants naturally produce to protect themselves against viruses, bacteria and fungi and may play an important nutritional role in human health. It is estimated that more than 5,000 individual phytochemicals have been identified in fruits, vegetables, herbs and grains. Being an important part of human diet, phytochemicals and their physiological effects have been thoroughly investigated. Phytochemicals can be classified as carotenoids, phenolics, alkaloids, nitrogen-containing compounds, and organosulfur compounds. The most studied of the phytochemicals are the phenolics and carotenoids [27].

Phytochemicals have three major physiological effects, namely antioxidant [28, 29], anticarcinogenic [30, 31] and antimutagenic effects [31–35]. Phytochemicals are also active against some viruses; their activity against HIV has been tested in vitro [36]. Many of these polyphenols have been found to be more powerful antioxidants than vitamins C, E and β-carotene using an in vitro model for heart disease, namely the oxidation of low density lipoproteins (LDL) [29]. The natural combination of phytochemicals in fruits and vegetables is responsible for its potent antioxidant activity. Thus, plant consumption may provide protection against oxidative stress which is a pathogenic mechanism of both carcinogenesis and atherosclerosis [25].

Currently, there are no recommended dietary allowances for phytochemicals. The benefit of a diet rich in fruits and vegetables is attributed to the natural combination and the complex mixture of phytochemicals present in these and other whole foods [37–39]. Thousands of phytochemicals are present in whole foods. These compounds differ in molecular size, polarity, and solubility, which may affect the bioavailability and distribution of each phytochemical in different macromolecules, subcellular organelles, cells, organs, and tissues. These additive and synergic effects of phytochemicals in fruits and vegetables have been proposed for their antioxidant activities.

Numerous investigations have shown that the actions of the dietary supplements alone don't explain the observed health benefits of diets rich in fruits, vegetables and whole grains, because taken alone, the individual antioxidant studied in clinical trials do not have consistent preventive effects [17–20]. Therefore, consumers should obtain them from a wide variety of fruits, vegetables and whole grains for optimal health benefits [27].

In addition to the antioxidant vitamins, phenols and other phytochemicals, edible wild plants are rich sources of minerals. These inorganic micronutrients are needed in small amounts to assist in a variety of essential body functions. Many minerals are components of important molecules, such as hemoglobin, vitamins, hormones and enzymes. Some of them are required for the normal functioning of nerves and muscles. They regulate the acid-base balance of body fluids and they form a structural part of bone and cartilage [40–41]. However, unlike other nutrients, such as amino acids and fatty acids, minerals must be supplied from the diet, since the body cannot produce them.

Moreover, omega-3 fatty acids (their beneficial properties will be discussed later) could be supplied through the consumption of green vegetables [23].

Animal Products

The per capita consumption patterns of the four Maghreb countries regarding animal products are presented in figure 5. As it was observed for most of the previously examined food groups, the consumption of meat and eggs show quite a large variation among the Maghreb countries. Libya is the country with the highest per capita meat and eggs consumption (26.6 and 9.8 kg per year, respectively) followed by Tunisia (26 and 6.8 kg per year, respectively).

A closer look at meat intake (fig. 5) even shows some differences in the consumption patterns of various meat types within the Maghreb region. For example, Tunisians eat the highest amount of bovine meat (6.5 kg) and Libyans the lowest (1.3 kg). Mutton and goat meat consumption is high in Tunisia (7 kg) and lowest in Morocco (4 kg). Regarding poultry, Libya shows the highest consumption (18.3 kg) whereas Algeria (7.8 kg) the lowest. Pork is not consumed in these countries due to religious customs.

A very interesting point, concerning the data presented here, is the very large difference between the per capita consumption of meat, egg and fish in the Maghreb and some European Mediterranean countries (fig. 6). For example, total per capita meat consumption in France, Spain, Italy and Greece is (60.1, 55.6, 47.4 and 51.4 kg/person/year, respectively), whereas the average consumption in the Maghreb is 22.8 kg/person/year. The difference becomes considerably bigger if we compare the above value with the average meat

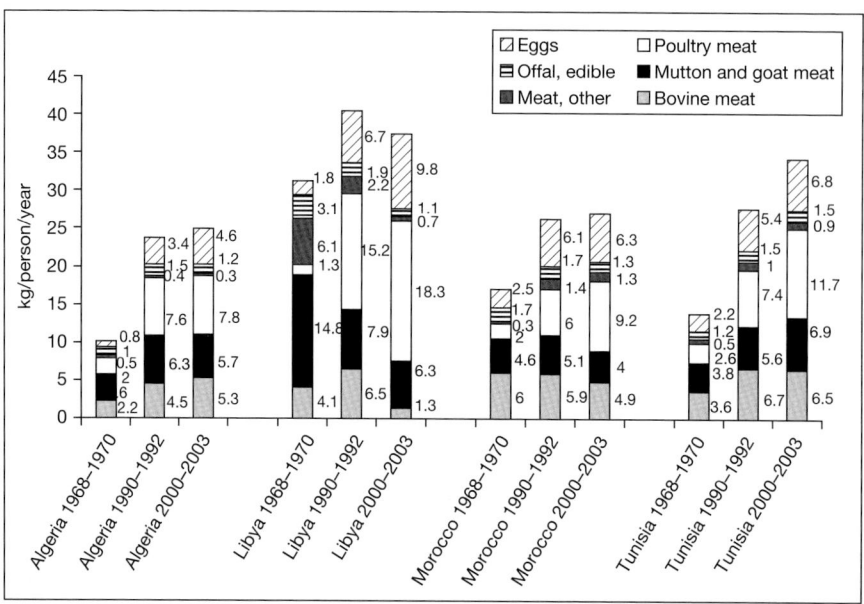

Fig. 5. Average per capita consumption (kg/person/year) of animal products for Algeria, Libya, Morocco and Tunisia for the years 1968–1970, 1990–1992 and 2000–2003. Values are shown on the right of each food category (FAO, statistics division).

consumption in the USA (93.2 kg for the same period). Egg consumption is about two times higher in Spain, France and Italy (13, 15.3 and 11.4 kg) than that in the Maghreb (6.8 kg on average).

Furthermore, the contribution of animal products to total dietary protein intake is quite low in the Maghreb. For example, meat proteins contribute about 10% on average to total protein intake. Milk proteins provide around 9%, while fish and seafood provide a very low amount of proteins 3%. Eggs are also a low-protein source since they provide about 2.5% of the total protein intake.

Although animal product consumption is very low in the Maghreb, there was a substantial increase in the quantities consumed the last 33 years. More specifically, Algerians consume about 10.8, Moroccans 6.5 and Tunisians 15.5 kg/person/year more meat than the quantities they used to eat 33 years ago, whereas Libyans consume almost the same quantity of meat that they used to eat. However, this increase in meat consumption seems to be closely related with a specific meat type. For example, per capita consumption of poultry has shown a remarkable increase. Algerians, Libyans, Moroccans and Tunisians in 2000–2003, ate 5.8, 17, 7.2 and 9 kg more poultry per year than they used to eat in 1968–1970 whereas beef, mutton and goat meat consumption has decreased

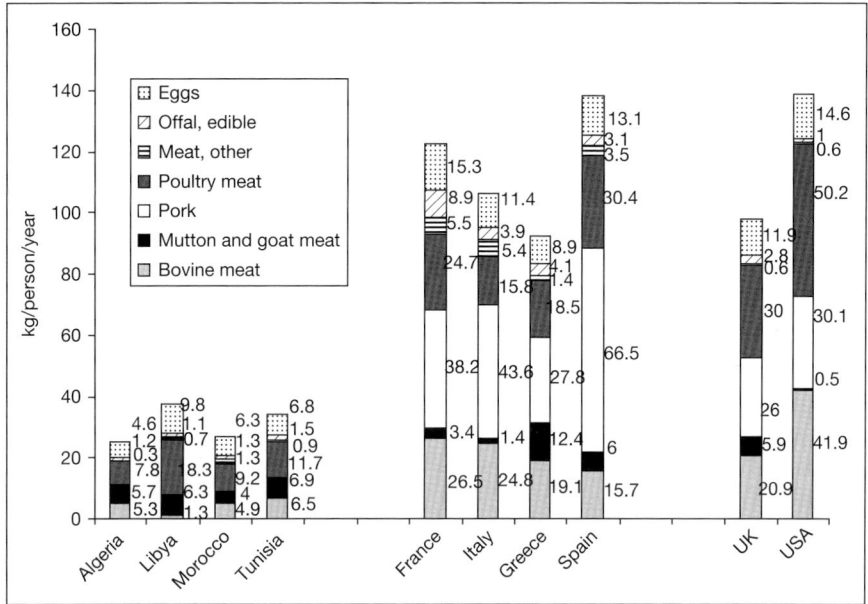

Fig. 6. Average per capita consumption (kg/person/year) of animal products for the Maghreb countries (Algeria, Libya, Morocco and Tunisia), some Mediterranean European countries, the United Kingdom and the USA for the period 2002–2003. Values are shown on the right of each food category (FAO, statistics division).

in Libya and Morocco by about 2.8 and 1.1 for beef meat and 8.5 and 0.6 kg for mutton and goat meat, respectively, during the last 33 years.

Egg consumption has also increased remarkably compared with the quantities consumed during 1968–1970. Egg consumption has increased almost 6 times in Algeria, 5.5 times in Libya, 2.5 in Morocco and 3 times in Tunisia.

Animal Fats and Vegetable Oils

A more detailed consideration of the per capita vegetable oil and animal fat intake, for the period 2000–2003, reveals some differences regarding the consumption patterns of the four countries (fig. 7). Although Moroccans have the lowest total oil and fat intake (according to fig. 1), they are the first in animal fat consumption (fig. 7). More specifically, they consume about 1.6 kg more animal fat per year compared with Algerians, 1.8 kg compared with Libyans and 1.2 kg compared with Tunisians. This low value for Moroccan total fat and

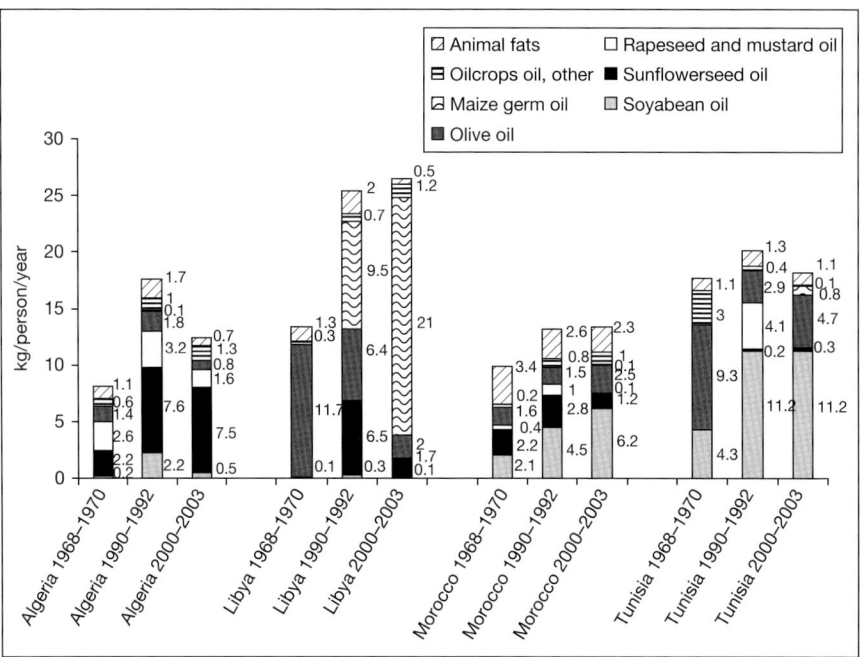

Fig. 7. Average per capita consumption (kg/person/year) of vegetable oil and animal fat for Algeria, Libya, Morocco and Tunisia for the years 1968–1970, 1990–1992 and 2000–2003. Values are shown on the right of each food category (FAO, statistics division).

oil consumption (fig. 1) is due to the much lower vegetable oil intake (they consume 1.7, 8.6 and 15 kg/person/year less vegetable oil than the Algerians, Tunisians and Libyans, respectively).

In addition, an even more detailed examination of the various types of vegetable oils consumed reveals some large differences regarding the consumption patterns of the Maghreb countries. For example in Algeria, about 60% of the total vegetable oil intake is sunflower oil. In contrast, sunflower oil consumption in Tunisia is negligible. Regarding soybean oil, Tunisia is the country with the highest consumption with 11.2 kg per capita intake (about 57% of the total oil consumed), whereas in Libya the amount consumed (0.1 kg) is very low. An important observation, concerning Libya, is that it is the only Maghreb country where maize oil is consumed which represents almost 80% of the total oil supply. Additionally, Libyans and Tunisians do not consume any rape and mustard oil whereas in Algeria the amount consumed accounts for 12.5% on the total vegetable oil supply. Quite unexpectedly, olive oil consumption in the Maghreb is very low. More specifically, olive oil per capita consumption is about 1 kg in Algeria, 2 kg in Libya, 2.5 kg in Morocco and 4.7 kg in Tunisia contributing thus to total supply 6.2, 7.7, 22.5 and 24%, respectively.

Another interesting point, concerning the dietary habits of the European Mediterranean countries (discussed above) and the Maghreb, is that of olive oil consumption, which is much higher in Spain, Italy and Greece. In more detail, total per capita olive oil consumption in Spain, Italy and Greece is 1.6, 11.7, 13.1 and 15.6 kg, respectively, accounting for 42.5, 48.7 and 63.2% of the total oil supply, respectively. However, olive oil consumption in the Maghreb (2.5 kg in average) is still higher than that in France, the UK and the USA (1.6, 0.8 and 0.7 kg, respectively).

Figure 7 also shows significant changes regarding consumption of vegetable oils in 1968–1970 and in 2000–2003 in the Maghreb. Vegetable oil intake in 2000–2003 is much higher (in all four Maghreb countries) than 33 years ago. More specifically, per capita vegetable oil consumption has increased by 3.1 kg in Tunisia, 4.2 kg in Morocco, 5.2 kg in Algeria and 13.9 kg in Libya since 1970. In more detail, sunflower oil consumption has increased in Algeria, and the same trend has been observed for soybean oil consumption showing a per capita increase of 0.3 kg in Algeria, 4.1 kg in Morocco and 6.9 kg in Tunisia. During 1970, rapeseed and mustard oil consumption was negligible in all the Maghreb countries, with the exception of Algeria where the per capita consumption was 2.6 kg. In 1990–1992, Tunisians and Moroccans consumed 4.1 and 1 kg, respectively, of rapeseed and mustard oil whereas in Algeria there was a 1.6-kg increase in consumption of these oils. In 2000–2003 these oils consumption decreased in Algeria (1.6 kg) and disappeared in Morocco, Libya and Tunisia. Another decrease was noticed regarding olive oil in Algeria, Libya and Tunisia, whereas in Morocco there was an increase of about 1 kg. The amount of olive oil consumed has decreased by 0.6, 9.7 and 4.6 kg, respectively, in the above-mentioned countries. Regarding animal fats, the amounts consumed in 2000–2003 are lower in Algeria (0.4 kg), Libya (0.8 kg) and Morocco (1.1 kg) whereas in Tunisia it remained the same (1.1 kg) in comparison with the quantities consumed during 1968–1970.

Nutritional Aspects

The current interest in the amount of fat in the diet is due to the relationship between fat consumption and the development of certain diseases. More specifically, the differences in mortality from coronary heart disease (CHD) between countries are related to the differences in fat consumption [42, 43]. The Seven Countries Study [44] established a positive correlation between the percentage of saturated fat in the diet and mortality due to CHD. The Lyon Diet Heart Study clearly showed that adopting a modified Cretan Mediterranean-type diet reduced the incidence of cardiac death by about 70% and other cardiac complications by about 50% [45]. The 'experimental' diet, a modified diet of Crete, was low in saturated and *trans* fatty acids with a ratio of omega-6:omega-3 = 4:1. It was rich in fruits and vegetables (compared with the control group) and also rich in oleic acid, omega-3 fatty acids, fiber, vitamins of the B group and various antioxidants including vitamins C and E, trace elements and flavonoids, whereas the control diet was close to the Step I American Heart Association diet.

Dietary sources of saturated fats are either animal fats (for example about 70% of the fatty acids in butter are saturated) or tropical oils (such as palm oil, coconut oil and palm kernel oil) [46]. Moreover, Buzina et al. [8] showed a negative correlation between coronary mortality and the proportion of monounsaturated fatty acids in the diet. Olive oil is a very rich source of monounsaturated fatty acids since it contains 80% oleic acid (C18:1ω9) [47]. Canola oil is another rich source (it contains 60% monounsaturated fatty acids). Furthermore, there is evidence that high intake of omega-6 polyunsaturated fatty acids, which are found in vegetable oils can lead to tumors in animals and to increase platelet aggregation in humans [48]. Some oils rich in omega-6 fatty acids are sunflower and soybean oil, which contain about 60% and 50% omega-6 fatty acids, respectively [46]. Recently, the omega-3 fatty acids, and in particular the ratio of omega-6 to omega-3 fatty acids [47, 48] have attracted great interest due to their association with low CHD and cancer rates. Some oils with a low ratio of omega-6 to omega-3 fatty acids are flaxseed, walnut, and canola oil. Olive oil is very low in omega-6 fatty acids (it contains about 6–8% omega-6 and 0.3–1.3% omega-3) which gives it a favorable ratio of omega-6 to omega-3 fatty acids. In addition, it is rich in antioxidants and in a substance called 'squalene', which has anti-inflammatory properties, slows blood clot formation and lowers cholesterol. Hence, the above composition in combination with its high content in monounsaturated fatty acids, places olive oil in a unique and superior position of all other oils [49].

The conclusion which could be drawn from the above is that low intake of saturated fats; high intake of monounsaturated fatty acids and low intake of polyunsaturated omega-6 fatty acids (related to omega-3) could be beneficial for health. On this basis, the Maghreb diet which is very low in animal fat (saturated fat) could potentially be healthy. However, the intake of monounsaturated fatty acids is not particularly high due to the low consumption of olive oil. Additionally, most of the fatty acids consumed are omega-6 polyunsaturated since their source is mainly sunflower and soybean oils. Therefore, some beneficial changes regarding the fat composition of the Maghreb diet should include an increase in the amount of monounsaturated fatty acids as well as a decrease in the quantity of omega-6 followed by an increase of the omega-3 fatty acids. This could be achieved by the substitution of other vegetable oils with olive oil, rape seed and mustard oils since their consumption increases the intake of monounsaturated fatty acids without any significant elevation of the omega-6 unsaturated fatty acids.

The Maghreb Diet and Cancer

Epidemiological studies have indicated that a relationship exists between certain diets and some types of cancer in a population [48]. It is sometimes thought that food and nutrition affect cancer risk only inasmuch as diets may contain certain specific carcinogenic substances. While various carcinogens have been identified in foods and drinks, these appear to contribute only slightly to the overall impact of diet on cancer risk [50]. However, the most important effects of diet may be mediated by actions that inhibit the cancer process.

More specifically, according to the American Cancer Society (ACS) recommendations, consumption of 400 g/day or more (or provide 7% or more of total energy) of a variety of vegetables and fruits may, by itself, decrease the overall cancer incidence by at least 20%. Diets high in vegetables and/or fruits may protect against cancers of the mouth and pharynx, esophagus, lung, stomach, colon, larynx, pancreas, breast and bladder. Furthermore, the ACS suggested that the level of dietary fat intake should be no more than 30% of total energy intake in order to prevent cancer of colon, breast and other cancers. There is also a universal agreement that the dietary level of saturated fat should be greatly reduced to 6–8% of energy intake, along with the reduction of dietary cholesterol. Moreover, 45–60% of total energy should be provided by starchy or protein-rich foods of plant origin. Finally, the consumption of alcohol is not recommended.

Cancer mortality in the countries of the Maghreb is particularly low in comparison with the USA, UK and even with some European Mediterranean countries (fig. 8). In more detail, the world standardized mortality cancer rate (per 100,000 population) in 2002 for the male population was 73.1, 83.4, 80.2 and 97.3 in Algeria, Libya, Morocco and Tunisia, respectively (Globocan database) [51]. The female population suffered less from cancer during the same period since; the world standardized mortality cancer rate was 68 in Algeria, 64.7 in Libya, 65.6 in Morocco and 59.5 in Tunisia.

The above rate for the male population was 162.3 in UK, 152.6 in USA, 173.6 in Spain, 170.9 in Italy, 191.7 in France and 148.2 in Greece. The world standardized numbers for the female populations of the above countries were 122.7, 111.9, 81.8, 95.2, 96.3 and 81.9, respectively.

The percent contribution of specific cancer death for the male and female Maghreb population (calculated as average for the four Maghreb countries) are

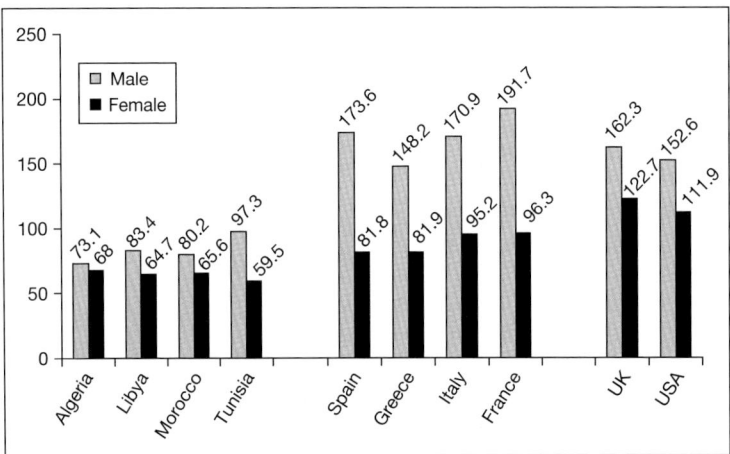

Fig. 8. World standardized mortality cancer rate (per 100,000 population) in the Maghreb countries (Algeria, Libya, Morocco and Tunisia), some Mediterranean European countries, the United Kingdom and the USA for the years 2002. Values are shown on the right of each food category (Globocan database, WHO).

presented in figures 9 and 10, respectively. As it can be seen from figure 9, lung cancer is the main cause of death of the male population followed by bladder cancer. For the female population (fig. 10), breast and cervix uteri cancers are the main causes of cancer deaths. Mortality from colon and rectum cancer, which have been very much connected with diet, is low for both male and female Maghreb populations (6.7 and 7.1%, respectively) compared with North America (10.1% for males and 11% for females), western Europe (11.3% for males and 14.6% for females) and even with southern Europe (10.4% for males and 12.9% for females).

Taking into account the recommendations of the ACS regarding the consumption of fruits and vegetables (400 g/day or 146 kg/year), this consumption in the four Maghreb countries, during 2000–2003, was equal to or above the recommended amount (fig. 1). Additionally, during the same period, the contribution of dietary fat to total energy intake in the Maghreb is in accordance with the recommendation made by the ACS. In more detail, fat contribution to total energy is 16.1% in Algeria, 25.3% in Libya, 13.6% in Morocco and 20% in Tunisia (the calculations were based on the assumption that 1 g of fat contains 9 cal). In addition animal fat percent contribution to total energy is 3.8% in Algeria, 5.2% in Libya, 4.9% in Morocco and 5% in Tunisia. These values also fall within the recommended range for animal fat contribution to energy intake since they are all quite less than 6%. Moreover, in the Maghreb, 50.5–61.9%

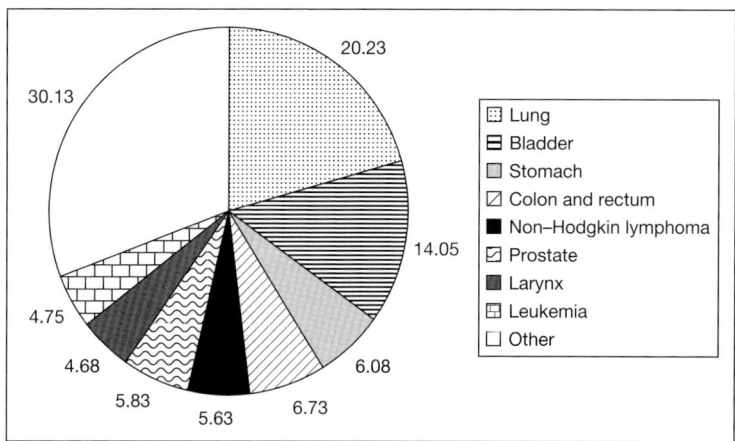

Fig. 9. Percent contribution of specific cancer deaths to total cancer mortality for the Maghreb male population in 2002 (values are averages of mortalities in Algeria, Libya, Morocco and Tunisia) (Globocan database, WHO).

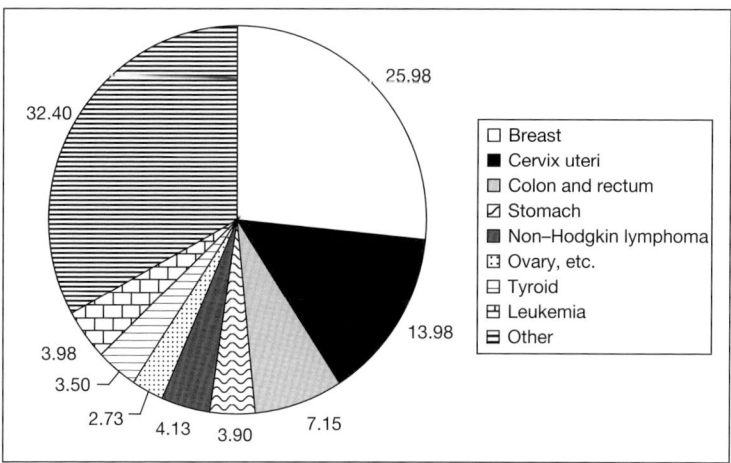

Fig. 10. Percent contribution of specific cancer deaths to total cancer mortality for the Maghreb female population in 2002 (values are averages of mortalities in Algeria, Libya, Morocco and Tunisia) (Globocan database, WHO).

(fig. 2) of total energy is provided by cereals, something that is also in accordance with the ACS recommendations.

The conclusion which could be drawn from the above, taking also into account the negligible alcohol consumption, is that the diet of the Maghreb could be protective against cancer. The above is supported by the low mortality observed in this region.

Conclusion

In conclusion, the Maghreb diet could be characterized as being a diet particularly high in cereals since they provide more than 50% of the dietary energy and protein intake. Cereals are also a very rich fiber source. The Maghreb diet is also rich in fruits and vegetables and thus rich in vitamins, antioxidants and fiber, all of which are health protective. In addition, the diet of the Maghreb is low in total fats (they provide less than 30% of the total energy), low in saturated fats (less than 6% of the total energy) with low amounts of added fats, predominantly vegetable oils. However, olive oil consumption is particularly low since sunflower oil and soybean oil are the main vegetable oils consumed. It is thus relatively low in saturated and monounsaturated fats and high in polyunsaturated fatty acids and in particular omega-6. Animal product (meat, egg, and fish) consumption is also very low. High levels of proteins from animal products may not only injure the walls of the coronary arteries; which can start the buildup of cholesterol; they can also promote blood clots; which can be the ultimate cause of a heart attack.

In all countries examined, per capita dietary energy supply increased considerably, during the 33-year period between 1968–1970 and 2000–2003. The relative contribution of vegetable oils to total energy supply has also increased remarkably throughout these periods (with the exception of olive oil which has decreased). In contrast, animal fat contribution has either remained stable or slightly decreased during the same period. Beneficial health changes include the rise in the consumption of vegetable products and fish. However, during the same period, meat, milk and egg consumption have also increased although their per capita consumption is still low in comparison with other Mediterranean countries.

Despite the overall changes regarding dietary patterns, the Maghreb diet could be protective against cancer and other chronic diseases.

References

1 Simopoulos AP, Nestel PJ (eds): Genetic Variation and Dietary Response. World Rev Nutr Diet. Basel, Karger, 1997, vol 80, pp 1–170.
2 Simopoulos AP: Genetic variation and nutrition. Nutr Rev 1999;57:S10–S19.
3 De Caterina R, Madonna R, Hassan J, Procopio AD: Nutrients and gene expression; in Simopoulos AP, Pavlou KN (eds): Nutrition and Fitness: Diet, Genes, Physical Activity and Health. World Rev Nutr Diet. Basel, Karger, 2001, vol 89, pp 12–22.

4   Simopoulos AP: The role of fatty acids in gene expression: health implications. Ann Nutr Metab 1996;40:303–311.
5   Leaf A, Kang JX: omega-3 fatty acids and cardiovascular disease; in Simopoulos AP, Pavlou KN (eds): Nutrition and Fitness: Diet, Genes, Physical Activity and Health. World Rev Nutr Diet. Basel, Karger, 2001, vol 89, pp 161–172.
6   Katan MB, Zock PL, Mensink RP: Dietary oils, serum lipoproteins, and coronary heart disease. Am J Clin Nutr 1995;61(suppl 1):1368–1373.
7   La Vecchia C, Harris RE, Wynder EL: Comparative epidemiology of cancer between the United States and Italy. Cancer Res 1988;48:7285–7293.
8   Buzina R, Suboticanec K, Saric M: Diet patterns and health problems: diet in southern Europe. Ann Nutr Metab 1991;35(suppl 1):32–40.
9   Serra-Majem L, Ferro-Luzzi A, Bellizzi M, Salleras L: Nutrition policies in Mediterranean Europe. Nutr Rev 1997;35(suppl 2):42–57.
10 Ferro-Luzzi A, Sette S: The Mediterranean diet: an attempt to define its present and past composition. Eur J Clin Nutr 1989;43(suppl 2):13–29.
11 Simopoulos AP: The Mediterranean diets: What is so special about the diet of Greece? The scientific evidence. J Nutr 2001;131:3065S–3073S.
12 Kromhout D, Bosschieter EB, Coulander CL: Dietary fibre and 10-years mortality from coronary heart disease, cancer and all causes. The Zutphen study. Lancet 1982;ii:508–521.
13 Goulder TJ, Alberti KG, Jenkins DJA: Effect of added fiber on the glucose and metabolic response to a mixed meal in normal and diabetic subjects. Diabetes Care 1978;264/532–537.
14 Ames BN, Shigenana MK, Hagen TM: Oxidants, antioxidants and degenerative diseases of aging. Proc Natl Acad Sci USA 1993;90:7915–7922.
15 Gey KF: The antioxidant hypothesis of cardiovascular disease: epidemiology and mechanisms. Bioch Soc Trans 1990;18:1041–1045.
16 Steinberg D, Parthasarathy S, Carew TE, Khoo JC, Witztum JL: Beyond cholesterol: modifications of low-density lipoprotein that increase its atherogenicity. N Engl J Med 1989;320:915–924.
17 Ommen GS, Goodman GE, Thomquist MD, Barnes J, Cullen MR: Effects of a combination of β-carotene and vitamin A on lung cancer and cardiovascular disease. N Engl J Med 1996;334:1150–1155.
18 Stephens NG, Parsons A, Schofield PM, Kelly F, Cheeseman K, Mitchinson MJ: Randomized controlled trial of vitamin E in patients with coronary heart disease: Cambridge Heart Antioxidant Study (CHAOS). Lancet 1996;347:781–786.
19 Yusuf S, Dagenias G, Pogue J, Bosch J, Sleight P: Vitamin E supplementation and cardiovascular events in high-risk patients. The Heart Outcomes Prevention Evaluation Study Investigators. N Engl J Med 2000;342:154–160.
20 Gruppo Italiano per lo Studio della Sopravivenza nell Infarto miocardico (GISSI): Dietary supplementation with vitamin E after myocardial infarction: Results of GISSI-Prevenzione trial. Lancet 1999;354:447–455.
21 Simopoulos AP: Preface; In Simopoulos AP (ed): Plants in Human Health and Nutrition Policy. World Rev Nutr Diet. Basel, Karger, 2003, vol 91, pp vii–xiii.
22 Halliwell B, Gutteridge JMC: Free Radicals in Biology and Medicine, ed 2. New York, Oxford University Press, 1989.
23 Simopoulos AP, Norman HA, Gillapsy JE: Purslane in human nutrition and its potential for world agriculture; in Simopoulos AP (ed): Plants in Human Nutrition. World Rev Nutr Diet. Basel, Karger, 1995, vol 77, pp 47–74.
24 Swanson C: Vegetables, Fruits, and Cancer Risk: The Role of Phytochemicals; in Bidlack WR, Omaye ST, Meskin MS, Jahner D (eds): Phytochemicals. A New Paradigm. Lancaster, Technomic Publishing, 1998, vol 15, pp 1–12.
25 German JB, Dillard CJ: Phytochemicals and targets of chronic disease; in Bidlack WR, Omaye ST, Meskin MS, Jahner D (eds): Phytochemicals. A New Paradigm. Lancaster, Technomic Publishing, 1998, vol 15, pp 13–32.
26 Demo A, Petrakis C, Kefalas P, Boskou D: Nutrient antioxidants in some herbs and Mediterranean plant leaves. Food Res Int 1998;31:351–354.

27 Liu RH: Potential synergy of phytochemicals in cancer prevention: mechanism of action. Am Soc Nutr Sci 2004;3479S–3485S.
28 Frankel S, Favero A, La Vacchia C, Negri E, Kinsella JE: Inhibition of oxidation of human low density lipoprotein by phenolic substances in red wine. Lancet 1993;341:454–457.
29 Vinson JA, Dabbagh YA, Serry MM, Cai S: Plant polyphenols exhibit lipoprotein-bound antioxidant activity using an in vitro oxidation model heart disease. J Agric Food Chem 1995;43: 2798–2799.
30 Rose DP, Boyar AP, Wynder EL: International comparison of mortality rates for cancer of breast, ovary, prostate and colon and per capita food consumption. Cancer 1986;58:2363–2371.
31 Franceschi S, Favero A, La Vacchia C, Negri E, Conti E, Montella M, Giacosa A, Monni O, Decarli A: Food groups and risk of colorectal cancer in Italy. Int J Cancer 1997;72:56–61.
32 Smart RC, Huang MT, Chang RL, Sayer JM, Jerina DM, Conney A: Disposition of naturally occurring antimutagenic plant phenol, ellagic acid and its synthetic derivatives 3-O-decylellagic acid and 3,3'-di-O-methylellagic acid in mice. Carcinogenesis 1986;7:1663–1667.
33 Knekt P, Jarvinen R, Seppanen R, Hellovaara M, Teppo L, Pukkala E, Aromaa A: Dietary flavonoids and the risk of lung cancer and other malignant neoplasms. Am J Epidemiol 1997;146: 223–230.
34 Stefani ED, Boffetta P, Deneo-Pellegrini H, Mendilaharsu M, Carzoglio JC, Ronco A, Olivera L: Dietary antioxidants and lung cancer risk: A case-controlled study in Uruguay. Nutr Cancer 1999;34:100–110.
35 Fotsis T, Pepper MS, Aktas E, Breit S, Rasku S, Adlercreutz H, Wahala K, Montesano R, Schweigerer L: Flavonoids, dietary-derived inhibitors of cell proliferation and in vitro angiogenesis. Cancer Res 1997;57:2916–2921.
36 Nakashima H, Murakami T, Yamamoto N, Sakagami H, Tanumo S, Hatano T, Yoshida T, Okudo T: Inhibition of human immunodeficiency viral replication by tanins and related compounds. Antiviral Res 1992;18:91–103.
37 Sun J, Chu YF, Wu X, Liu RH: Antioxidant and antiproliferative activities of fruits. J Agric Food Chem 2002;50:7449–7454.
38 Chu YF, Sun J, Wu X, Liu RH: Antioxidant and antiproliferative activities of vegetables. Food Chem 2002;50:6910–6916.
39 Eberhardt MV, Lee CY, Liu RH: Antioxidant activity of fresh apples. Nature 2000;405:903–904.
40 Berry GS, Gaupaul HS: Biology of Ourselves. A Study of Human Biology. Etobicoke, Wiley Canada, 1982, vol 14.
41 Watkins B: Fatty acids modulate bone formation and cartilage function. International Society for the Study of Fatty Acids and Lipids (ISSFAL). ISSFAL Newslett 1997;4:15–21.
42 De Lorgeril M, Renaud S, Mamelle N, Salen P, Martin JL, Monjaud I, Guidollet J, Touboul P, Delaye J: Mediterranean α-linolenic acid-rich diet in the secondary prevention of coronary heart disease. Lancet 1994;343:1454–1459.
43 Kafatos A, Diacatou A, Voukiklaris G, Nikolakakis N, Kounali D, Mmalakis G, Dontas AS: Heart disease risk factor status and dietary changes in the Cretan population over the past 30 years: The seven countries study. Am J Clin Nutr 1997;65:1882–1886.
44 Keys A: A Multivariate Analysis of Diet and Coronary Heart Disease. Cambridge, Harvard University Press, 1980, pp 1–67.
45 De Lorgeril M, Salen P: Modified Cretan Mediterranean diet in the prevention of coronary heart disease and cancer; in Simopoulos AP, Visoli F (eds): Mediterranean Diets. World Rev Nutr Diet. Basel, Karger, 2000, vol 87, pp 1–23.
46 Simopoulos AP: omega-3 fatty acids in health and disease and in growth and development. Am J Clin Nutr 1991;54:438–463.
47 Simopoulos AP, Robinson J: The Omega Diet. The Lifesaving Nutritional Program Based on the Diet of the Island of Crete. New York, Harper Collins, 1999.
48 Findanza F: Nutrition and cancer: general considerations; in Zpia V (ed): Advances in Nutrition and Cancer. New York, Plenum Press, 1993, pp 65–67.
49 Simopoulos AP: The Mediterranean food guide: Greek column rather than Egyptian pyramid. Nutr Today 1995;30:54–61.

50 The American Cancer Society 1996 Advisory Committee on Diet, Nutrition and Cancer Prevention: Guidelines on diet, nutrition and cancer prevention: Reducing the risk of cancer with healthy food choices and physical activity. CA Cancer J Clin 1996;325–341.
51 World Health Organisation: Globocan I. Cancer and Mortality Worldwide in 2002.

Sabrina Zeghichi-Hamri
Laboratoire Nutrition, Vieillissement et Maladies Cardiovasculaires (NVMCV)
UFR de Médecine, Domaine de la Merci
FR–38056 La Tronche (France)
Tel. +33 476 63 71 52, Fax +33 476 63 71 52, E-Mail zeghichi@yahoo.fr

Antioxidants in the Mediterranean Diets: An Update

Paola Bogani, Francesco Visioli

Institute of Pharmacological Sciences, University of Milan, Milan, Italy

Dietary intake of fruits and vegetables is strongly and inversely associated with the risk of developing cancers and coronary heart disease (CHD) [1]. Indeed, low amounts of these foods in the diet doubles the risk of most cancers and significantly increases the risk for developing CHD [2]. However, in the USA, only 9% of the population includes the recommended five servings per day of fruits and vegetables in their diet. Conversely, the traditional Mediterranean diets include a significantly larger amount of plant foods; this notable difference between the two eating styles has been associated with a lower risk of developing the above-mentioned diseases [3]. As described below, the involvement of excessive free radical production and the great number of epidemiological studies linking antioxidant intake with a reduced incidence of certain diseases indicate that dietary antioxidants play a protective role [4–6].

Because diets in the Mediterranean are (or were) characterized by abundant plant foods (fruits, vegetables, breads, nuts, seeds; wine and olive oil), researchers and epidemiologists have attributed a great deal of protective activities to antioxidants. However, most of the evidence comes from epidemiological observations and in vitro studies. This chapter will indicate the need for controlled human studies, including selected examples that will eventually clarify the role of minor components – including antioxidants – in cardioprotection and chemoprevention.

Oxidation Processes and Human Pathology

Much has been said about the involvement of reactive oxygen species (ROS) in the onset of several pathologies. Antioxidants are, indeed, necessary for counteraction of excessive production of ROS. ROS include free radicals such as superoxide ($O_2^{\bullet-}$) and hydroxyl radical ($HO^{\bullet}$) and nonradicals such as hydrogen peroxide (H_2O_2) and ozone (O_3), just to name a few.

It is important to note, at this juncture, that production of ROS in the body is a physiological consequence of the reaction of some molecules, e.g. adrenaline, dopamine and some components of the cytochrome P450 transport chain, with atmospheric oxygen. Some ROS (superoxide, hydrogen peroxide and hypochlorous acid in particular) are made deliberately as part of the phagocytic defense mechanisms against foreign bodies. Another important source of ROS is the oxygen we breathe: it has been estimated that the human body can produce over 2 kg of $O_2^{\bullet-}$ per year, as a by-product of everyday breathing. However, problems arise when the production of ROS exceeds the antioxidant capacity of the body. When this occurs, several molecules in the human body can react with ROS and become oxidatively modified. The participation of excessive ROS production in the origin of several clinical conditions is now supported by experimental data [5].

The features setting the Mediterranean diets apart from other diets are illustrated in the various chapters of this book, but the abundance of fresh fruits and vegetables and the use of olive oil instead of hard fat are key factors for which the Mediterranean diets are renowned. Fruits, vegetables, and olive oil (vide infra) are rich in antioxidants that may therefore contribute to the observed protection from CHD [7].

Still, intervention studies performed with supplements have yielded mixed results. Descriptive, case-control, and prospective studies have shown a protection against cardiovascular events, whereas randomized trials have failed to confirm these results. Other trials are underway and will hopefully shed light on the contribution of antioxidant vitamins to a lower incidence of CHD.

Cancer

Oxidative DNA damage increases the risk of mutagenesis, especially if such DNA lesion is carried over during cell division [8]. It should also be noted that ROS, in particular hydrogen peroxide, are tight regulators of cell replication [8] and exert important signal transduction activities [9]. Consequently, excessive cell proliferation might be inhibited by decreasing oxidant-induced cell division [8, 10]. In addition, vitamin and mineral deficiencies can lead to DNA damage [11] and most in vitro studies are supportive of this antioxidant theory. However, in addition to demonstrations of oxidative stress inherent to cell culture [12, 13], data from Halliwell et al. [13] indicate formation of hydrogen peroxide induced by polyphenolic compounds added to the cell media, suggesting that interpretation of some data on chemopreventive potential of phenolic antioxidants might be a consequence of artifacts, namely the creation of a pro rather than an antioxidant environment.

Most research on the chemopreventive properties of antioxidants is based on their activities toward oxidant-induced DNA damage, rather than on lipid peroxidation. However, the formation of adducts between lipoperoxidation products, namely 4-hydroxy-2-nonenal, has also been implicated in carcinoma formation [10]. Hence, there is potential for antioxidants that have only been studied with respect to lipid peroxidation to also prevent DNA damage. Accordingly, epidemiological studies are 'overwhelmingly consistent in showing protective effects of antioxidant nutrients (most of which inhibit lipid peroxidation but have not been tested on DNA damage) in cancers of the stomach, esophagus, oral cavity, and lung' [2].

Even though the vast majority of in vitro studies demonstrated antioxidant, and hence potentially chemopreventive activities of Mediterranean oligonutrients, their pro-oxidant or pro-carcinogenic potential should not be overlooked. For example, both vitamin E and carotenoids have been shown to act as pro-oxidants under certain conditions [14, 15]. Another typical Mediterranean oligonutrient, indole-3-carbinol, abundant in cruciferous vegetables such as broccoli, can also promote or enhance carcinogenesis, depending on the experimental conditions [16]. Hence, although the rationale behind the antioxidant/chemoprevention theory and the biochemical evidence – derived from in vitro experiments – that support it are quite strong, it appears premature, based on available data, to make bold statement on the in vivo chemopreventive properties of individual food items or their components. In summary, further work is needed to clarify this important issue but, be it as it may, the protection afforded by a healthful, balanced diet, rather than that supposedly provided by supplements, appears to be naturally superior in cancer-fighting effectiveness.

Mediterranean Antioxidants: Selected Examples

As fully discussed in the appropriate chapters of this book, the abundance of legumes, fruits and vegetables, and the use of olive oil as the principal source of fat, distinguish the Mediterranean diets from other types of diets. Hence, the antioxidant compounds provided by these classes of foods can be conveniently divided into antioxidant vitamins and of antioxidants other than vitamins. The most recent findings on the effects of such compounds on human health will be further discussed.

Table 1. Biological activities of lycopene in human studies

Activity	References
Antioxidant activity (protection against free radicals, DNA damage, oxidative stress)	[33, 34, 71–86]
Absorption and metabolism	[32, 87–90]
Anticancer potential	[91]
Immune function	[36, 92, 93]

Is Lycopene the 'Active Ingredient' of Tomato?

Carotenoids such as lycopene, β-carotene, phytoene, and phytofluene, are present in considerable amounts both in fresh tomato (~3.5–5 mg/100 g) or its products, e.g. puree (~20 mg/100 g) and paste (~45 mg/100 g). In addition to carotenoids, tomato and its products contain several compounds such as vitamin C, folate, polyphenols, etc. that, at least in vitro, modulate radical-mediated oxidative damage that contribute to the initiation and progression of chronic disease processes [17]. Interest in tomato and its components stems from the firm evidence of decreased incidence of certain types of cancer and other degenerative diseases associated with tomato intake [17].

Among the various species, lycopene accounts for more than 50% of plasma carotenoids [18] and is also present in other human tissues such as skin, adipose tissue, liver, testes, adrenal gland, as well as being abundant in buccal mucosal cells and lymphocytes [17]. Phytoene and phytofluene are also present in human plasma, in concentrations of about 0.1–0.2 μmol/l [19], although only few studies report their concentration in human cells and tissues. It is noteworthy that lycopene is also abundant in the prostate and that high intakes of lycopene are inversely associated with prostate cancer incidence [20]. On the other hand, the effects of lycopene on cardiovascular disease are still equivocal. In particular, while low adipose tissue lycopene levels have been associated with increased risk of myocardial infarction in the multicenter EURAMIC study [21], there are studies where the association of lycopene intake with atherosclerosis risk [22], incidence of myocardial infarction [23], or intima-media thickness [24, 25] is not significant (though Gianetti et al. [26] did report a significant inverse correlation between serum lycopene concentrations and intima-media thickness). Intervention studies have shown a lipid lowering effect of lycopene in doses of 60 mg/day [27] or 20–150 mg/day [28], while its effects on LDL oxidation are still controversial [29]. A summary of human studies of lycopene is shown in table 1.

The consumption of tomatoes and tomato products (which is highest in Greece [30]) has been shown to increase serum lycopene levels [28, 31]. Also, lycopene bioavailability is higher when it is ingested via cooked food, e.g. tomato sauce or pizza, than from raw tomato [32].

To further investigate the contribution of lycopene to cardioprotection and chemoprevention, we carried out intervention trials with tomato and its products, providing healthy volunteers with moderate (7–8 mg/day) amounts of lycopene through whole tomato, puree, and paste. Surrogate markers of cardiovascular disease were evaluated and correlated with lycopene consumption. Albeit no increase in plasma antioxidant capacity was recorded, in line with other observations, lower isoprostane excretion and higher resistance of LDL to oxidation was found after supplementation [33, 34]. Interestingly, tomato administration produced lymphocyte DNA resistance to oxidation, suggesting that the cancer-preventive effects of tomato consumption might indeed be mediated by lycopene and other carotenoids [33, 34]. To ascertain the role of lycopene in chemoprevention, we undertook a cross-over, placebo-controlled intervention trial with a soft drink (Lyc-o-mato®) formulated with a lycopene oleoresin that also includes phytoene and phytofluene (5.7, 3.7 and 2.7 mg, respectively, in addition to 1 mg of β-carotene and 1.8 mg α-tocopherol/250 ml). We demonstrated that consumption of Lyc-o-mato increases plasma and lymphocyte carotenoid content and the antioxidant defense system of lymphocytes [35]. Moreover, Lyc-o-mato® supplementation is able to decrease tumor necrosis factor-α (TNF-α) production by whole blood (by 34.4%), suggesting anti-inflammatory effects in vivo [36].

In turn, this nutraceutical might constitute an additional or alternative source of bioactive carotenoids. Wherever feasible, future controlled studies with lycopene and other carotenoids will clarify the extent of their contribution to the chemopreventive properties of the Mediterranean diets.

Olive Oil and Red Wine: Do We Have Solid Human Evidence?

Olive Oil
Olive oil is the principal source of fat in the Mediterranean diet. In the past few years, researchers have been intensively studying the biological properties of olive oil minor components, some of which (oleuropein, hydroxytyrosol) have recently become commercially available. It must be noted, though, that only olive oil marketed as 'extra virgin', i.e. the one with a degree of acidity lower than 0.8% according to the current regulations, contains substantial amounts of phenolic compounds. In addition to a large number of in vitro studies, some animal studies and accumulating human trials are indicating that extra

Table 2. Biological properties of olive oil phenolics

Model	Activity	References
In vitro	Antioxidant activity	[94–115]
	Increased NO production	[116]
	Anti-inflammatory activity	[117–122]
	Antiatherogenic activity	[123–125]
	Metabolism	[41, 126]
	Cytostatic activity	[127, 128]
	Antimicrobial activity	[128, 129]
Animal	Chemoprevention	[130, 131]
	Antioxidant activity	[132–135]
	Anti-inflammatory effect	[136]
	Inhibition of progression of aortic lesions	[137, 138]
	Antithrombotic effect	[139]
	Absorption and metabolism	[43, 140–145]
Human	Blood lipid modulation and eicosanoid production	[146–150]
	Decreased oxidative stress	[151–159]
	Modulation of postprandial lipemia	[44, 46, 160–163]
	Improved vasomotion	[164]
	Absorption and metabolism	[37, 39, 40, 43, 44, 165, 166]

virgin olive oil modulates surrogate markers or properties of cardiovascular disease in humans (table 2).

One of the most important fields of research concerns the bioavailability and metabolism of olive oil phenolics. In the year 2000, we first demonstrated that olive oil phenolics are dose-dependently absorbed by humans and that they are excreted in the urine mostly as glucuronide conjugates; that study also demonstrated increased rate of conjugation with increasing amounts of phenolics administered with olive oil [37]. Other studies elucidated the metabolic pathways of hydroxytyrosol and oleuropein, which produce elevated quantities of homovanillyl alcohol and homovanilic acid [38, 39]. To date, the most complete study in this area is from Miro-Casas et al. [40], who developed a method to quantify hydroxytyrosol and its metabolites in plasma. In brief, absorption of hydroxytyrosol is nearly complete and its plasma half-life is reported to be 2.43 h.

At the cellular level, studies carried out in CACO-2 intestinal cells demonstrated that hydroxytyrosol is absorbed from the gut by passive diffusion [41]. Hydroxytyrosol conjugates undergo extensive hydrolysis in the stomach and oleuropein is degraded by the intestinal flora [42], hence explaining the high concentrations of hydroxytyrosol retrieved in the urine [43]. Finally, the

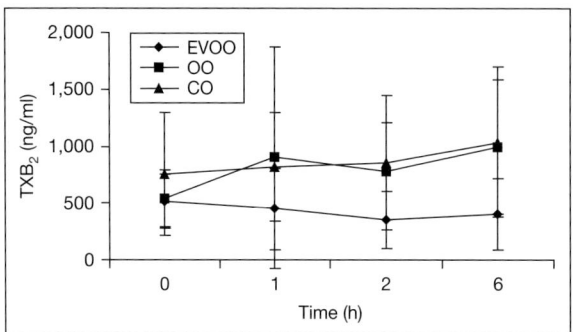

Fig. 1. Mean (± SD) serum postprandial concentrations of TXB_2. Twelve volunteers, following a Latin-square design, received in the morning 50 ml of extra virgin olive oil (EVOO, n = 12), corn oil (CO, n = 12) or olive oil (OO, n = 12). Blood aliquots at baseline (0 h), 2 and 6 h after meal were incubated for 1 h at 37°C, to stimulate TXB_2 production, which was evaluated by immunoassay (Cayman Chemical, Ann Arbor, Mich., USA). Significant differences between EVOO and OO and between EVOO and CO were recorded after 2 and 6 h from the ingestion. Differences between EVOO and other oils were assessed through analysis of covariance at time 2 and random effects regression for the entire period [46].

post-prandial absorption of olive oil phenolics and their incorporation into human lipoproteins was demonstrated [44, 45]. We have recently investigated the effects of olive oil phenols on post-prandial oxidative stress and inflammatory markers [46] (fig. 1).

It is noteworthy that hydroxytyrosol (previously also known as DOPET) is a derivative of dopamine metabolism, formed via monoamino oxidase-catalyzed deamination and subsequent reduction [47], and is found in the brain and other tissues. Hence, future investigations of the neuroprotective effects of hydroxytyrosol are warranted, also in light of the inverse association between olive oil (and monounsaturates) consumption and cognitive decline in the elderly [48]. While the high number of in vitro and animal studies provide useful information on the mechanisms of action and the in vivo activities of olive oil phenolics, human studies are required to support claims that olive oil is superior to seed oils in terms of healthful properties. Indeed, there are now approximately 15 controlled studies, the vast majority of which indicates that extra virgin olive oil does positively modulate surrogate markers of cardiovascular disease [49]. In this respect, human evidence for extra virgin olive oil is stronger that that obtained, as an example, for red wine or tea. Areas of future research will eventually elucidate the role of olive oil phenolics in chemoprevention and neuroprotection.

Table 3. Biological activities of resveratrol in humans

Activity	References
Metabolism and bioavailability	[56–59, 167]
Cardiovascular effects	
Antioxidant activities	[168]
Inhibition of platelet aggregation	[169, 170]
Anticancer potential	[171]

Wine

Moderate consumption of wine is typical of most meals of the Mediterranean areas. The hypothesis that wine could provide protection from CHD originates from the 'French paradox', i.e. the observation that in France, where the diet is rich in saturated fat – and the presence of other risk factors, such as smoke and high cholesterol levels, do not differ from those in neighboring countries in Southern Europe – the incidence of CHD is remarkably low [50]. Indeed, as opposed to most alcoholic beverages, wine, namely red wine, contains remarkable amounts of aromatic compounds, most of which are phenolic in nature [51]. This feature of red wine has been often emphasized to propose its superiority to other alcoholic beverages. It should be noted, however, that ethanol per se exerts physiological effects, such as increase in high-density lipoprotein (HDL) levels [52], inhibition of platelet aggregation [53], and increases endothelial nitric oxide production [54]. Finally, the central, namely anxiolytic activities of moderate ethanol intake might play an important role in the overall health status of the individual.

Of all the phenolic components of red wine, research has been concentrating on *trans*-resveratrol, a phytoalexin produced by grapes in response to fungi infection. Its levels in red wine, especially in that of high quality, are quite low [55] and, to date, only four studies have addressed its absorption and metabolism in humans [56–59]. The conclusion is that resveratrol as such is poorly absorbed and its circulating concentrations are unlikely to produce an effect in humans. Moreover, human-volunteer studies had thus far yielded mixed results (table 3), leaving an open question as to whether the decreased mortality from CHD observed in moderate drinkers is attributable to wine phytochemicals, to ethanol itself, or even the diet of wine consumers [60]. In summary, the 'alimentary' use of wine – i.e. wine as food – as in the case of the Mediterranean diets, should be cautiously encouraged, but the negative effects of binge drinking must not be overlooked.

Phenolic Antioxidants: Wild Plants and Endothelial Function

Endothelial dysfunction is a serious complication of atherosclerosis [61, 62] and is in part a consequence of oxidative stress, which plays a major role in its onset and maintenance [63, 64]. The downstream consequence of oxidative stress in the arterial wall is a reduced production/availability of the vasorelaxant factor nitric oxide (NO), which leads to the development of endothelial dysfunction [63, 65]. Accordingly, administration of some antioxidants, e.g. vitamin C and flavonoids from tea and wine, has been shown to ameliorate endothelial function and vasomotion [65, 66] and increasing evidence over the past decade shows that several dietary factors may partly modulate nitric oxide synthase (NOS) activity [67]. The project 'Local Food Nutraceuticals' was started in 2001 to investigate the effects of extracts obtained from selected, phenol-rich wild plants traditionally eaten in the Mediterranean area on the production of NO and prostacyclin by cultured aortic endothelial cells.

NO is an uncharged gaseous radical with a half-life between 3 and 6 s [68]. It plays a quintessential role in regulation of systemic vascular tone [64] and remodeling of the vascular wall [65]. The vasodilatory action of NO stems from its rapid diffusion and direct activation of soluble guanylyl cyclase forming cGMP which lowers intracellular calcium in the vascular smooth muscle (VSM), leading to relaxation of the muscle. Endothelial NO is formed by endothelial nitric oxide synthase (eNOS) via a five electron reduction of the terminal guanidino group of L-arginine yielding L-citrulline as a secondary product [64]. Thus, one of the most popular methods to indirectly detect NO production relies on the measurement of the conversion of L-arginine to L-citrulline, by using radioactive substrates.

In our studies, supplementation of porcine aortic endothelial cells (PAEC) with *Cynara cardunculus* or *Thymus pulegioides* extracts increases NO production. Moreover, enhanced secretion into the medium of prostacyclin, another important vasorelaxant factor, further confirms the vasomodulatory potential of these wild plants [69]. Recently, we further tested a *C. cardunculus* extract on isolated aortic rings and after supplementation to aged rats. The results confirm that the vasorelaxant properties of *C. cardunculus* are maintained in vivo, suggesting that part of the lower incidence of endothelial dysfunction and the higher vascular health observed in the Mediterranean area are to be attributed to the consumption of wild plants [70].

Conclusions

The involvement of ROS in several human pathologies is now well recognized. Conversely, antioxidant therapy has yet to be proved beneficial, partly in view of the mixed results of recent randomized trials. By contrast, epidemiological studies continue to link the above-mentioned dietary habits with a lower occurrence of cardiovascular events and cancers. It then appears that the intake and the interaction of several 'micronutrients' provided by a healthful diet, such as that in use in the Mediterranean area during the mid-1940s, is likely the link that affords protection from such pathologies [7]. In turn, the answer to the debate on the efficacy of antioxidant supplements is likely to be found in the adoption of a Mediterranean-style diet, in which the abundance of bioactive compounds provided by fruits, vegetables, wine, and olive oil grants a higher protection toward ROS-induced diseases.

Acknowledgments

The work from our laboratory described here was mostly supported by EU grant FAIR CT 97 3039, EU grant QLK-00173–2001 (Local Food Nutraceuticals) and grants from the Istituto Nutrizionale Carapelli. Tory Hagen and his laboratory at the Linus Pauling Institute always provide an excellent working environment.

References

1 Trichopoulou A, Costacou T, Bamia C, Trichopoulos D: Adherence to a Mediterranean diet and survival in a Greek population. N Engl J Med 2003;348:2599–2608.
2 Block G, Patterson B, Subar A: Fruit, vegetables, and cancer prevention: a review of the epidemiological evidence. Nutr Cancer 1992;18:1–29.
3 Parfitt VJ, Rubba P, Bolton C, Marotta G, Hartog M, Mancini M: A comparison of antioxidant status and free radical peroxidation of plasma lipoproteins in healthy young persons from Naples and Bristol. Eur Heart J 1994;15:871–876.
4 Aruoma OI: Free radicals, oxidative stress, and antioxidants human health and disease. JAOCS 1998;75:199–212.
5 Halliwell B: Antioxidants in human health and disease. Annu Rev Nutr 1996;16:33–50.
6 Visioli F, Borsani L, Galli C: Diet and prevention of coronary heart disease: the potential role of phytochemicals. Cardiovasc Res 2000;47:419–425.
7 The Local Food Consortium: Understanding local Mediterranean diets: a multidisciplinary pharmacological and ethnobotanical approach. Pharmacol Res 2005;52:353–366.
8 Ames BN, Shigenaga MK, Hagen TM: Oxidants, antioxidants, and the degenerative diseases of aging. Proc Natl Acad Sci USA 1993;90:7915–7922.
9 Poli G, Leonarduzzi G, Biasi F, Chiarpotto E: Oxidative stress and cell signalling. Curr Med Chem 2004;11:1163–1182.
10 Loo G: Redox-sensitive mechanisms of phytochemical-mediated inhibition of cancer cell proliferation (review). J Nutr Biochem 2003;14:64–73.
11 Ames BN: DNA damage from micronutrient deficiencies is likely to be a major cause of cancer. Mutat Res 2001;475:7–20.
12 Smith AR, Visioli F, Hagen TM: Vitamin C matters: increased oxidative stress in cultured human aortic endothelial cells without supplemental ascorbic acid. Faseb J 2002;16:1102–1104.
13 Halliwell B: Oxidative stress in cell culture: an under-appreciated problem? FEBS Lett 2003;540: 3–6.

14 Stocker R: The ambivalence of vitamin E in atherogenesis. Trends Biochem Sci 1999;24:219–223.
15 Paolini M, Cantelli-Forti G, Perocco P, Pedulli GF, Abdel-Rahman SZ, Legator MS: Co-carcinogenic effect of beta-carotene. Nature 1999;398:760–761.
16 Xu M, Schut HA, Bjeldanes LF, Williams DE, Bailey GS, Dashwood RH: Inhibition of 2-amino-3-methylimidazo[4,5-f]quinoline-DNA adducts by indole-3-carbinol: dose-response studies in the rat colon. Carcinogenesis 1997;18:2149–2153.
17 Rao AV, Rao LG: Lycopene and human health. Curr Topics Nutr Res 2004;2:127–136.
18 Johnson EJ: The role of carotenoids in human health. Nutr Clin Care 2002;5:56–65.
19 Hoppe PP, Kramer K, van den Berg H, Steenge G, van Vliet T: Synthetic and tomato-based lycopene have identical bioavailability in humans. Eur J Nutr 2003;42:272–278.
20 Giovannucci E, Rimm EB, Liu Y, Stampfer MJ, Willett WC: A prospective study of tomato products, lycopene, and prostate cancer risk. J Natl Cancer Inst 2002;94:391–398.
21 Kohlmeier L, Kark JD, Gomez-Gracia E, Martin BC, Steck SE, Kardinaal AF, Ringstad J, Thamm M, Masaev V, Riemersma R, Martin-Moreno JM, Huttunen JK, Kok FJ: Lycopene and myocardial infarction risk in the EURAMIC Study. Am J Epidemiol 1997;146:618–626.
22 D'Odorico A, Martines D, Kiechl S, Egger G, Oberhollenzer F, Bonvicini P, Sturniolo GC, Naccarato R, Willeit J: High plasma levels of alpha- and beta-carotene are associated with a lower risk of atherosclerosis: results from the Bruneck study. Atherosclerosis 2000;153:231–239.
23 Hak AE, Stampfer MJ, Campos H, Sesso HD, Gaziano JM, Willett W, Ma J: Plasma carotenoids and tocopherols and risk of myocardial infarction in a low-risk population of US male physicians. Circulation 2003;108:802–807.
24 Iribarren C, Folsom AR, Jacobs DR Jr, Gross MD, Belcher JD, Eckfeldt JH: Association of serum vitamin levels, LDL susceptibility to oxidation, and autoantibodies against MDA-LDL with carotid atherosclerosis: a case-control study. The ARIC Study Investigators. Atherosclerosis Risk in Communities. Arterioscler Thromb Vasc Biol 1997;17:1171–1177.
25 Bonithon-Kopp C, Coudray C, Berr C, Touboul PJ, Feve JM, Favier A, Ducimetiere P: Combined effects of lipid peroxidation and antioxidant status on carotid atherosclerosis in a population aged 59–71 y: The EVA Study. Etude sur le Vieillisement Arteriel. Am J Clin Nutr 1997;65: 121–127.
26 Gianetti J, Pedrinelli R, Petrucci R, Lazzerini G, De Caterina M, Bellomo G, De Caterina R: Inverse association between carotid intima-media thickness and the antioxidant lycopene in atherosclerosis. Am Heart J 2002;143:467–474.
27 Fuhrman B, Elis A, Aviram M: Hypocholesterolemic effect of lycopene and beta-carotene is related to suppression of cholesterol synthesis and augmentation of LDL receptor activity in macrophages. Biochem Biophys Res Commun 1997;233:658–662.
28 Rao AV, Agarwal S: Bioavailability and in vivo antioxidant properties of lycopene from tomato products and their possible role in the prevention of cancer. Nutr Cancer 1998;31:199–203.
29 Hininger IA, Meyer-Wenger A, Moser U, Wright A, Southon S, Thurnham D, Chopra M, Van Den Berg H, Olmedilla B, Favier AE, Roussel AM: No significant effects of lutein, lycopene or beta-carotene supplementation on biological markers of oxidative stress and LDL oxidizability in healthy adult subjects. J Am Coll Nutr 2001;20:232–238.
30 Al-Delaimy WK, van Kappel AL, Ferrari P, Slimani N, Steghens JP, Bingham S, Johansson I, Wallstrom P, Overvad K, Tjonneland A, Key TJ, Welch AA, Bueno-de-Mesquita HB, Peeters PH, Boeing H, Linseisen J, Clavel-Chapelon F, Guibout C, Navarro C, Quiros JR, Palli D, Celentano E, Trichopoulou A, Benetou V, Kaaks R, Riboli E: Plasma levels of six carotenoids in nine European countries: report from the European Prospective Investigation into Cancer and Nutrition (EPIC). Publ Health Nutr 2004;7:713–722.
31 Hadley CW, Clinton SK, Schwartz SJ: The consumption of processed tomato products enhances plasma lycopene concentrations in association with a reduced lipoprotein sensitivity to oxidative damage. J Nutr 2003;133:727–732.
32 Gartner C, Stahl W, Sies H: Lycopene is more bioavailable from tomato paste than from fresh tomatoes. Am J Clin Nutr 1997;66:116–122.
33 Visioli F, Riso P, Grande S, Galli C, Porrini M: Protective activity of tomato products on in vivo markers of lipid oxidation. Eur J Nutr 2003;42:201–206.

34 Riso P, Visioli F, Erba D, Testolin G, Porrini M: Lycopene and vitamin C concentrations increase in plasma and lymphocytes after tomato intake: effects on cellular antioxidant protection. Eur J Clin Nutr 2004;58:1350–1358.
35 Porrini M, Riso P, Brusamolino A, Berti C, Guarnieri S, Visioli F: Daily intake of a formulated tomato drink affects carotenoid plasma and lymphocyte concentrations and improves cellular antioxidant protection. Br J Nutr 2005;93:93–99.
36 Riso P, Visioli F, Grande S, Guarnieri S, Gardana C, Simonetti P, Porrini M: Effect of a tomato-based drink on markers of inflammation, immunomodulation, and oxidative stress. J Agric Food Chem 2006;54:2563–2566.
37 Visioli F, Galli C, Bornet F, Mattei A, Patelli R, Galli G, Caruso D: Olive oil phenolics are dose-dependently absorbed in humans. FEBS Lett 2000;468:159–160.
38 Caruso D, Visioli F, Patelli R, Galli C, Galli G: Urinary excretion of olive oil phenols and their metabolites in humans. Metabolism 2001;50:1426–1428.
39 Miro-Casas E, Covas MI, Fito M, Farre-Albadalejo M, Marrugat J, de la Torre R: Tyrosol and hydroxytyrosol are absorbed from moderate and sustained doses of virgin olive oil in humans. Eur J Clin Nutr 2003;57:186–190.
40 Miro-Casas E, Covas MI, Farre M, Fito M, Ortuno J, Weinbrenner T, Roset P, de la Torre R: Hydroxytyrosol disposition in humans. Clin Chem 2003;49:945–952.
41 Manna C, Galletti P, Maisto G, Cucciolla V, D'Angelo S, Zappia V: Transport mechanism and metabolism of olive oil hydroxytyrosol in CACO-2 cells. FEBS Lett 2000;470:341–344.
42 Corona G, Tzounis X, Assunta Dessi M, Deiana M, Debnam ES, Visioli F, Spencer JP: The fate of olive oil polyphenols in the gastrointestinal tract: Implications of gastric and colonic microflora-dependent biotransformation. Free Radic Res 2006;40:647–658.
43 Visioli F, Galli C, Grande S, Colonnelli K, Patelli C, Galli G, Caruso D: Hydroxytyrosol excretion differs between rats and humans and depends on the vehicle of administration. J Nutr 2003;133: 2612–2615.
44 Bonanome A, Pagnan A, Caruso D, Toia A, Xamin A, Fedeli F, Berra B, Zamburlini A, Ursini F, Galli G: Evidence of postprandial absorption of olive oil phenols in humans. Nutr Metab Cardiovasc Dis 2000;10:111–120.
45 Covas MI, de la Torre K, Farre-Albaladejo M, Kaikkonen J, Fito M, Lopez-Sabater C, Pujadas-Bastardes MA, Joglar J, Weinbrenner T, Lamuela-Raventos RM, de la Torre R: Postprandial LDL phenolic content and LDL oxidation are modulated by olive oil phenolic compounds in humans. Free Radic Biol Med 2006;40:608–616.
46 Bogani P, Galli C, Villa M, Visioli F: Postprandial anti-inflammatory and antioxidant effects of extra virgin olive oil. Atherosclerosis 2006;Epub ahead of print.
47 Lamensdorf I, Eisenhofer G, Harvey-White J, Hayakawa Y, Kirk K, Kopin IJ: Metabolic stress in PC12 cells induces the formation of the endogenous dopaminergic neurotoxin, 3,4-dihydroxyphenylacetaldehyde. J Neurosci Res 2000;60:552–558.
48 Solfrizzi V, Colacicco AM, D'Introno A, Capurso C, Torres F, Rizzo C, Capurso A, Panza F: Dietary intake of unsaturated fatty acids and age-related cognitive decline: an 8.5-year follow-up of the Italian Longitudinal Study on Aging. Neurobiol Aging 2006;27:1694–1704.
49 Perez-Jimenez F: International conference on the healthy effect of virgin olive oil. Eur J Clin Invest 2005;35:421–424.
50 Renaud S, de Lorgeril M: Wine, alcohol, platelets, and the French paradox for coronary heart disease. Lancet 1992;339:1523–1526.
51 Vinson JA, Jang J, Yang J, Dabbagh Y, Liang X, Serry M, Proch J, Cai S: Vitamins and especially flavonoids in common beverages are powerful in vitro antioxidants which enrich lower density lipoproteins and increase their oxidative resistance after ex vivo spiking in human plasma. J Agric Food Chem 1999;47:2502–2504.
52 Rotondo S, de Gaetano G: Protection from cardiovascular disease by wine and its derived products. Epidemiological evidence and biological mechanisms. World Rev Nutr Diet. Basel, Karger, 2000, vol 87, pp 90–113.
53 Salem RO, Laposata M: Effects of alcohol on hemostasis. Am J Clin Pathol 2005;123(suppl): S96–S105.

54 Venkov CD, Myers PR, Tanner MA, Su M, Vaughan DE: Ethanol increases endothelial nitric oxide production through modulation of nitric oxide synthase expression. Thromb Haemost 1999;81: 638–642.
55 Gambuti A, Strollo D, Ugliano M, Lecce L, Moio L: trans-Resveratrol, quercetin, (+)-catechin, and (−)-epicatechin content in south Italian monovarietal wines: relationship with maceration time and marc pressing during winemaking. J Agric Food Chem 2004;52:5747–5751.
56 Goldberg DM, Yan J, Soleas GJ: Absorption of three wine-related polyphenols in three different matrices by healthy subjects. Clin Biochem 2003;36:79–87.
57 Walle T, Hsieh F, DeLegge MH, Oatis JE Jr, Walle UK: High absorption but very low bioavailability of oral resveratrol in humans. Drug Metab Dispos 2004;32:1377–1382.
58 Meng X, Maliakal P, Lu H, Lee MJ, Yang CS: Urinary and plasma levels of resveratrol and quercetin in humans, mice, and rats after ingestion of pure compounds and grape juice. J Agric Food Chem 2004;52:935–942.
59 Vitaglione P, Sforza S, Galaverna G, Ghidini C, Caporaso N, Vescovi PP, Fogliano V, Marchelli R: Bioavailability of trans-resveratrol from red wine in humans. Mol Nutr Food Res 2005;49:495–504.
60 Johansen D, Friis K, Skovenborg E, Gronbaek M: Food buying habits of people who buy wine or beer: cross-sectional study. BMJ 2006;332:519–522.
61 Vita JA, Keaney JF Jr: Endothelial function: a barometer for cardiovascular risk? Circulation 2002;106:640–642.
62 Assanelli D, Bonanome A, Pezzini A, Albertini F, Maccalli P, Grassi M, Archetti S, Negrini R, Visioli F: Folic acid and vitamin E supplementation effects on homocysteinemia, endothelial function and plasma antioxidant capacity in young myocardial-infarction patients. Pharmacol Res 2004;49:79–84.
63 Cai H, Harrison DG: Endothelial dysfunction in cardiovascular diseases. Circ Res 2000;87:840–844.
64 Thomas SR, Chen K, Keaney JF Jr: Oxidative stress and endothelial nitric oxide bioactivity. Antioxid Redox Signal 2003;5:181–194.
65 Schulz E, Anter E, Keaney JF: Oxidative stress, antioxidants, and endothelial function. Curr Med Chem 2004;11:1093–1104.
66 Carr A, Frei B: The role of antioxidants in preserving the biological activity of endothelium-derived nitric oxide. Free Radic Biol Med 2000;28:1806–1814.
67 Wu G, Meininger CJ: Regulation of nitric oxide synthesis by dietary factors. Annu Rev Nutr 2002;22:61–86.
68 Moncada S, Palmer RM, Higgs EA: Nitric oxide: physiology, pathophysiology, and pharmacology. Pharmacol Rev 1991;43:109–142.
69 Grande S, Bogani P, de Saizieu A, Schueler G, Galli C, Visioli F: Vasomodulating potential of Mediterranean wild plant extracts. J Agric Food Chem 2004;52:5021–5026.
70 Rossoni G, Grande S, Galli C, Visioli F: Wild artichoke prevents the age-associated loss of vasomotor function. J Agric Food Chem 2005;53:10291–10296.
71 Bub A, Barth SW, Watzl B, Briviba K, Rechkemmer G: Paraoxonase 1 Q192R (PON1–192) polymorphism is associated with reduced lipid peroxidation in healthy young men on a low-carotenoid diet supplemented with tomato juice. Br J Nutr 2005;93:291–297.
72 Collins JK, Arjmandi BH, Claypool PL, Perkins-Veazie P, Baker RA, Clevidence BA: Lycopene from two food sources does not affect antioxidant or cholesterol status of middle-aged adults. Nutr J 2004;3:15.
73 Walrand S, Farges MC, Dehaese O, Cardinault N, Minet-Quinard R, Grolier P, Bouteloup-Demange C, Ribalta J, Winklhofer-Roob BM, Rock E, Vasson MP: In vivo and in vitro evidences that carotenoids could modulate the neutrophil respiratory burst during dietary manipulation. Eur J Nutr 2005;44:114–120.
74 Briviba K, Schnabele K, Rechkemmer G, Bub A: Supplementation of a diet low in carotenoids with tomato or carrot juice does not affect lipid peroxidation in plasma and feces of healthy men. J Nutr 2004;134:1081–1083.
75 Astley SB, Hughes DA, Wright AJ, Elliott RM, Southon S: DNA damage and susceptibility to oxidative damage in lymphocytes: effects of carotenoids in vitro and in vivo. Br J Nutr 2004;91:53–61.
76 Kiokias S, Gordon MH: Dietary supplementation with a natural carotenoid mixture decreases oxidative stress. Eur J Clin Nutr 2003;57:1135–1140.

77 Porrini M, Riso P, Oriani G: Spinach and tomato consumption increases lymphocyte DNA resistance to oxidative stress but this is not related to cell carotenoid concentrations. Eur J Nutr 2002;41:95–100.
78 Mecocci P, Polidori MC, Cherubini A, Ingegni T, Mattioli P, Catani M, Rinaldi P, Cecchetti R, Stahl W, Senin U, Beal MF: Lymphocyte oxidative DNA damage and plasma antioxidants in Alzheimer disease. Arch Neurol 2002;59:794–798.
79 Bohm F, Edge R, Burke M, Truscott TG: Dietary uptake of lycopene protects human cells from singlet oxygen and nitrogen dioxide-ROS components from cigarette smoke. J Photochem Photobiol B 2001;64:176–178.
80 Briviba K, Kulling SE, Moseneder J, Watzl B, Rechkemmer G, Bub A: Effects of supplementing a low-carotenoid diet with a tomato extract for 2 weeks on endogenous levels of DNA single strand breaks and immune functions in healthy non-smokers and smokers. Carcinogenesis 2004;25: 2373–2378.
81 Bub A, Barth S, Watzl B, Briviba K, Herbert BM, Luhrmann PM, Neuhauser-Berthold M, Rechkemmer G: Paraoxonase 1 Q192R (PON1–192) polymorphism is associated with reduced lipid peroxidation in R-allele-carrier but not in QQ homozygous elderly subjects on a tomato-rich diet. Eur J Nutr 2002;41:237–243.
82 Pellegrini N, Riso P, Porrini M: Tomato consumption does not affect the total antioxidant capacity of plasma. Nutrition 2000;16:268–271.
83 Porrini M, Riso P: Lymphocyte lycopene concentration and DNA protection from oxidative damage is increased in women after a short period of tomato consumption. J Nutr 2000;130:189–192.
84 Polidori MC, Mecocci P: Plasma susceptibility to free radical-induced antioxidant consumption and lipid peroxidation is increased in very old subjects with Alzheimer disease. J Alzheimers Dis 2002;4:517–522.
85 Polidori MC, Cherubini A, Stahl W, Senin U, Sies H, Mecocci P: Plasma carotenoid and malondialdehyde levels in ischemic stroke patients: relationship to early outcome. Free Radic Res 2002;36:265–268.
86 Polidori MC, Savino K, Alunni G, Freddio M, Senin U, Sies H, Stahl W, Mecocci P: Plasma lipophilic antioxidants and malondialdehyde in congestive heart failure patients: relationship to disease severity. Free Radic Biol Med 2002;32:148–152.
87 Bugianesi R, Salucci M, Leonardi C, Ferracane R, Catasta G, Azzini E, Maiani G: Effect of domestic cooking on human bioavailability of naringenin, chlorogenic acid, lycopene and beta-carotene in cherry tomatoes. Eur J Nutr 2004;43:360–366.
88 Edwards AJ, Vinyard BT, Wiley ER, Brown ED, Collins JK, Perkins-Veazie P, Baker RA, Clevidence BA: Consumption of watermelon juice increases plasma concentrations of lycopene and beta-carotene in humans. J Nutr 2003;133:1043–1050.
89 Riso P, Brusamolino A, Scalfi L, Porrini M: Bioavailability of carotenoids from spinach and tomatoes. Nutr Metab Cardiovasc Dis 2004;14:150–156.
90 Olmedilla B, Granado F, Southon S, Wright AJ, Blanco I, Gil-Martinez E, van den Berg H, Thurnham D, Corridan B, Chopra M, Hininger I: A European multicentre, placebo-controlled supplementation study with alpha-tocopherol, carotene-rich palm oil, lutein or lycopene: analysis of serum responses. Clin Sci (Lond) 2002;102:447–456.
91 Kim HS, Bowen P, Chen L, Duncan C, Ghosh L, Sharifi R, Christov K: Effects of tomato sauce consumption on apoptotic cell death in prostate benign hyperplasia and carcinoma. Nutr Cancer 2003;47:40–47.
92 Watzl B, Bub A, Briviba K, Rechkemmer G: Supplementation of a low-carotenoid diet with tomato or carrot juice modulates immune functions in healthy men. Ann Nutr Metab 2003;47: 255–261.
93 Hughes DA, Wright AJ, Finglas PM, Polley AC, Bailey AL, Astley SB, Southon S: Effects of lycopene and lutein supplementation on the expression of functionally associated surface molecules on blood monocytes from healthy male nonsmokers. J Infect Dis 2000;182(suppl 1): S11–S15.
94 Manna C, D'Angelo S, Migliardi V, Loffredi E, Mazzoni O, Morrica P, Galletti P, Zappia V: Protective effect of the phenolic fraction from virgin olive oils against oxidative stress in human cells. J Agric Food Chem 2002;50:6521–6526.

95 Deiana M, Rosa A, Cao CF, Pirisi FM, Bandino G, Dessi MA: Novel approach to study oxidative stability of extra virgin olive oils: importance of alpha-tocopherol concentration. J Agric Food Chem 2002;50:4342–4346.
96 Deiana M, Aruoma OI, Bianchi ML, Spencer JP, Kaur H, Halliwell B, Aeschbach R, Banni S, Dessi MA, Corongiu FP: Inhibition of peroxynitrite dependent DNA base modification and tyrosine nitration by the extra virgin olive oil-derived antioxidant hydroxytyrosol. Free Radic Biol Med 1999;26:762–769.
97 Leenen R, Roodenburg AJ, Vissers MN, Schuurbiers JA, van Putte KP, Wiseman SA, van De Put FH: Supplementation of plasma with olive oil phenols and extracts: influence on LDL oxidation. J Agric Food Chem 2002;50:1290–1297.
98 Fito M, Covas MI, Lamuela-Raventos RM, Vila J, Torrents L, de la Torre C, Marrugat J: Protective effect of olive oil and its phenolic compounds against low density lipoprotein oxidation. Lipids 2000;35:633–638.
99 Stupans I, Kirlich A, Tuck KL, Hayball PJ: Comparison of radical scavenging effect, inhibition of microsomal oxygen free radical generation, and serum lipoprotein oxidation of several natural antioxidants. J Agric Food Chem 2002;50:2464–2469.
100 Hashimoto T, Ibi M, Matsuno K, Nakashima S, Tanigawa T, Yoshikawa T, Yabe-Nishimura C: An endogenous metabolite of dopamine, 3,4-dihydroxyphenylethanol, acts as a unique cytoprotective agent against oxidative stress-induced injury. Free Radic Biol Med 2004;36:555–564.
101 Manna C, Galletti P, Cucciolla V, Montedoro G, Zappia V: Olive oil hydroxytyrosol protects human erythrocytes against oxidative damages. J Nutr Biochem 1999;10:159–165.
102 Visioli F, Bellomo G, Montedoro G, Galli C: Low density lipoprotein oxidation is inhibited in vitro by olive oil constituents. Atherosclerosis 1995;117:25–32.
103 Grignaffini P, Roma P, Galli C, Catapano AL: Protection of low-density lipoprotein from oxidation by 3,4-dihydroxyphenylethanol. Lancet 1994;343:1296–1297.
104 Masella R, Vari R, D'Archivio M, Di Benedetto R, Matarrese P, Malorni W, Scazzocchio B, Giovannini C: Extra virgin olive oil biophenols inhibit cell-mediated oxidation of LDL by increasing the mRNA transcription of glutathione-related enzymes. J Nutr 2004;134: 785–791.
105 Visioli F, Vinceri FF, Galli C: 'Waste waters' from olive oil production are rich in natural antioxidants. Experientia 1995;51:32–34.
106 Saija A, Trombetta D, Tomaino A, Lo CR, Princi P, Uccella N, Bonina F, Castelli F: 'In vitro' evaluation of the antioxidant activity and biomembrane interaction of the plant phenols oleuropein and hydroxytyrosol. Int J Pharm 1998;166:123–133.
107 Speroni E, Guerra M, Minghetti A: Oleuropein evaluated in vitro and in vivo as an antioxidant. Phytother Res 1998;12:S98–S100.
108 Visioli F, Bellomo G, Galli C: Free radical-scavenging properties of olive oil polyphenols. Biochem Biophys Res Commun 1998;247:60–64.
109 Pellegrini N, Visioli F, Buratti S, Brighenti F: Direct analysis of total antioxidant activity of olive oil and studies on the influence of heating. J Agric Food Chem 2001;49:2532–2538.
110 Lavelli V: Comparison of the antioxidant activities of extra virgin olive oils. J Agric Food Chem 2002;50:7704–7708.
111 Gorinstein S, Martin-Belloso O, Katrich E, Lojek A, Ciz M, Gligelmo-Miguel N, Haruenkit R, Park YS, Jung ST, Trakhtenberg S: Comparison of the contents of the main biochemical compounds and the antioxidant activity of some Spanish olive oils as determined by four different radical scavenging tests. J Nutr Biochem 2003;14:154–159.
112 Pellegrini N, Serafini M, Colombi B, Del Rio D, Salvatore S, Bianchi M, Brighenti F: Total antioxidant capacity of plant foods, beverages and oils consumed in Italy assessed by three different in vitro assays. J Nutr 2003;133:2812–2819.
113 Valavanidis A, Nisiotou C, Papageorgiou Y, Kremli I, Satravelas N, Zinieris N, Zygalaki H: Comparison of the radical scavenging potential of polar and lipidic fractions of olive oil and other vegetable oils under normal conditions and after thermal treatment. J Agric Food Chem 2004;52: 2358–2365.
114 Salami M, Galli C, De Angelis L, Visioli F: Formation of F2-isoprostanes in oxidized low density lipoprotein: inhibitory effect of hydroxytyrosol. Pharmacol Res 1995;31:275–279.

115 Moreno JJ: Effect of olive oil minor components on oxidative stress and arachidonic acid mobilization and metabolism by macrophages RAW 264.7. Free Radic Biol Med 2003;35:1073–1081.
116 Visioli F, Bellosta S, Galli C: Oleuropein, the bitter principle of olives, enhances nitric oxide production by mouse macrophages. Life Sci 1998;62:541–546.
117 Petroni A, Blasevich M, Salami M, Papini N, Montedoro GF, Galli C: Inhibition of platelet aggregation and eicosanoid production by phenolic components of olive oil. Thromb Haemost 1995;78:151–160.
118 Miles EA, Zoubouli P, Calder PC: Differential anti-inflammatory effects of phenolic compounds from extra virgin olive oil identified in human whole blood cultures. Nutrition 2005;21:389–394.
119 de la Puerta R, Ruiz-Gutierrez V, Hoult JR: Inhibition of leukocyte 5-lipoxygenase by phenolics from virgin olive oil. Biochem Pharmacol 1999;57:445–449.
120 Kohyama N, Nagata T, Fujimoto S, Sekiya K: Inhibition of arachidonate lipoxygenase activities by 2-(3,4-dihydroxyphenyl)ethanol, a phenolic compound from olives. Biosci Biotechnol Biochem 1997;61:347–350.
121 Miles EA, Zoubouli P, Calder PC: Effects of polyphenols on human Th1 and Th2 cytokine production. Clin Nutr 2005;24:780–784.
122 Beauchamp GK, Keast RS, Morel D, Lin J, Pika J, Han Q, Lee CH, Smith AB, Breslin PA: Phytochemistry: ibuprofen-like activity in extra-virgin olive oil. Nature 2005;437:45–46.
123 Carluccio MA, Siculella L, Ancora MA, Massaro M, Scoditti E, Storelli C, Visioli F, Distante A, De Caterina R: Olive oil and red wine antioxidant polyphenols inhibit endothelial activation: antiatherogenic properties of mediterranean diet phytochemicals. Arterioscler Thromb Vasc Biol 2003;23:622–629.
124 Turner R, Etienne N, Alonso MG, de Pascual-Teresa S, Minihane AM, Weinberg PD, Rimbach G: Antioxidant and anti-atherogenic activities of olive oil phenolics. Int J Vitam Nutr Res 2005;75:61–70.
125 Dell'agli M, Fagnani R, Mitro N, Scurati S, Masciadri M, Mussoni L, Galli GV, Bosisio E, Crestani M, De Fabiani E, Tremoli E, Caruso D: Minor components of olive oil modulate proatherogenic adhesion molecules involved in endothelial activation. J Agric Food Chem 2006;54:3259–3264.
126 Edgecombe SC, Stretch GL, Hayball PJ: Oleuropein, an antioxidant polyphenol from olive oil, is poorly absorbed from isolated perfused rat intestine. J Nutr 2000;130:2996–3002.
127 Saenz MT, Garcia MD, Ahumada MC, Ruiz V: Cytostatic activity of some compounds from the unsaponifiable fraction obtained from virgin olive oil. Farmaco 1998;53:448–449.
128 Tranter HS, Tassou SC, Nychas GJ: The effect of the phenolic compound, oleuropein, on growth and enterotoxin B production by *Staphylococcus aureus*. J Appl Bacteriol 1993;74:253–259.
129 Bisignano G, Tomaino A, Lo Cascio R, Crisafi G, Uccella N, Saija A: On the in-vitro antimicrobial activity of oleuropein and hydroxytyrosol. J Pharm Pharmacol 1999;51:971–974.
130 Budiyanto A, Ahmed NU, Wu A, Bito T, Nikaido O, Osawa T, Ueda M, Ichihashi M: Protective effect of topically applied olive oil against photocarcinogenesis following UVB exposure of mice. Carcinogenesis 2000;21:2085–2090.
131 Perino G, Conti B, Ciliberti A, Maltoni C: Incidence of pancreatic tumors and tumor precursors in Sprague-Dawley rats after administration of olive oil. Ann NY Acad Sci 1988;534:604–617.
132 Wiseman SA, Tijburg LB, van De Put FH: Olive oil phenolics protect LDL and spare vitamin E in the hamster. Lipids 2002;37:1053–1057.
133 Alarcon de la Lastra C, Barranco MD, Martin MJ, Herrerias J, Motilva V: Extra-virgin olive oil-enriched diets reduce indomethacin-induced gastric oxidative damage in rats. Dig Dis Sci 2002;47:2783–2790.
134 Coni E, Di Benedetto R, Di Pasquale M, Masella R, Modesti D, Mattei R, Carlini EA: Protective effect of oleuropein, an olive oil biophenol, on low density lipoprotein oxidizability in rabbits. Lipids 2000;35:45–54.
135 Wiseman SA, Mathot JN, de Fouw NJ, Tijburg LB: Dietary non-tocopherol antioxidants present in extra virgin olive oil increase the resistance of low density lipoproteins to oxidation in rabbits. Atherosclerosis 1996;120:15–23.
136 Martinez-Dominguez E, de la Puerta R, Ruiz-Gutierrez V: Protective effects upon experimental inflammation models of a polyphenol-supplemented virgin olive oil diet. Inflamm Res 2001;50:102–106.

137 Aguilera CM, Ramirez-Tortosa MC, Mesa MD, Ramirez-Tortosa CL, Gil A: Sunflower, virgin-olive and fish oils differentially affect the progression of aortic lesions in rabbits with experimental atherosclerosis. Atherosclerosis 2002;162:335–344.

138 Gonzalez-Santiago M, Martin-Bautista E, Carrero JJ, Fonolla J, Baro L, Bartolome MV, Gil-Loyzaga P, Lopez-Huertas E: One-month administration of hydroxytyrosol, a phenolic antioxidant present in olive oil, to hyperlipemic rabbits improves blood lipid profile, antioxidant status and reduces atherosclerosis development. Atherosclerosis 2006;188:35–42.

139 Brzosko S, De Curtis A, Murzilli S, de Gaetano G, Donati MB, Iacoviello L: Effect of extra virgin olive oil on experimental thrombosis and primary hemostasis in rats. Nutr Metab Cardiovasc Dis 2002;12:337–342.

140 Bai C, Yan X, Takenaka M, Sekiya K, Nagata T: Determination of synthetic hydroxytyrosol in rat plasma by GC-MS. J Agric Food Chem 1998;46:3998–4001.

141 Ruiz-Gutierrez V, Juan ME, Cert A, Planas JM: Determination of hydroxytyrosol in plasma by HPLC. Anal Chem 2000;72:4458–4461.

142 Tan HW, Tuck KL, Stupans I, Hayball PJ: Simultaneous determination of oleuropein and hydroxytyrosol in rat plasma using liquid chromatography with fluorescence detection. J Chromatogr [B] 2003;785:187–191.

143 D'Angelo S, Manna C, Migliardi V, Mazzoni O, Morrica P, Capasso G, Pontoni G, Galletti P, Zappia V: Pharmacokinetics and metabolism of hydroxytyrosol, a natural antioxidant from olive oil. Drug Metab Dispos 2001;29:1492–1498.

144 Tuck KL, Freeman MP, Hayball PJ, Stretch GL, Stupans I: The in vivo fate of hydroxytyrosol and tyrosol, antioxidant phenolic constituents of olive oil, after intravenous and oral dosing of labeled compounds to rats. J Nutr 2001;131:1993–1996.

145 Tuck KL, Hayball PJ, Stupans I: Structural characterization of the metabolites of hydroxytyrosol, the principal phenolic component in olive oil, in rats. J Agric Food Chem 2002;50:2404–2409.

146 Oubina P, Sanchez-Muniz FJ, Rodenas S, Cuesta C: Eicosanoid production, thrombogenic ratio, and serum and LDL peroxides in normo- and hypercholesterolaemic post-menopausal women consuming two oleic acid-rich diets with different content of minor components. Br J Nutr 2001;85:41–47.

147 Marrugat J, Covas MI, Fito M, Schroder H, Miro-Casas E, Gimeno E, Lopez-Sabater MC, Farre M: Effects of differing phenolic content in dietary olive oils on lipids and LDL oxidation: a randomized controlled trial. Eur J Nutr 2004;43:140–147.

148 Leger CL, Carbonneau MA, Michel F, Mas E, Monnier L, Cristol JP, Descomps B: A thromboxane effect of a hydroxytyrosol-rich olive oil wastewater extract in patients with uncomplicated type I diabetes. Eur J Clin Nutr 2005;59:727–730.

149 Berbert AA, Kondo CR, Almendra CL, Matsuo T, Dichi I: Supplementation of fish oil and olive oil in patients with rheumatoid arthritis. Nutrition 2005;21:131–136.

150 Serrano-Martinez M, Palacios M, Martinez-Losa E, Lezaun R, Maravi C, Prado M, Martinez JA, Martinez-Gonzalez MA: A Mediterranean dietary style influences TNF-alpha and VCAM-1 coronary blood levels in unstable angina patients. Eur J Nutr 2005;44:348–354.

151 Ramirez-Tortosa MC, Suarez A, Gomez MC, Mir A, Ros E, Mataix J, Gil A: Effect of extra-virgin olive oil and fish-oil supplementation on plasma lipids and susceptibility of low-density lipoprotein to oxidative alteration in free-living spanish male patients with peripheral vascular disease. Clin Nutr 1999;18:167–174.

152 Ramirez-Tortosa MC, Urbano G, Lopez-Jurado M, Nestares T, Gomez MC, Mir A, Ros E, Mataix J, Gil A: Extra-virgin olive oil increases the resistance of LDL to oxidation more than refined olive oil in free-living men with peripheral vascular disease. J Nutr 1999;129:2177–2183.

153 Masella R, Giovannini C, Vari R, Di Benedetto R, Coni E, Volpe R, Fraone N, Bucci A: Effects of dietary virgin olive oil phenols on low density lipoprotein oxidation in hyperlipidemic patients. Lipids 2001;36:1195–1202.

154 Vissers MN, Zock PL, Leenen R, Roodenburg AJ, van Putte KP, Katan MB: Effect of consumption of phenols from olives and extra virgin olive oil on LDL oxidizability in healthy humans. Free Radic Res 2001;35:619–629.

155 Vissers MN, Zock PL, Wiseman SA, Meyboom S, Katan MB: Effect of phenol-rich extra virgin olive oil on markers of oxidation in healthy volunteers. Eur J Clin Nutr 2001;55:334–341.

156 Nagyova A, Haban P, Klvanova J, Kadrabova J: Effects of dietary extra virgin olive oil on serum lipid resistance to oxidation and fatty acid composition in elderly lipidemic patients. Bratisl Lek Listy 2003;104:218–221.
157 Haban P, Klvanova J, Zidekova E, Nagyova A: Dietary supplementation with olive oil leads to improved lipoprotein spectrum and lower n–6 PUFAs in elderly subjects. Med Sci Monit 2004;10:PI49–P154.
158 Salvini S, Sera F, Caruso D, Giovannelli L, Visioli F, Saieva C, Masala G, Ceroti M, Giovacchini V, Pitozzi V, Galli C, Romani A, Mulinacci N, Bortolomeazzi R, Dolara P, Palli D: Daily consumption of a high-phenol extra-virgin olive oil reduces oxidative DNA damage in postmenopausal women. Br J Nutr 2006;95:742–751.
159 Visioli F, Caruso D, Galli C, Viappiani S, Galli G, Sala A: Olive oils rich in natural catecholic phenols decrease isoprostane excretion in humans. Biochem Biophys Res Commun 2000;278: 797–799.
160 Soares MJ, Cummings SJ, Mamo JC, Kenrick M, Piers LS: The acute effects of olive oil v. cream on postprandial thermogenesis and substrate oxidation in postmenopausal women. Br J Nutr 2004;91:245–252.
161 Piers LS, Walker KZ, Stoney RM, Soares MJ, O'Dea K: The influence of the type of dietary fat on postprandial fat oxidation rates: monounsaturated (olive oil) vs. saturated fat (cream). Int J Obes Relat Metab Disord 2002;26:814–821.
162 Nicolaiew N, Lemort N, Adorni L, Berra B, Montorfano G, Rapelli S, Cortesi N, Jacotot B: Comparison between extra virgin olive oil and oleic acid rich sunflower oil: effects on postprandial lipemia and LDL susceptibility to oxidation. Ann Nutr Metab 1998;42:251–260.
163 Weinbrenner T, Fito M, Farre Albaladejo M, Saez GT, Rijken P, Tormos C, Coolen S, De La Torre R, Covas MI: Bioavailability of phenolic compounds from olive oil and oxidative/antioxidant status at postprandial state in healthy humans. Drugs Exp Clin Res 2004;30:207–212.
164 Ruano J, Lopez-Miranda J, Fuentes F, Moreno JA, Bellido C, Perez-Martinez P, Lozano A, Gomez P, Jimenez Y, Perez Jimenez F: Phenolic content of virgin olive oil improves ischemic reactive hyperemia in hypercholesterolemic patients. J Am Coll Cardiol 2005;46:1864–1868.
165 Miro-Casas E, Farre AM, Covas MI, Rodriguez JO, Menoyo CE, Lamuela RR, de la Torre R: Capillary gas chromatography-mass spectrometry quantitative determination of hydroxytyrosol and tyrosol in human urine after olive oil intake. Anal Biochem 2001;294:63–72.
166 Vissers MN, Zock PL, Roodenburg AJ, Leenen R, Katan MB: Olive oil phenols are absorbed in humans. J Nutr 2002;132:409–417.
167 Soleas GJ, Yan J, Goldberg DM: Ultrasensitive assay for three polyphenols (catechin, quercetin and resveratrol) and their conjugates in biological fluids utilizing gas chromatography with mass selective detection. J Chromatogr [B] 2001;757:161–172.
168 Bhavnani BR, Cecutti A, Gerulath A, Woolever AC, Berco M: Comparison of the antioxidant effects of equine estrogens, red wine components, vitamin E, and probucol on low-density lipoprotein oxidation in postmenopausal women. Menopause 2001;8:408–419.
169 Wang Z, Zou J, Huang Y, Cao K, Xu Y, Wu JM: Effect of resveratrol on platelet aggregation in vivo and in vitro. Chin Med J (Engl) 2002;115:378–380.
170 Wang Z, Huang Y, Zou J, Cao K, Xu Y, Wu JM: Effects of red wine and wine polyphenol resveratrol on platelet aggregation in vivo and in vitro. Int J Mol Med 2002;9:77–79.
171 Levi F, Pasche C, Lucchini F, Ghidoni R, Ferraroni M, La Vecchia C: Resveratrol and breast cancer risk. Eur J Cancer Prev 2005;14:139–142.

Francesco Visioli
University of Milan, Department of Pharmacological Sciences
Via Balzaretti 9
IT–20133 Milan (Italy)
Tel. +39 02 50318280, Fax +39 02 700426106, E-Mail francesco.visioli@unimi.it

Olive Oil

Dimitrios Boskou

Aristotle University of Thessaloniki, School of Chemistry, Laboratory of Food Chemistry and Technology, Thessaloniki, Greece

In the realm of the traditional food arena, olive oil and its products are a dominant class that continues to grow. Olive oil is an integral ingredient of the diet of the countries surrounding the Mediterranean Sea. It has always been the main source of fat in the cuisine of these countries. In the past few years, however, olive oil has been gaining interest among consumers of Northern Europe, the USA, Australia and other countries, although these new consumers are not always familiar with the properties and characteristics of this valuable natural product. The growing enthusiasm about the 'Mediterranean diet' and olive oil is mainly due to the belief that there is a positive role of this diet in the prevention of certain diseases and in particular of coronary heart disease. The prevailing theories concerning the demonstrated success of the Mediterranean diet in protecting against ischemic heart disease relate the health benefits to (a) the consumption of lesser amounts of saturated fats; (b) the consumption of greater amounts of monounsaturated fatty acids due to olive oil, and (c) the intake of omega-3 fatty acids from fish, wild plants, nuts and legumes.

Benefits of the Mediterranean diet have also been connected to bioactive compounds such as vitamins and natural antioxidants. The latter are a big category of organic compounds, which comprises flavonoids, hydroxycinnamic acids and other phenolic acids, and polar phenols. Such compounds occur naturally in fruits, vegetables, nuts, seeds, whole grain products, herbal teas, wine and olive oil. The nonglyceridic fraction of the latter is a rich source of antioxidant phenols.

Olive oil has been used for centuries for culinary purposes, but it has been relatively recently the subject of thorough research. Chemical and analytical work to elucidate the structure and to quantify minor constituents is now progressing rapidly and it is hoped that the precise information about actual composition and levels of key functional components, mainly polar phenols, will be properly used in future studies to be set up for the evaluation of olive oil's beneficial effect on health.

What differentiates olive oil chemically from fats used in other diets will be described in this chapter. Some culinary applications in the Mediterranean area will also be discussed with emphasis on chemical composition and the presence of functional and other minor ingredients, such as sterols, carotenoids, beta-tocopherol and polar phenolic compounds.

Olive Oil Composition

The composition of olive oil is primarily triacylglycerols and secondarily free fatty acids and some 0.5–1.5% nonglyceridic constituents. Extra virgin olive oil has maximum acidity in terms of oleic acid, 0.8 g/100 g; virgin olive oil, 2 g/100 g. Extensive information for the chemistry and composition of olive oil is provided in the reviews by Boskou [1, 2], and also in the International Olive Oil Council (IOOC) Standards [3], the Codex Alimentarius Standards [4] and the European Commission Regulations [5].

Fatty Acids and Triacylglycerols
The major fatty acids of olive oil are: palmitic 7.5–20%, stearic 0.5–5%, palmitoleic 0.3–3.5%, oleic 55–83%, linoleic 3.5–21% and linolenic 0.0–1%. Other fatty acids can also be found in trace amounts: myristic ≤0.05%, heptadecanoic ≤0.3%, heptadecenoic ≤0.3%, arachidic ≤0.6%, eicosanoic ≤0.4%, behenic ≤0.2%, lignoceric ≤0.2%. This composition differentiates olive oil from other edible vegetable oils, with the exception of high oleic sunflower oil and hazelnut oil which have a similar fatty acid profile.

The fatty acid composition of olive oil depends on the zone of production, the variety, the latitude, the climatic conditions, and the maturity of the fruit. Spanish, Italian, and Greek olive oils are low in linoleic and palmitic acids and have a higher percentage of oleic acid. Olive oils from Tunisia have a high linoleic and palmitic acid content and a lower oleic acid content. Expansion of olive oil tree cultivation in countries such as Australia, New Zealand, and South Africa created the need for a more general survey by the IOOC on the fatty acid composition of virgin olive oil produced around the world. A revision of Codex Alimentarius standards, in order to be more representative of global production, is expected.

The triacylglycerol profile of olive oil is also different from profiles of other vegetable oils such as maize, cotton seed, sunflower seed, soybean, rapeseed oil, etc. The major triacylglycerols found in olive oil are OOO, POO, OOL, POL and SOO (O = oleic acid; P = palmitic acid; S = stearic acid; L = linoleic acid;

Ln = linolenic acid). Smaller amounts of OLO, POP, PLO, POS, OLnL, LOL, OLnO, PLL, PLnO and LLL are also encountered [5]. Like other vegetable oils, olive oil has a high concentration of unsaturated fatty acids and a low concentration of palmitic and stearic acid in position 2 of the triacylglycerol molecule. Fully saturated triacylglycerols and triunsaturated triacylglycerols with three linolenic acids in all the three positions have not been detected.

Slight deviations from the 1,3-random, 2-random distribution of fatty acids in the glycerol moiety of olive oil triacylglycerols have been observed by Santinelli et al. [6] and Vlahov et al. [7]. At the 2-position lower amounts of oleic acid and higher amounts of linoleic acid were found in comparison to those expected from the calculations based on the theoretical random patterns.

Triacylglycerols determined by high-performance liquid chromatography (HPLC) are used to check authenticity of olive oil. Trilinolein or equivalent chain number (ECN) 42 triacylglycerols is the sum of LLL, PoPoPo, SLLn, PoPoL, PPoL, PPoLn, OLLn, PLLn, and PoOLn (Po = palmitoleic acid). This sum is compared to theoretically calculated values based on the fatty acid composition and distribution patterns.

Partial Glycerides

Monoacyl- and diacylglycerols are always present in small quantities in olive oil. The presence of partial glycerides is due either to incomplete biosynthesis of triacylglycerols or hydrolysis. In virgin olive oil, the concentration of diacylglycerols (DG) is in the range of 1–2.8% [8, 9]. Monoacylglycerols occur in much smaller quantities (less than 0.25%). During storage 1,2-diacylglycerols isomerize to the more stable diacylglycerols. This change is a good index for the age and quality of the oil [10, 11].

Free Fatty Acids

The limit for the free fatty acids content, expressed as oleic acid %, is different for each type of olive oil (see 'Quality and Genuineness').

Minor Constituents

The various classes of minor constituents can be divided into two classes: those which are fatty acid derivatives and compounds with different chemical structure. Phospholipids, waxes, and sterylesters belong to the first class. Hydrocarbons, aliphatic alcohols, free sterols, tocopherols, pigments, and polar phenols such as hydroxytyrosol to the second class.

Hydrocarbons

Squalene (2,6,10,15,19,23,hexamethyl,2,6,10,14,18,22-tetracosahexaene) is a highly unsaturated aliphatic hydrocarbon with important biological properties.

It is a metabolic precursor of cholesterol and other sterols. As an oxygen carrier, it has been extensively researched and found to play a key role in maintaining health [12, 13]. Today there are claims that squalene can enhance the quality of life, if taken continuously, and that its consumption is beneficial for patients with heart disease, diabetes, arthritis, hepatitis, and other diseases. Squalene is found in large quantities in shark liver oil and occurs also in small amounts in olive oil (approximately 0.5%), wheat germ oil, bran oil, and yeast. The presence of squalene in olive oil probably makes a significant contribution to the health effects of the latter. A chemopreventive effect of squalene on colon cancer has been reported by Rao et al. [14].

Smith et al. [15] studied the inhibition of 4-(methylnitrosamino)-1-(3-pyridyl)-1-butanone-induced lung tumorigenesis by dietary olive oil and squalene in the mouse. The squalene diet decreased significantly lung hyperplasia. These findings support the hypothesis that squalene possesses chemopreventive activity, further suggesting that frequent olive oil consumption may be a protective factor against lung or colon cancer. The abstract of a patent published in 1999 [16] indicates that a functional food can be prepared by mechanical extraction of grain germs (wheat germ or maize germ) with extra virgin olive oil. Obviously the inventor aims at combining beneficial effects of the minor constituents present in the oils such as tocopherols and squalene.

Squalene has been reported to possess weak antioxidant properties and may have a protective role toward alpha-tocopherol oxidation [17]. Squalene content is dramatically reduced during the process of refining.

The other important hydrocarbon of olive oil is beta-carotene. This is discussed in the 'Carotenoids' section. Trace amounts of other hydrocarbons are also present; they are diterpene or triterpene hydrocarbons, isoprenoid polyolefins and n-paraffins [18].

Sterols

Phytosterols are functional ingredients. They have an absorption level 20 times lower than that of cholesterol; the latter is absorbed in the digestive system in significant amounts [19]. This difference in absorption affects the availability of phytosterols and cholesterol and has nutritional implications. It is known since the 1950's that phytosterols inhibit cholesterol absorption in the body during digestion. Erickson [20] prepared the first hypocholesteremic product based on sterols. It was a shortening suitable for cooking and frying, which contained an oil base with 1.5–3.0% beta-sitosterol or stigmasterol oleate. Recently, methods have been developed for manufacturing sterol esters, which are added to spreads like margarine. These spreads have a cholesterol-lowering effect and they are considered as a type of 'functional food'.

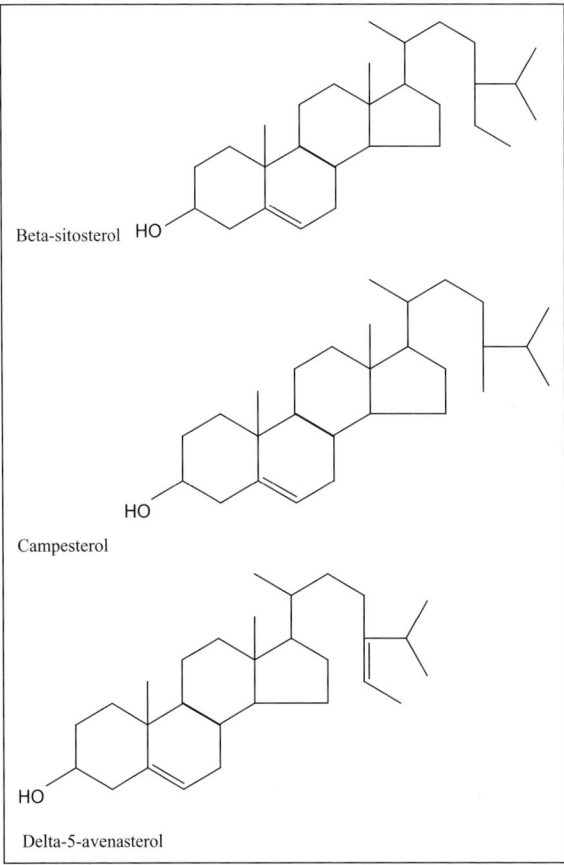

Fig. 1. The main desmethylsterols present in olive oil.

Four classes of sterols occur in olive oil, common sterols (4-alpha-desmethylsterols), 4-alpha-methylsterols, triterpene alcohols (4,4-dimethylsterols), and triterpene dialcohols.

Common Sterols (4-Alpha-Methylsterols). This is the major class in olive oil. Usual values reported for this class are 1,000–2,000 mg/kg. Lampante oils may have higher levels [5].

Part of total sterols is present as esters with fatty acids but also as steryl-glycosides. The main components of this sterol fraction are beta-sitosterol, campesterol and delta-5-avenasterol (fig. 1) [1, 5]. Other sterols or stanols present in smaller quantities or in trace amounts are stigmasterol, cholesterol, brassicasterol, chlerosterol, ergosterol, sitostanol, campestanol, delta-7-avenasterol, delta-7-cholestanol, delta-7-campesterol, delta-7-stigmasterol, delta-5,23-stigmastadienol, delta-5,24-stigmastadienol, delta-7,22-ergostadienol, delta-7,24-ergostadienol, 24-methylene-cholesterol, and 22,23-dihydrobrassicasterol. Refining causes a loss of sterols as high as 25%.

The level and composition of sterol is affected by the cultivar, crop year, ripeness and storage of the fruit, geographical origin and processing.

Virgin olive oil shows a remarkable resistance to oxidation and polymerization during domestic deep-frying of potatoes or in other uses at frying temperatures [21, 22]. Compared to other vegetable oils such as sunflower, cotton seed oil, corn oil and soybean oil, olive oil shows a significantly lower rate of alteration, as demonstrated by measurements of viscosity, total polar compounds, and loss of tocopherols. This increased stability to thermal oxidation explains why this oil can be used for repeated frying operations before reaching the rejection point of approximately 27% total polar compounds.

A possible explanation for the resistance of olive oil to rapid deterioration at elevated temperatures might be the presence of natural antioxidants. Delta-5-avenasterol is probably responsible for this resistance, because it has an ethylidene group in the side chain. Sterols with this structural feature retard oxidative polymerization in heated triacylglycerols [23, 24].

4-Alpha-Methylsterols. 4-Alpha-methylsterols present in olive oil in small amounts are also found as free sterols and esters [25, 26]. The main constituents of this sterol fraction are obtusifoliol, gramisterol, cycloeucalenol, and citrostadienol [1]. The level of total 4-alpha-methylsterols varies from 50 to 360 mg/kg.

Triterpene Alcohols. This class of minor components is also very complex. The main triterpene alcohols are beta-amyrin, butyrospermol, 24-methylene cycloartanol, and cycloartenol. Others found in minute quantities are cyclobranol, cycloradol, dammaradienol, germaniol, 24-methylene-24-dihydroparkeol, taraxerol, alpha-amyrin,7,4-tirucallodienol, parkeol, and tirucallol [27]. Triterpene alcohols are present in the free and esterified form. Total triterpene alcohol levels have been found to vary between 350 and 1,500 mg/kg [25, 28–31].

Triterpene Dialcohols. Virgin olive oil contains erythrodiol (homo-olestranol, 5α-olean-12-ene-3β,28-diol) and uvaol (o^{12}-ursen-3β,28-diol) at levels usually lower than 50 mg/kg. Solvent extracted oil has a higher content [5].

Fatty Alcohol, Waxes and Diterpene Alcohols

Aliphatic and aromatic alcohols occur in olive oil in the free and esterified form. The most important are fatty alcohols and diterpene alcohols. Alkanols and alkenols with less than ten carbon atoms like benzyl alcohol and 2-phenyl ethanol have been reported to be constituents of the volatile fraction. Fatty alcohols are mainly linear saturated alcohols with more than 20 carbon atoms such as docosanol, tetracosanol, hexacosanol, and octacosanol [2, 32]. The level of fatty alcohols depends on the cultivar, crop year, fruit ripeness, and processing. Among the various homologues, tetracosanol and hexacosanol were found to be present at higher levels. Esters of fatty alcohols with fatty acids (waxes) are important minor constituents because they are used as a criterion to differentiate various olive oil types [5].

Diterpene Alcohols

Phytol and geranylgeraniol are two acyclic diterpenoids present in the aliphatic alcohol fraction of olive oil in the free and esterified form [2]. Levels of geranylgeraniol are used in the calculation of the Alcoholic Index, a useful parameter for detecting extracted olive oil in virgin olive oil.

Tocopherols

Tocopherols are important fat-soluble vitamins. They contribute to the stability of an oil and they also have a beneficial biological role as quenchers of free radicals in vivo. Dietary benefits of olive oil are partly attributed to its fatty acid composition and partly to the presence of alpha-tocopherol and other natural antioxidants. Alpha-tocopherol acts not only as a free radical trapping agent but also as a singlet oxygen quencher. This protective effect against photo-oxidation is enhanced by the presence of beta-carotene.

Research on the levels of tocopherols in virgin olive oils indicated that this depends on the cultivar and technological factors. Application of good manufacturing practice and quality control have a positive impact on tocopherol levels, which are today much higher than the mean value of 100 mg/kg reported in the past [33, 34]. This is important, taking into consideration the biological properties of alpha-tocopherol.

Data for Italian and Spanish oils show a rather wide range of tocopherol levels (55–350 mg/kg) [28, 35–40]. Compared to them, Greek oils have alpha-tocopherol levels that are among the highest. For the crop seasons 1994–1995, 1995–1996 and 1996–1997, Psomiadou et al. [41] reported values of alpha-tocopherol of 127–370, 98–333 and 100–365 mg/kg, respectively. From the four known E-vitamers, alpha-tocopherol comprises 90% of the total tocopherol content.

Alpha-tocopherol is found in the free form. Low amounts of the homologues beta-tocopherol (approx. 10 mg/kg), delta-tocopherol (approx. 10 mg/kg) and gamma-tocopherol (approx. 20 mg/kg) are usually reported. Refining and hydrogenation cause losses of tocopherols.

Blekas et al. [42] examined the effect of alpha-tocopherol and its concentration on olive oil triglyceride stability. They found that this phenol acts as an antioxidant at all levels but the antioxidant effect is greater at low concentrations (100 mg/kg) than at higher concentrations (500–1,000 mg/kg). In the presence of more effective antioxidants such as ortho-diphenols, alpha-tocopherol did not show any significant antioxidant activity during the period of low peroxide accumulation, but acted well when the primary oxidation products reached a critical point. An extension of this study [43] indicated that o-diphenols are consumed first. Morello et al. [44], however, states that the compound is consumed from the beginning. In all cases, alpha-tocopherol contributes to the stability of the oil and retains its protective effect at levels of acidity and peroxide value near the regulatory limits.

Volatile and Aroma Compounds

Volatile compounds present in olive oil have been reported by many investigators [45–53]. More than 250 constituents have been identified. These are mainly hydrocarbons, alcohols, aldehydes, ketones, acids, esters, ethers, and furan derivatives.

Some of the volatile compounds are odorless (hexane, octane), while others make a very small contribution to the flavor at the concentrations they are found. Guth and Grosch [47] and Blekas and Guth [54] indicated that a rather limited number of compounds in the complex mixtures of volatiles causes the characteristic odours of various olive oils. Certain compounds are responsible for important flavor attributes, for example: (z)-3-hexenal for the 'green, apple like' odor; hexanal for the 'grassy' odor; ethyl-2-methylpropanate and ethyl-2-methylbutanoate for the 'fruity' odor; and heptanal, various octenals, nonenals, and decenals for the 'fatty' odor.

Approximately 20 compounds contribute to the sensory defects [48, 54, 55].

Other Minor Constituents

Triterpene Acids

Hydroxy pentacyclic triterpene acids are important olive fruit constituents. They are biologically active compounds. They are also present at trace amounts in olive oil [2]. Oleanolic (3β-hydroxyolean-12-en-28-oic acid) and maslinic acid (2α, 3β-dihydroxyolean-12-en-28-oic acid) are the main triterpene acids present in virgin olive oil, because they occur in the olive husk and a small quantity may be extracted during processing. Both compounds and traces of ursolic acid (3β-hydroxyurs-12-en-28-oic acid) are also located in the reticular lipid layer of olive skin (fig. 2).

Phospholipids

Experimental work for the identification of phospholipids in olive oil is rather limited. Phosphatidylcholine, phospatidylethanolamine, phosphatitylinositol and phosphatidylserine were reported to be the main phospholipids

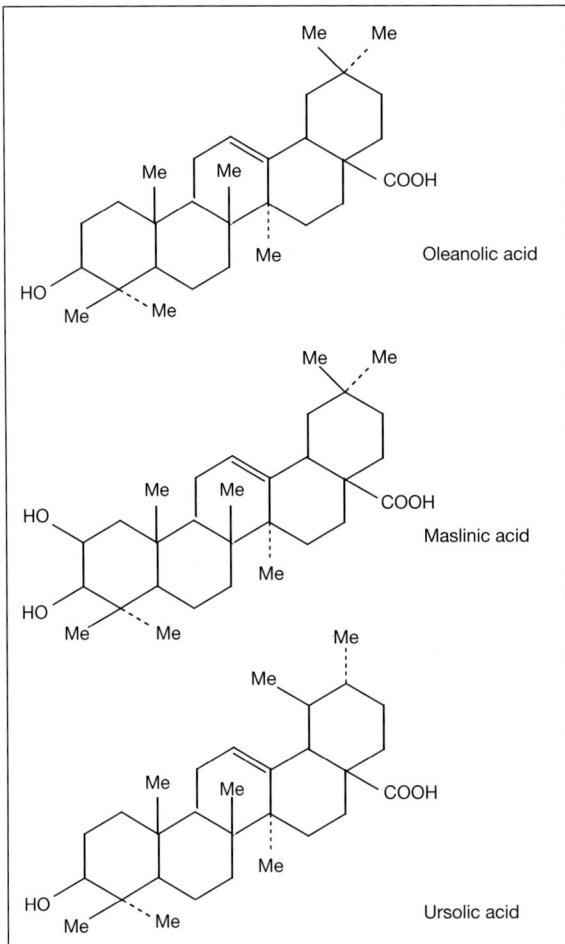

Fig. 2. Triterpene acids present in olive oil.

present in olive oil [56]. The fatty acid composition was found to be similar to that of triacylglycerols.

In a recent report Boukhcinas et al. [57] identified glycerophospholipids present in olive oil by liquid chromatography-mass spectrometry (LC-MS). Phosphatidylethanolamine, phosphatidylcholine, phosphatidylinositol, phosphatidic acid, and also phosphatidylglycerol were the phospholipids identified and quantified. Phosphatidylserine was not detected. However, the study was based only on one sample from the retail market.

The level of phospholipids may be important because these compounds have an antioxidant activity. According to Pokorny and Korczak [58] they may act as synergists (regeneration of antioxidants such as alpha-tocopherol or other phenols) or as metal scavengers. At high levels, however, phospholipids may cause foaming or darkening during frying. The possible contribution of phospholipids to the oxidative stability of olive oil has not been studied. Koidis and Boskou [59] determined phosphorous in cloudy olive oils, filtered oils, and refined oils. Values obtained were in the range of 1–6 mg P/kg oil (n = 26), corresponding to approximately 20–156 mg P/kg oil. The higher level of phospholipids in the unfiltered oils may be an additional antioxidant factor to phenols. These veiled oils were found to be more stable to oxidation and this was attributed to the higher levels of polar phenols [60].

Proteins
Minute quantities of proteins may be detected mainly in unfiltered oils [59].

Polar Phenolic Compounds

Epidemiological and laboratory studies conducted in the last 30 years suggest that the consumption of olive oil provides health benefits that are related to its fatty acid composition and the presence of minor constituents [61]. An important class of bioactive minor constituents are polar phenols, known also as olive oil 'polyphenols'. The term polyphenols is conventional since not all of them are polyhydroxy compounds.

Polar phenolics present in olive oil, in addition to their bioactivity, are also important for the keepability (shelf life) and flavor of the oil. Chemically, they belong to the following classes [2, 62–66] (fig. 3):

- *Phenolic acids* (4-hydroxybenzoic acid, protocatechuic acid, syringic acid, 4-hydroxyphenylacetic acid, homovanillic acid, o- and p-coumaric acids, caffeic acid, ferulic acid, sinapic acid, gallic acid).
- *Tyrosol, hydroxytyrosol and their derivatives* (oleuropein, ligstroside, aglycones of oleuropein and ligstroside, deacetoxy and dialdehydic forms of the aglycones, hydroxytyrosol acetate).
- *Flavones* (luteolin, apigenin).
- *Lignans* (pinoresinol, acetoxypinoresinol, syringaresinol).
- *Hydroxy-isochromans.*

Litridou et al. [67] reported the presence of an ester of tyrosol with a dicarboxylic acid. The total polar phenol content and o-diphenols was higher in the less polar part of the methanol-water extracts. Glycosides were found to be present only in trace amounts. García et al. [64] and Tovar et al. [68] determined the dialdehydic forms of elenolic acid linked to hydroxytyrosol and tyrosol, 1-acetoxy-ethyl-1,2-dihydroxybenzene (hydroxytyrosol acetate),

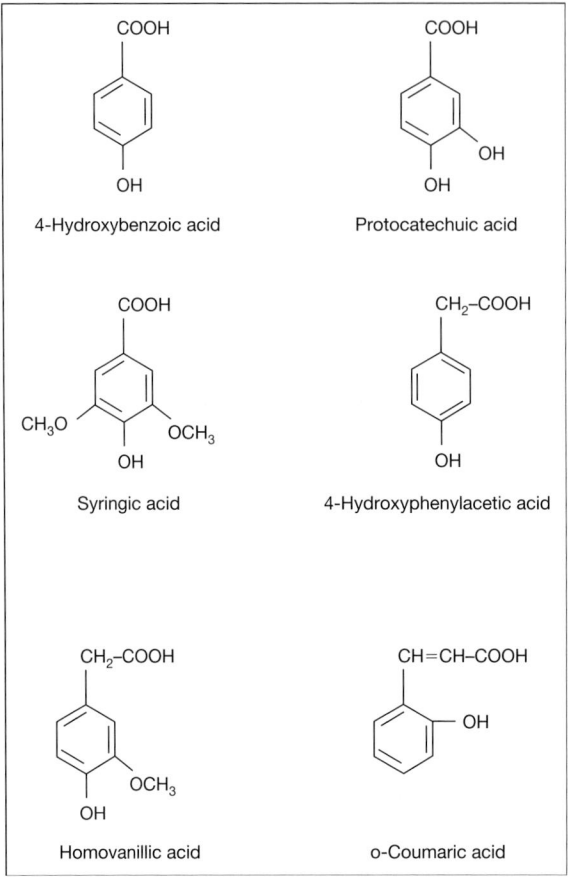

Fig. 3. Polar phenols present in olive oil.

1-acetoxypinoresinol, pinoresinol, oleuropein aglycone, luteolin, and ligstroside aglycone as phenols with the higher concentration. Oleocanthal, a compound present mainly in freshly pressed extra virgin olive oil, was found to have the same pharmacological activity as the anti-inflammatory drug Ibuprofen [69].

The total polar phenolic compound content differs from oil to oil. Levels are usually between 100 and 300 mg/kg, but wider ranges (50–1000 mg/kg) have also been reported.

Polyphenols and Keepability (Shelf Life)

A high polyphenol content is beneficial for the shelf life of the oil, as indicated by a good correlation of stability and total polyphenol content [70, 71].

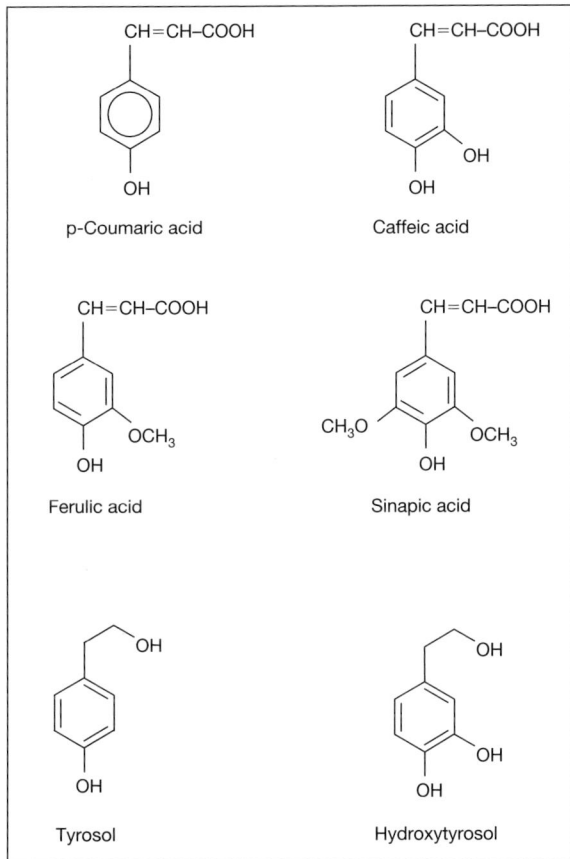

Fig. 3. (continued)

Hydroxytyrosol and mainly aglycone forms of oleuropein make a significant contribution to the antioxidant effect [72].

Polyphenols and Sensory Properties

If not excessive, the bitter taste of virgin olive oil is considered a positive attribute and related to the concentration of polar phenolic compounds [73, 74]. For the bitterness, the dialdeydic and aldeydic forms of decarboxymethyl-oleuropein and ligstroside aglycones were found to be mainly responsible. According to Andrewes et al. [75], who also studied the relation between sensory characteristics and individual phenols, the deacetoxy-ligstroside aglycone has a strong burning pungent sensation at the back of the throat. The acetoxy-oleuropein

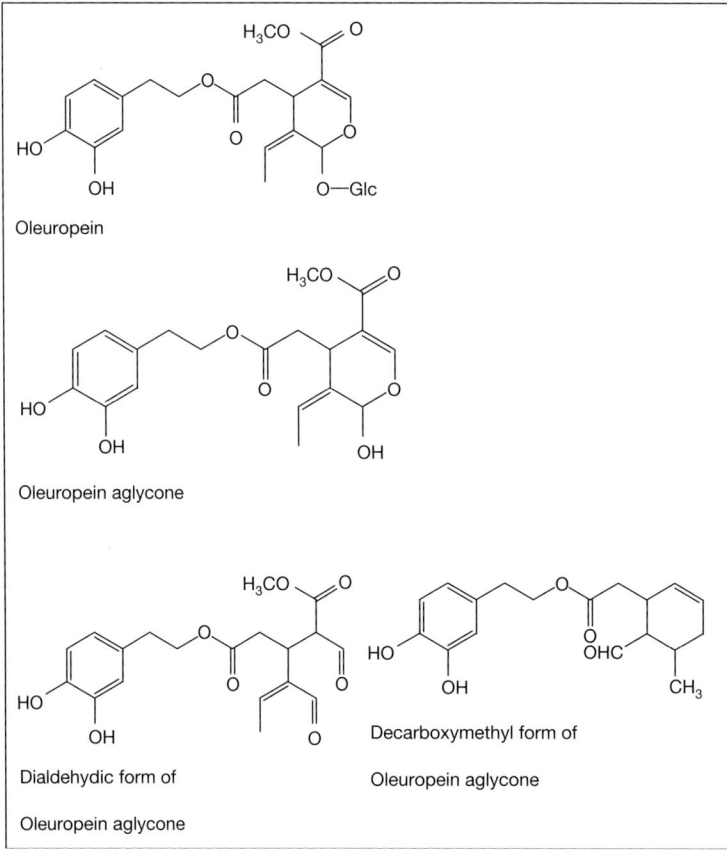

Fig. 3. (continued)

aglycone has a slight burning taste and the sensation is perceived mainly on the tongue. Tyrosol was found to be bitter but not astringent. The authors concluded that pungent virgin olive oils have a higher deacetoxy-ligstroside aglycone level. The bitter and pungent taste of olive oils has also been evaluated by Beauchamp et al. [69] and Mateos et al. [76].

Antioxidant Properties

The number of publications related to the biological role of olive oil and its minor constituents is increasing continuously. The accumulated data suggest that olive oil polar phenols contribute to the health benefits attributed to the Mediterranean diet. The latter is believed to be linked to a lower incidence of coronary heart disease, prostate and colon cancer [77–80]. The potential of

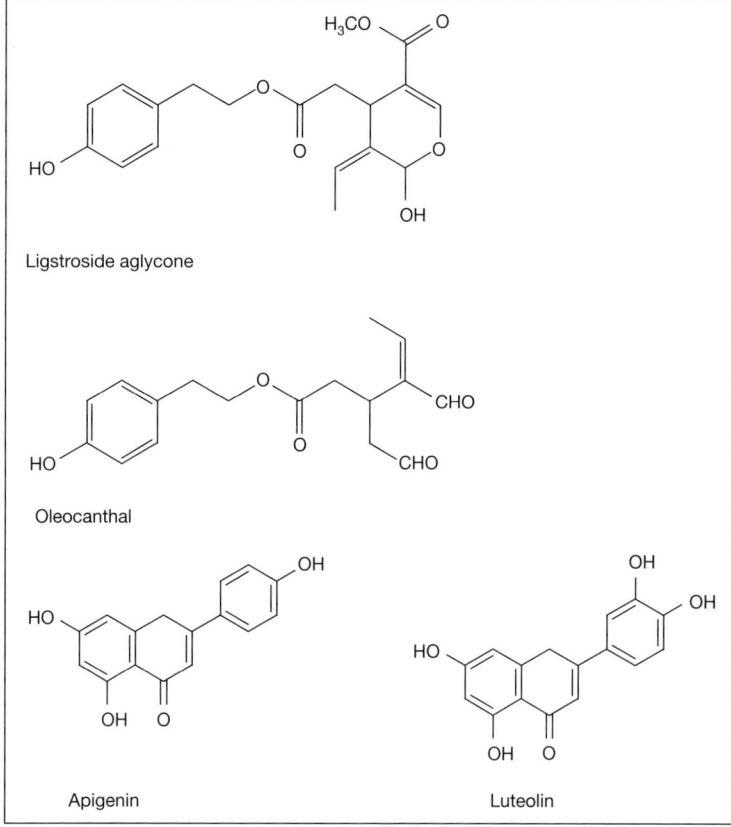

Fig. 3. (continued)

olive oil phenols to scavenge synthetic radicals, peroxy radicals, superoxide radicals and hypochlorous acid and to reduce damage due to hydrogen peroxide and peroxynitrate has been discussed in reviews authored by Tuck and Hayball [81], Visioli et al. [82] and Boskou et al. [83].

Low-Density Lipoprotein Oxidation. The in vivo lipoprotein oxidation is considered a dominant risk factor for the development of atherosclerosis [84, 85]. Phenolic compounds present in olive oil are potent in vitro inhibitors of low-density lipoprotein (LDL) oxidation. This was demonstrated in a series of papers by Visioli and Galli [82]. Still, the effect of olive oil phenols in vivo on the oxidizability of LDL is not yet clear [86].

Visioli's work, concentrated mainly on hydroxyltyrosol and its derivatives, stimulated experimental studies with other olive oil bioactive phenols.

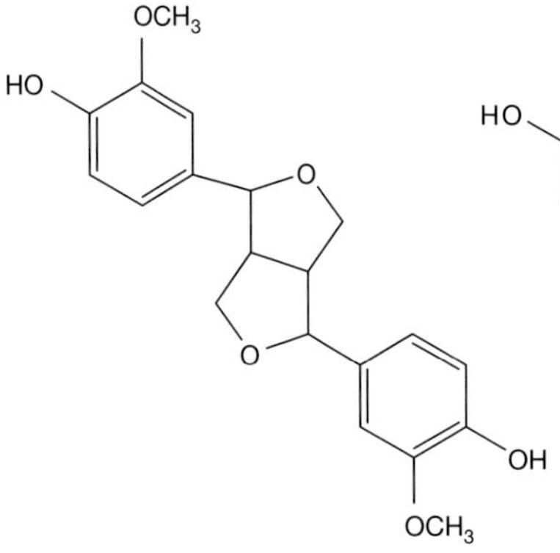

Pinoresinol

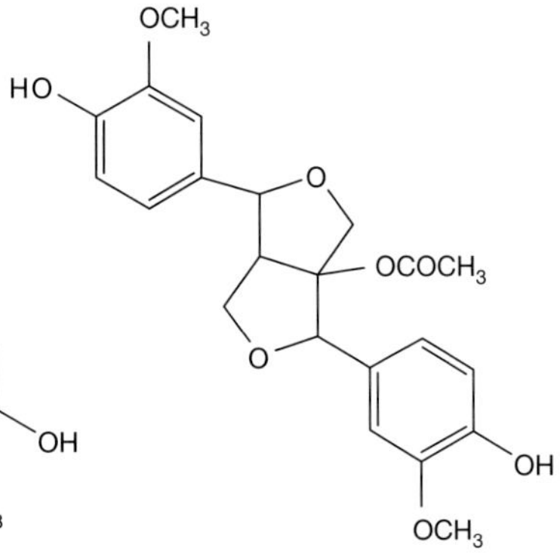

Acetoxypinoresinol

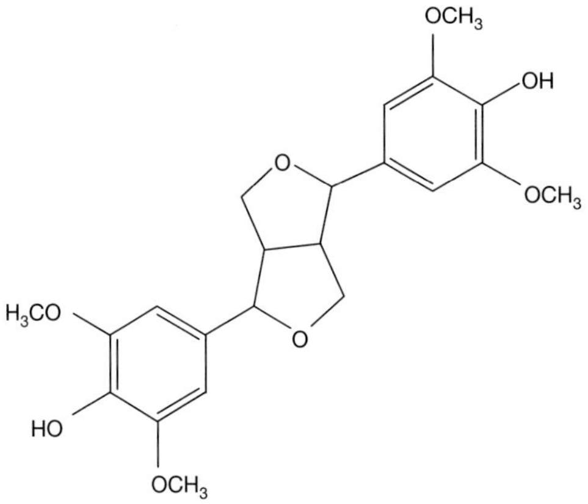

Syringaresinol

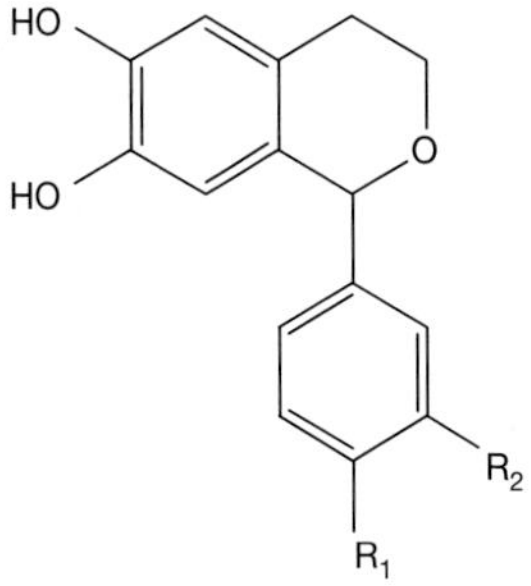

1-phenyl-6,7-dihydroxy-isochroman $R_1=H, R_2=H$

Fig. 3. (continued)

Nardini et al. [87] studied the activity of caffeic and other hydroxycinnamic acids on in vitro LDL oxidation with Cu^{2+}. Protocatechuic acid was studied by Masella et al. [88], who used macrophage-like cells in the LDL model oxidation.

Coni et al. [89] conducted an in vivo study with rabbits fed special diets containing olive oil and oleuropein. The biochemical parameters measured in the rabbit plasma and the isolated LDL verified the antioxidant efficiency of oleuropein.

Masella et al. [90] studied the effect of dietary intake of extra virgin olive oil on the oxidative susceptibility of LDL, isolated from the plasma of hyperlipidemic patients. The intake of extra virgin olive oil did not affect LDL fatty acid composition but significantly reduced the formation of LDL oxidation products induced by $CuSO_4$. These results are attributed to the presence of phenolic antioxidants in olive oil.

Fito et al. [91] indicated that inhibition of LDL oxidation in vitro is enhanced by olive oil phenols.

Isoprostane Formation. The isoprostanes, prostaglandin-like compounds formed from peroxidation of long-chain PUFA, are used as biochemical markers for the assessment of oxidant stress and lipid peroxidation [84]. Visioli et al. [92] evaluated in humans the antioxidant activity of phenols with a catecholic structural feature. Human volunteers were administered olive oil with varying levels of o-diphenols. Isoprostane 8-iso-PGF_{2a} was determined in the urine by mass spectrometry after incubation with β-glucuronidase. It was concluded that the administration of hydroxytyrosol and oleuropein aglycones results in a dose-dependent reduction of the urinary formation of isoprostanes.

Scavenging of Radicals and Other Reactive Species. Free radical scavenging activity of hydroxytrosol and its derivatives using 1,7-diphenyl-2-picrylhydrazyl radical (DPPH•.) was measured by Visioli et al. [93], Saija et al. [94], Gordon et al. [95], Tuck et al. [96], and Lavelli [97]. Tuck et al. [96] studied the scavenging activity not only of hydroxytyrosol but also of its metabolites in rats (homovanillic acid, homovanillic alcohol, glucuronide conjugate, and sulphate conjugate). The glucuronide was found to be a more potent antioxidant compared to hydroxytyrosol itself. Saija et al. [94], in addition to the DPPH test, conducted additional measurements to obtain more information for the scavenging activity of hydroxytyrosol and oleuropein against peroxyl radicals near the membrane surface and within the membranes, using a model system consisting of dipalmitoylphosphatidylcholine/linoleic acid unilamellar vesicles and a water soluble azo compounds and free radical generator.

The radical scavenging capacity of the major phenols present in olive oil was also measured by Briante et al. [98], who used the stable red radical cation DMPD•+. The same authors attempted to differentiate phenols on the basis of their ability to scavenge radicals and to chelate metal ions. In order to evaluate olive oil as a source of antioxidants, many researchers used ORAC (oxygen radical absorbance capacity) value determination, an indication of the capacity to protect against oxidation by peroxyl radicals [99].

Pellegrini et al. [100] determined TRAP (total-radical trapping antioxidant parameter), TEAC (trolox equivalent antioxidant capacity), and FRAP (ferric-reducing antioxidant capacity) in plant food beverages and various edible oils including olive oil in an attempt to obtain additional information, necessary to investigate the relation between antioxidant intake and diseases related to oxidative stress.

Scavenging of Reactive Nitrogen Species. Deiana et al. [101] found that hydroxytyrosol was very protective against peroxynitrite dependent nitration of tyrosine and DNA damage by peroxynitrite in vitro.

Scavenging activities of the major olive oil phenols against reactive nitrogen species (nitric oxide, peroxinitrite) were studied by De la Puerta et al. [102]. Caffeic acid, oleuropein, and hydroxytyrosol reduced the amount of nitric oxide formed by sodium nitroprusside and were also found to have the ability to reduce chemically generated peroxinitrite.

Quality and Genuineness

Good quality olive oil means an oil with chemical, organoleptic, nutritional and culinary characteristics that give the product a market value satisfying the consumers and the producers. The quest of quality is based on the applications of clearly defined rules during growing and processing of olives and retail packing of oil. The final product should comply with the established characteristics, whose traceability can be documented [103].

Consumers are now more aware of the potential health benefits of virgin olive oil and their choice is high quality oil that preserves the flavor and its minor constituents. Due to significant differences in the prices there is always a temptation for fraudulent action, such as mixing virgin olive with cheap vegetable oils or olive oils of inferior quality. In the last two decades, many methodologies have been developed to detect possible frauds, based mainly on gas chromatography, HPLC and spectrometry. Some of these analytical techniques have been incorporated into the standards of the European Union Commission regulations. Others, not yet adopted, may be used to support non-conclusive results from official analyses or for a rapid assessment of quality or identity.

Definitions [3–5]
Extra virgin olive oil. Virgin olive oil having free acidity, as % of oleic acid, up to 0.8, and the other characteristics according to regulations in force.

Virgin olive oil. Virgin olive oil having free acidity, as % of oleic acid, up to 2.0, and the other characteristics according to regulations in force.

Ordinary Virgin Olive Oil. Virgin olive oil having free acidity, as % of oleic acid, up to 3.3, and the other characteristics according to regulations in force. (Note: EU regulations do not include this category.)

Virgin Lampante Olive Oil. Virgin olive oil having free acidity, as % of oleic acid, greater than 3.3, and the other characteristics according to regulations in force.

Refined Olive Oil. Olive oil obtained from virgin olive oil refining that preserves its natural glyceridic composition, having free acidity, as % of oleic acid, up to 0.3, and the other characteristics according to regulations in force.

Olive Oil. Oil obtained by blending refined olive oil and virgin olive oil having free acidity, as % of oleic acid, up to 1.0, and the other characteristics according to regulations in force.

Crude Pomace Olive Oil. Oil extracted from olive pomace by means of a solvent having the characteristics according to regulations in force.

Refined Olive Pomace Oil. Oil obtained from crude olive pomace oil by refining that preserves its natural glyceridic composition, having free acidity, as % of oleic acid, up to 0.3, and the other characteristics according to regulations in force.

Olive Residue Oil. Oil obtained by blending refined olive residue oil and virgin olive oil having free acidity, as % of oleic acid, up to 1.0, and the other characteristics according to regulations in force.

Characteristics of Extra Virgin Olive Oil (EVOO) and Virgin Olive Oil (VOO)

Free acidity (as oleic acid %).	EVOO ≤ 0.8	VOO ≤ 2
Peroxide value (mEq oxygen/kg oil)	EVOO ≤ 20	VOO ≤ 20
Specific spectrophotometric constants		
K232	EVOO ≤ 2.50	VOO ≤ 2.60
K270	EVOO ≤ 0.22	VOO ≤ 0.25
Delta K	EVOO ≤ 0.001	VOO ≤ 0.001

These constants are related to the presence of conjugated dienes and trienes formed during autoxidation and treatment. Delta K is calculated from the specific absorbances at 270 nm.

Organoleptic Assessment

Md defect (median of predominant defect)	EVOO 0	VOO ≤ 2.5
Md fruity (median of fruity)	EVOO >0	VOO >0

The medians are calculated from the intensities assigned by the tasters on a scale and are compared to levels adopted for each grade.

Metals

Iron should not exceed 3 mg/kg and copper 0.1 mg/kg. These transition metals should be kept at the lowest possible levels because they are pro-oxidant.

Moisture and Volatile Matter
EVOO ≤0.2%   VOO ≤0.2%
Fatty acid composition   Myristic acid   EVOO ≤0.05%   VOO ≤0.05%
                         Linolenic acid   EVOO ≤1%   VOO ≤1%
                         Arachidic acid   EVOO ≤0.6%   VOO ≤0.6%
                         Eicosenoic acid EVOO ≤0.04%   VOO ≤0.04%
                         Behenic acid   EVOO ≤0.02%   VOO ≤0.02%

The accepted ranges for the fatty acids are based on a joint position on the revision of the Codex Alimentarius Standard for olive oil. The harmonization occurred in 2003 [102]. The limits may be slightly changed in the near future when a worldwide survey of olive oil production arranged by the IOOC is over and the new data are examined by the Codex Alimentarius Committee on Fats and Oils.

Trans Unsaturated Fatty Acids (% of Total Fatty Acids)
Total *trans* monoenes   EVOO ≤0.05   VOO ≤0.05
Total *trans* polyenes   EVOO ≤0.05   VOO ≤0.05

Virgin olive oil contains only *cis* isomers of unsaturated fatty acids. A partial isomerization takes place in the refining process.

Saturated Fatty Acids at 2-Position
EVOO ≤1.5%   VOO ≤1.5%

During biosynthesis of triacylglycerols very low amounts of saturated fatty acids are esterified at position 2 of the glycerol moiety. This is the basis for the detection of adulteration with chemically prepared oils from refining by-products. In the synthetic oils the 1,3-random-2-random distribution cannot be reproduced.

Delta CN 42 Values
EVOO ≤0.2   VOO ≤0.2
Sterol composition

	% of total sterols	
	EVOO	VOO
Cholesterol	≤0.5	≤0.5
Brassicasterol	≤0.1	≤0.1
Campesterol	≤0.4	≤0.4
Beta-sitosterol	≤93	≤93
Delta-7-stigmasterol	≤0.5	≤0.5

The sterol profile is quite characteristic of each botanical species. Therefore, the analysis of the sterol fraction is useful in the detection of olive oil adulteration with foreign oils; beta-sitosterol percentage is calculated from the peaks of delta-5,23-stigmastadienol, chlerosterol, beta-sitosterol, sitostanol, delta-5-avenasterol and delta-5,24-stigmastadienol.

Erythrodiol and Uvaol (% of Total Sterols)
EVOO ≤0.45   VOO ≤0.45
High levels of the two diols, waxes and aliphatic alcohols are indicative of the presence of oil obtained by extraction from the olive residues, since these compounds accumulate in the skin of the fruit.

Waxes
EVOO ≤250 mg/kg (the sum of   VOO ≤250 mg/kg.
C40+ C42 +C44 + C46)

Stigmastadiene
EVOO ≤0.15 mg/kg   VOO ≤0.15 mg/kg
Unsaturated hydrocarbons with a steroidal structure are formed by dehydration of sterols during refining. These limits are useful in detecting the presence of oils subjected to bleaching and thermal treatment.

Other Properties Used to Evaluate Quality not Included in International Standards
Polar phenolic compounds are important for the keepability (shelf life) of the oil (see 'Relative' section).

Partial glycerides are also useful to check quality and freshness. The ratio of 1,3-diacylglycerols is considered a good parameter, as fresh virgin olive oil contains initially mainly 1,2-diglycerides. During preservation 1,3-diglycerides are formed.

Refining may cause isomerization of triterpene alcohols, due to the opening of the C3 carbon atom and translocation of the double bond. The detection of the formed isomers may be used to detect the addition of refined oil to virgin olive oil.

Positive and negative sensory attributes are related to the presence of certain volatiles. Some aldehydes such as haxanal and nonanal and the ratios of *trans*-2-hexenal to hexanal are used to assess quality.

Olive Oil Extraction

Processing of olives has undergone serious changes in the last 30–40 years. In this period there has been a gradual transition from the traditional mills to the three-phase and later to the two-phase centrifugal systems. The big change was in the production capacity and the improvement of the oil quality by minimizing the length of time from the picking to the crushing. Other technological innovations in the olive oil industry aim at obtaining oil which retains as much as possible minor constituents, such as phenolic antioxidants.

Traditional Mills. The olives are crushed by millstones. The resultant mash is spread on round mats. The latter are stacked one upon the other and pressed by a heavy beam. The products, oil, pomace, and waste water are separated in clarifiers.

To obtain good quality olive oil in this machinery, the fruits should not be stored for a long time in the mill yard as the time that elapses between harvesting and crushing is critical, and the mats carefully cleaned.

The method has a by-product, pomace, which is used for the recovery of olive residue oil, and a waste product, water. The latter creates problems of sustainability because it generates a residue which has to be treated to avoid environmental contamination.

Three-Phase Decanters. Horizontal centrifuges or decanters (as they are also known) consist of cylindrical-conical bowls, with a hollow similarly shaped, and helical blades. Due to the difference in the speed at which the bowl rotates and the hollow gyrates, the pomace is thrown to one end of the centrifuge, while the oil and water are pushed to the other. The oil and water are then separated in vertical centrifuges. The pomace is used for the production of olive residue oil (olive pomace oil).

In the three-phase systems the solid phase is separated from the liquid phase by diluting the past with water. The amount of water added is critical for the extraction yields.

Two-Phase Decanters. The distinguishing characteristic of the two-phase system is that it uses a centrifugal system in a way that produces oil and a different waste product, a wet pomace (alperujo), a combination of pomace and waste water. Water is not added and the oil has a higher content of phenolic compounds.

Percolation (Selective Filtration). This system is one of the best, since it operates at room temperature without the addition of water. The oil phase is separated from the paste because of the difference in the interfacial tension of the oil and vegetation water. This is obtained through a steel plate that is continuously plunged and withdrawn from the paste. As the extraction of the oil is not complete, the system is usually combined with a centrifuge. Thus, two fractions are obtained, one from the percolation and the other from the centrifugation of the remaining past.

Olive Oil Production and Consumption. Traditional and Modern Use

Olive Oil Production
Olive oil world production is approximately 2.8 million tones. Its share in the world edible vegetable oils market is 3.5%. Half of this production originates

from Spain (approximately 1.15 million tons). Italy is the second world producer with an average of 500 thousand tons and Greece the third (340 thousand tons). Other important olive oil-producing countries are Tunisia, Syria, Turkey, and Morocco. In a small scale, olive oil is also produced in Algeria, Portugal and Jordan. There are much smaller amounts of production in Argentina, Croatia, Israel, Lebanon, Libya, Palestine, France, Cyprus, Mexico, and the USA. The five member states of the European Union (Spain, Italy, Greece, France, and Portugal) share jointly some 75–80% of the world production. A share of 15–20% belongs to other non EU members and the rest, somewhat less than 5%, to the rest of the world [IOOC, various documents]. In Australia a production of 6,750 tons is expected for the year 2006 [104].

Consumption Trends

Olive oil is the Mediterranean region's principal source of fat and has been characteristically used for decades in place of animal fats and seed oils of Northern European countries. Greece has the highest per capita consumption (approximately 19 kg/year) [105] followed by Italy and Spain (approximately 12 kg/year), Portugal, Syria, Jordan, and Tunisia. In France and in the countries of central and northern Europe consumption of olive oil is very low. In the last 15 years a significant increase in olive oil intake has occurred. New consumers in these countries share the highest percentage. Collected data also indicate that there is significant annual growth rate in a group of countries including USA, Australia, Japan, and Brazil.

Traditional and Modern Use

A Greek poet, Ulysses Elytis, has said that 'cooking should be in absolute harmony with the natural and cultural environment. It should be inspired by the environment but also serve it faithfully.'

Thus, when one stares at some parts of the Mediterranean region, e.g. the Aegean Sea, one can only think of a cuisine which is simple, light, placid, with well-defined tastes and full of harmony. A contrast to the cuisine of the countries of Northern Europe, which tends to be very rich and sophisticated, based on too much skillfulness, and aiming at demonstrating grandeur.

Olive oil has a remarkable stability and can be stored for almost 2 years. The resistance to oxidation is combined with many unique characteristics due to differences of olives from which the oil is obtained and the mode of extraction. These qualities offer opportunities for a variety of culinary applications with none or very little processing.

Olive oil contributes remarkable complex flavors that are reflected throughout the whole dish. A good quality olive oil blends perfectly with greens. Traditional vegetable dishes are prepared with seasonal vegetables, various greens, parsley and grains. Although very old, these recipes contain wisely balanced ingredients and meet health criteria as defined by modern science.

In vegetarian dishes, olive oil with herbal hues are usually preferred. For salads, a pronounced hint of apple is suitable, while for grilled meats a peppery flavor is desirable. Other dishes such as pies, mayonnaise, fried eggs, etc., require different hues for those who can go deep into sensorial characteristics like mouthful, bouquet, taste, aftertaste, etc., and have developed their own personal preferences. 'Freshly cut grass flavor', 'flowery aroma', 'pepperiness' and other such comments are very likely to be heard not only in oil-tasting parties but even in common discussions of consumers with a sophisticated palate.

The exquisite taste of olive oil is very often complemented by the sharp taste of vinegar or lemon or tomato. A simple traditional salad dressing is an instantly beaten mixture of olive oil and lemon juice, a rich source of both lipid-soluble and water-soluble vitamins. Attempts are now being made to stabilize such dressings with gums [106].

In salads or in cooking, olive oil is usually mixed with herbs and spices, which are also an important element of the Mediterranean diet. Herbs like oregano or rosemary or thyme or other plants of the *Lamiaceae* family are rich sources of phenolic compounds with strong antioxidant activity. These herbs maintain the nutritional value of the food and enhance the shelf life of the food product [107, 108].

Antoun and Tsimidou [109] prepared gourmet olive oils, which contained dry oregano and rosemary. Such oils, containing small amounts of the herbs, not only satisfied sensory requirements, even among non-olive oil consumers, but also had an improved resistance to autoxidation. This is obviously due to the contribution of antioxidants present in the herbs like rosemaric acid, caffeic acid, carnosol, rosmanol, carnosic acid, carvacrol, thymol and others.

Positive and Negative Attributes. The International Olive Oil Council in its Trade Standards defines 3 positive attributes: bitter, fruity and pungent; and 11 negative attributes: fusty, musty, muddy, sediment, winey-vinegary, rancid, heated or burnt, hay or woody, greasy, vegetable water, brine and earthy. These properties may be processing defects; others are due to storage and packaging.

Some of the positive attributes can be declared in the label of the packaged olive oil according to Regulation EC 1019/02. This, however, has to wait until July 2006, when the International Olive Oil Council finalizes the sensory evaluation methods (Regulation EC 1750/2004).

New Applications

Olive oil is added to margarines and hypocholesteremic spreads, butter, creams, pastes prepared from nuts, and reduced-fat mayonnaise. The level of replacement of other fats by olive oil is not well known, as most of these applications are patented. In a recent report, Ansomera and Astiarazan [110] proposed the use of olive oil in fermented sausages to obtain better stability during storage and improved ratios of mono- and di-unsaturated fatty acids to saturated fatty acids.

Olive Oil in Frying. Olive oil shows a remarkable resistance during domestic deep frying of potatoes or in other uses at frying temperatures [111–112]. When compared to other vegetable oils, such as sunflower, cotton seed, corn and soybean oil, olive oil has a significantly lower rate of deterioration. This increased stability to thermal oxidation explains why the oil can be used for repeated fryings.

The explanation for the resistance of olive oil to rapid deterioration at elevated temperatures is its fatty acid composition and the presence of natural antioxidants, such as tocopherols, squalene and delta-5-avenasterol [1, 2]. The polar antioxidants found in virgin olive oil may also make a contribution to the increased stability and polymerization.

These properties of olive oil are obviously known to the people of the Mediterranean basin who traditionally use good quality olive oil for frying, but always for a limited number of fryings. According to Varela [113] and Varela and Ruiz Roso [114], deep frying in olive oil offers a means to improve the lipid intake profile, since during the frying operation important changes occur in fat composition because of the fat penetration into the fried food (a favorable change in the polyunsaturated plus monounsaturated fatty acids to saturated fatty acids ratio when meat is cooked). A better combination is to cook fish in olive oil (a combination of the nutritional benefits of the oil and the omega-3 fatty acids) [115, 116].

Loss of Phenols. The level of phenols in heated olive oil is important since these compounds are considered components with an important biological role. Phenolics such as hydroxytyosol and its derivatives deteriorate relatively rapidly [111, 117]. Lignans are more stable. As a result of the loss of phenols during heating, the antioxidant activity of the oil, determined by the ABTS radical decolorization assay or the DPPH radical test, diminishes [118, 119].

Loss of the antioxidant capacity of olive oil and other vegetable oils due to heating at frying temperatures were also reported by Quils et al. [120] and Carlos Espin et al. [121]. Kalantzakis et al. [122] examined the loss of antioxidant capacity, evaluated by the DPPH decolorization test, and the polar transformation products formed from various vegetable oils heated at 180°C for 10 h. It was observed that olive oil lost its radical scavenging capacity at a shorter time of heating in relation to soybean, sunflower, cottonseed oil, and a commercial frying oil. However, olive oil reached the level of 25% total polar compounds (rejection point) after 10 h of heating, while all the other oils reached this upper limit in shorter periods.

It can be concluded that olive oil as a frying medium has a remarkable stability and a resistance to oxidative polymerization. When, however, health effects are expected from the presence of natural antioxidants, the number of heating operations should be restricted to a minimum.

Cloudy and Unfiltered Oil

When freshly prepared, olive oil is in a form of emulsion-dispersion, which can persist for months before complete deposition of a residue. Small quantities of cloudy (veiled) oil (the fresh olive juice) are sold to consumers who prefer this type as more 'green' and richer in flavor. The oil is usually sold in bulk to the consumers directly from the mills. Unfiltered oils are virgin olive oils not filtered through filter paper or diatomaceous earth, but bottled only after settling. There are many firms specializing in the trade of packed unfiltered raw olive oil with varying flavoring characteristics (sweet, fruity, peppery, etc.). The usual practice is with oils of early harvest from green olives. Very often the oils are advertised as 'stone made' or 'cold pressed' to stress that olives have been processed in the traditional mode at low temperature. The product is considered ideal for use in restaurants and other 'fine-eating' establishments.

Veiled oils were found to have longer induction periods compared to filtered oils. In a recent study, Tsimidou et al. [60] found a higher total phenolic compounds content in veiled oils in relation to the filtered; this may explain partly the higher stability.

Freshly prepared virgin olive oil contains oleocanthal, a tyrosol derivative (the deacetoxy, dialdehydic form of ligstroside aglycone) which is related to the stinging sensation in the back of the throat [75]. This compound was recently synthesized and found to have the same pharmacological properties as Ibuprofen, a nonsteroidal anti-inflammatory drug [69]. This finding may add to the popularity of pungent olive oil, but for the proper evaluation of the biological role of this and other phenols more work is needed for the levels in olive oil and bioavailability.

Conclusions

Olive oil, a food staple in the warmer regions around the Mediterranean Sea, is now becoming more popular throughout Europe and in the USA, Canada, Australia and other countries. This is mostly due to the promotion of the health benefits of Mediterranean dietary patterns. Olive oil, a basic constituent of the Mediterranean diet, is rich in monounsaturated fatty acids and has a resistance to oxidative changes because of its moderate unsaturation and the presence of nutrient and non-nutrient antioxidants. There is also increasing evidence that some of its constituents, mainly phenolic antioxidants, inhibit or modulate oxygen-related reactions and have substantial favorable effect against oxidative injury. It is therefore important to understand better the nature of the nonglyceride components of olive oil and to improve methods to quantify functional ingredients.

The production of high quality virgin olive oil with a sufficient level of biophenols can be guaranteed by present day chemical knowledge and the combination of tradition and technology. Chemical and analytical work related to important minor constituents of olive oil is progressing rapidly. However, the available knowledge on the metabolic fate of the various bioactive phenolic compounds is not yet complete. Absorption and bioavailability studies show that tyrosol and hydroxytyrosol can be retrieved in plasma and urine after olive oil intake, but very little is known about aglycones (the main constituents of the olive oil polar fraction), their hydrolysis products, and possible interactions with other food components. Thus, new information is expected for the levels of bioactive compounds and their metabolic fate from studies to be initiated, taking into consideration the accumulated knowledge on olive oil composition.

References

1   Boskou D: Olive Oil: Chemistry and Technology. Champaign, AOCS Press, 1996.
2   Boskou D: Olive oil; in Gunstone F (ed): Vegetable Oils in Food Technology. Oxford, CRC Press, 2002, pp 244–277.
3   International Olive Oil Council: Trade standards applying to olive oil and olive pomace oil. COI/T.15/NC, No 3, 2003.
4   Codex Alimentarius Standard for olive oils and olive pomace oils, CODEX STAN 33–33–1981 (Rev 2–2003).
5   Commission of the European Communities. Regulation No 2568/91: Official Journal of the European Communities L 248, 1991, regulation 282/98. Official Journal of the European Communities, L 28/5,1998, regulation 1989/03. Official Journal of the European Communities L 295, 2003.
6   Santinelli F, Damiani P, Christie WW: The triacylglycerol structure of olive oil determined by silver ion high performance liquid chromatography in combination with stereospecific analysis. J Am Oil Chem Soc 1992;69:552–556.
7   Vlahov G: ^{13}C nuclear magnetic resonance spectroscopy to check 1,3-random, 2-random pattern of fatty acid distribution in olive oil triacylglycerols. Spectroscopy 2005;19:109–117.
8   Frega N, Bocci F, Lercker G: Free fatty acids and diacylglycerols as quality parameters for extra virgin olive oil. Riv Ital Sost Grasse 1993;70:153–156.
9   Kiosseoglou V, Kouzounas P: The role of diglycerides, monoglycerides and free fatty acids in olive oil minor surface-active lipid interaction with proteins at oil-water interface. J Disp Sci Techn 1993;14:527–531.
10 Pérez-Camino C, Moreda W, Cert A: Effects of olive fruit quality and oil storage practices on the diacylglycerol content of virgin olive oils. J Agric Food Chem 2001;49:699–704.
11 Spyros A, Philippidis A, Dais P: Kinetics of diglyceride formation and isomerization in virgin olive oils by employing ^{31}P NMR spectroscopy: formulation of a quantitative measure to assess olive oil storage history. J Agric Food Chem 2004;52:157–164.

12 Anon: Biological role and practical use of squalene and squalane, 1996. http://www.squalene.com/what.htm.
13 Anon: Southernblue 1997. http://www.southernblue.com.au/squalene.htm.
14 Rao C, Newmark H, Reddy B: Chemopreventive effect of squalene on colon cancer. Carcinogenesis 1998;19:287–290.
15 Smith T, Yang G, Seril D, et al: Inhibition of 4-(methylnitrosamino)-1-(3-pyridyl)-1-butanone-induced lung tumorigenesis by dietary olive oil and squalene. Carcinogenesis 1998;19:703–706.
16 Eyres L: Patent Abstracts, Lipid Technology, Jan1999, p 22.
17 Psomiadou E, Tsimidou M: On the role of squalene in olive oil stability. J Agric Food Chem 1999;47:4025–4032.
18 Lanzón A, Albi T, Cert A, et al: The hydrocarbon fraction of virgin olive oil and changes resulting from refining. J Am Oil Chem Soc 1994;71:285–291.
19 Vuostito BA, Miettinen TA: Absorption, metabolism and serum concentration of cholesterol in vegetarians: effect of cholesterol feedings. Am J Clin Nutr 1994;59:1325–1331.
20 Erickson BA: Hypocholesteremic shortening. Ger Offen 1971;2:035–069.
21 Andrikopoulos NK, Tzamtzis VA, Giannopoulos GA, Kalantzopoulos GK, Demopoulos CA: Deterioration of some vegetable oils. I. During heating or frying of several foods. Rev Fr Corps Gras 1989;36:127–129.
22 Romero A, Questa C, Sanchez-Muniz FJ: Behavior of extra virgin olive oil in potato frying: thermooxidative alteration of the fat content in the fried food. Grasas Aceites 1998;49:370–375.
23 Boskou D, Morton ID: Effect of sterols on the rate of deterioration of heated oils. J Sci Food Agric 1976;27:928–932.
24 Blekas G, Boskou D: Effect of esterified sterols on the stability of heated oils; in Charalambous G (ed): The Shelf Life of Food and Beverages. Amsterdam, Elsevier, 1986, pp 641–645.
25 Kiosseoglou V, Vlachopoulou I, Boskou D: Esterified 4-monomethyl- and 4,4-dimethyl-sterols in some vegetable oils. Grasas Aceites 1987;38:102–103.
26 Chryssafidis D, Magos P, Kiosseoglou V: Composition of total and esterified 4α-monomethylsterols and triterpene alcohols in virgin olive oil. J Sci Food Agric 1992;58:581–583.
27 Itoh T, Yoshida K, Yatsu T: Triterpene alcohols and sterols of Spanish olive oil. J Am Oil Chem Soc 1981;58:545 550.
28 Cert A, Alba J, Pérez-Camino C: Influence of extraction methods on the characteristics and minor components of extra virgin olive oil. Olivae 1999;79:41–50.
29 Ranalli A, Ferrante M, De Mattia G, et al: Analytical evaluation of virgin olive oil of first and second extraction. J Agric Food Chem 1999;47:417–424.
30 Aparicio R, Luna G: Characterisation of monovarietal virgin olive oils. Eur J Lipid Sci Technol 2002;104:614–627.
31 Boskou D, Stefanou G, Konstandinidis M: Tetracosanol and hexacosanol content of Greek olive oils. Grasas Aceites 1983;34:402–404.
32 Reiter B, Lorbeer E: Analysis of the wax ester fraction of olive oil and sunflower oil by gas chromatography and gas chromatography-mass spectrometry. J Am Oil Chem Soc 2001;78:881–888.
33 Gunstone F, Harwood J, Padley F (eds): The Lipid Handbook, ed 2. London, Chapman & Hall, 1994.
34 Belitz H-D, Grosch W, Schieberle P (eds): Food Chemistry, ed 3. Berlin, Springer, 2004.
35 Conte L, Caboni M, Lercker G: Olive oils produced in Romagne. Note 1. Oils from Lamone river valley. Riv Ital Sost Grasse 1993;70:157–160.
36 Fedeli E, Cortesi N: Quality, origin and technology of virgin olive oils. Riv Ital Sost Grasse 1993;70:419–426.
37 Esti M, Cinquanta L, Carrone A, et al: Anti-oxidative compounds and quality parameters in virgin olive oils produced in Molise. Riv Ital Sost Grasse 1996;73:147–150.
38 Cert A, Alba J, León-Camacho M, et al: Effects of talk addition and operating mode on the quality and oxidative stability of virgin olive oils obtained by centrifugation. J Agric Food Chem 1996;44:3930–3934.
39 Manzi P, Panfili G, Esti M, et al: Natural antioxidants in the unsaponifiable fraction of virgin olive oils from different cultivars. J Sci Food Agric 1998;77:115–120.

40 Salvador M, Aranda F, Fregapane G: Chemical composition of commercial Cornicabra virgin olive oils from 1995/96 and 1996/97 crops. JAOCS 1998;75:1305–1311.
41 Psomiadou E, Tsimidou M, Boskou D: α-Tocopherol content of Greek virgin olive oils. J Agric Food Chem 2000;48:1770–1775.
42 Blekas G, Tsimidou M, Boskou D: Contribution of alpha-tocopherol to olive oil stability. Food Chem 1995;52:289–294.
43 Blekas G, Boskou D: Antioxidant activity of 3,4-dihydrophenylacetic acid and a-tocopherol on the triglyceride matrix of olive oil: effect of acidity. Grasas Aceites 1998;49:34–37.
44 Morello J, Motilva M, Tovar M: Changes in commercial virgin olive oil (cv. Arbequina) during storage, with special emphasis on the phenolic fraction. Food Chem 2004;85:357–364.
45 Montedoro G, Bertuccioli M, Anichini F: In Charalambous G (ed): Flavor of Foods and Beverages. St. Louis, Academic Press, 1978, pp 247–281.
46 Olías J, Gutiérrez F, Dobarganes C: Volatile components in the aroma of virgin olive oil. IV. Their evolution and influence in the aroma during the fruit ripening process in the 'Picual' and 'Hojiblanca' varieties. Grasas Aceites 1980;31:391–402.
47 Guth H, Grosch W: A comparative study of the potent odorants of different virgin olive oils. Fat Sci Technol 1991;93:335–339.
48 Angerosa F, Basti C: The volatile composition of samples from the blend of monovarietal olive oils and from the processing of mixtures of olive fruits. Eur J Lipid Sci Technol 2003;105: 327–332.
49 Reiners J, Grosch W: Odorants of virgin olive oils with different flavor profiles. J Agric Food Chem 1998;46:2754–2763.
50 Bortolomeazzi R, Berno P, Pizzale L: Sesquiterpene, alkene, and alkane hydrocarbons in virgin olive oils of different varieties and geographical origins. J Agric Food Chem 2001;49:3278–3283.
51 Cavalli J-F, Fern andez X, Lizzani-Cuvelier L: Characterization of volatile compounds of French and Spanish virgin olive oils by HS-SPME: identification of quality-freshness markers. Food Chem 2004;88:151–157.
52 Vichi S, Castellote A, Pizzale L, et al: Analysis of virgin olive oil volatile compounds by headspace solid-phase microextraction coupled to gas chromatography with mass spectrometric and flamme ionization detection. J Chromatogr 2003;83:19–33.
53 Morales M, Luna G, Aparicio R: Comparative study of virgin olive oil sensory defects. Food Chem 2005;91:293–301.
54 Blekas G, Guth H: Evaluation and quantification of potent odorants of Greek virgin olive oil; in Charalambous G (ed): Food Flavors: Generation, Analysis and Process Influence. Amsterdam, Elsevier Sciences, 1995, pp 419–427.
55 Sanchez Saez J, Herce Garraleta M, Balea Otero T: Identification of cinnamic acid ethyl ester and 4-vinylphenol in off-flavour olive oils. Anal Chim Acta 1991;247:295–297.
56 Alter M, Gutfinger T: Phospholipids in several vegetable oils. Riv Ital Sost Grasse 1982;59:14–18.
57 Boukhchina S, Sebai K, Cherif A, et al: Identification of glycerophospholipids in rapeseed, olive, almond and sunflower oils by LC-MS and LC-MS-MS. Can J Chem 2004;82:1210–1215.
58 Pokorny J, Korczak J: In Pokorny J, Yanishlieva N, Gordon M (eds): Antioxidants in Food. Boca Raton, CRC Press, 2001, pp 311–330.
59 Koidis A, Boskou D: The contents of protein and phospholipids of cloudy (veiled) virgin olive oils. Eur J Lipid Sci Technol 2006;108:323–328.
60 Tsimidou M, Georgiou A, Koidis A, et al: Loss of stability of 'veiled' (cloudy) virgin olive oils in storage. Food Chem 2005;93:377–383.
61 IOOC Scientific Seminar, State of the art in olive oil, nutrition and health. Consensus statement, March, 2005.
62 Owen R, Mier W, Giacosa A: Identification of lignans as major components in the phenolic fraction of olive oil. Clin Chem 2000;46:976–988.
63 Mateos R, Espartero J, Trujillo M: Determination of phenols, flavones and lignans in virgin olive oil by solid phase extraction and HPLC with diode array ultraviolet detection. J Agric Food Chem 2001;49:2185–2192.
64 Garcia A, Brenes M, Martinez F: HPLC evaluation of phenols in virgin olive oil during extraction at laboratory and industrial scale. J Am Oil Chem Soc 2001;78:625–629.

65 Bianco A, Coccioli F, Guiso M: Presence in olive oil of a new class of phenolic compounds: hydroxyl-isochromans. Food Chem 2001;77:405–411.
66 Christoforidou S, Dais P, Tseng L-H: Separation and identification of phenolic compounds in olive oil by coupling high-performance liquid chromatography with postcolumn solid-phase extraction to nuclear magnetic resonance spectroscopy (LC-SPE-NMR). J Agric Food Chem 2005;53:4667–4679.
67 Litridou M, Linssen J, Schols H, Bewrgmans M, Posthumus M, Tsimidou M, Boskou D: Phenolic compounds of virgin olive oils: fractionation by solid phase extraction and antioxidant activity assessment. J Sci Food Agric 1997;74:169–174.
68 Tovar M, Motilva M, Romero M: Changes in the phenolic composition of virgin olive oil from young trees (*Olea europae* L. cv. Arbequina) grown under linear irrigation strategies. J Agric Food Chem 2001;41:5502–5508.
69 Beauchamp G, Keast R, Morel D: Ibuprofen-like activity in extra virgin olive oil. Nature 2005;437:45–46.
70 Tsimidou M, Papadopoulos G, Boskou D: Phenolic compounds and stability of virgin olive oil. Food Chem 1992;45:141–144.
71 Monteleone E, Caporale G, Carlucchi A: Optimization of extra virgin olive oil quality. J Sci Food Agric 1998;77:31–37.
72 Gutierrez-Rosales F, Arnaud T: Contribution of polyphenols on the oxidative stability of virgin olive oil. Proceedings 24th World Congress ISF, Berlin, 2001, pp 61–62.
73 Angerosa F, Mostallino R, Basti C: Influence of malaxation temperature and time on the quality of virgin olive oils. Food Chem 2001;72:19–28.
74 Gutierrez-Rosales F, Rios J, Gomez-Rey M: Main polyphenols in the bitter taste of virgin olive oil. Structural confirmation by on line HPLC electrospray ionization mass spectrometry. J Agric Food Chem 2003;51:6021–6025.
75 Andrewes P, Busch J, De Joode T, Groenewegen A, Alexandre H: Sensory properties of virgin olive oil polyphenols: identification of deacetoxy-ligstroside aglycon as a key contributor to pungency. J Agric Food Chem 2003;51:1415–1420.
76 Mateos R, Cert A, Perez-Camino C, et al: Evaluation of virgin oil bitterness by quantification of secoiridoid derivatives. J Am Oil Chem Soc 2004;81:71–76.
77 Assmann G, Wahrburg U: Scientific basis for olive oil, monounsaturated fatty acids, antioxidants and LDL oxidation. 1999.
78 http:/europa.eu.int/comm./dg06/prom/olive/medinfo.
79 Keys A: Mediterranean diet and public health: personal reflections. Am J Clin Nutr 1995;61: 1321S–1323S.
80 Wahrburg U, Kratz M, Cullen P: Mediterranean diet, olive oil and health. Eur J Lipid Sci Technol 2002;104:698–705.
81 Tuck KL, Hayball PJ: Major phenolic compounds in olive oil: metabolism and health effects. J Nutr Biochem 2002;13:636–644.
82 Visioli F, Bogani P, Grande S, Galli C: Olive oil and oxidative stress. Grasas Aceites 2004;55: 66–75.
83 Boskou D, Blekas G, Tsimidou M: Phenolic compounds in olive oil and olives. Curr Top Nutraceut Res 2005;3:125–136.
84 Salonen JT: Markers of oxidative damage and antioxidant protection: assessment of LDL oxidation. Free Rad Res 2000;33:541–546.
85 Aviram M: Review of human studies and oxidative damage and antioxidant protection related to cardiovascular diseases. Free Rad Res 2000;33:S85–S97.
86 Vissers N, Zock PL, Katan MB: Bioavailability and antioxidant effects of olive oil phenols in humans. Eur J Clin Nutr 2004;58:955–965.
87 Nardini M, D'Aquino M, Tomassi G, Gentili V, Di Felice M, Scaccini C: Inhibition of human low density lipoprotein oxidation by caffeic acid and other hydroxyl-cinnamic acid derivatives. Free Rad Biol Med 1955;12:541–552.
88 Masella R, Vari R, D'Archivio M, Di Benedetto R, Matarrese P, Malorni W, Scazzocchio B, Giovannini C: Extra virgin olive oil biophenols inhibit cell-mediated oxidation of LDL by increasing the mRNA transcription of glutathione-related interaction. J Nutr 2004;134:785–791.

89 Coni E, Di Benedetto R, Di Pasquale M, Masella R, Modesti D, Mattei R Carlini EA: Protective effect of oleuropein, an olive oil biophenol, on low density lipoprotein oxidizability in rabbits. Lipids 2000;35:45–54.
90 Masella R, Giovanini C, Vari R, Di Benedetto R, Coni E, Volpe R, Fraone N, Bucci: Effects of dietary virgin olive oil phenols on low density lipoprotein oxidation in hyperlipidemic patients. Lipids 2001;36:1195–1202.
91 Fito M, Covas ML, Lamuela-Raventos RM: Protective effect of olive oil and its phenolic compounds against low density lipoprotein oxidation. Lipids 2000;35:633–638.
92 Visioli F, Caruso D, Galli C, Viappiani S, Galli G, Sala A: Olive oil rich in natural catecholic phenols decrease isoprostane excretion in humans. Biochem Biophys Res Commun 2000;278:797–799.
93 Visioli F, Bellomo G, Galli C: Free radical scavenging properties of olive oil polyphenols. Biochem Biophys Res Commun 1998;247:60–64.
94 Saija A, Trombetta D, Tomaino A, Lo Cascio R, Princi P, Ucella N, Bonina F, Castelli F: In vitro evaluation of the antioxidant activity and biomembrane interaction of the plant phenols oleuropein and hydroxytyrosol. Int J Pharmaceut 1998;166:123–133.
95 Gordon MH, Paiva-Martins F, Almeida M: Antioxidant activity of hydroxytyrosol acetate compared with that of other olive oil polyphenols. J Agric Food Chem 2001;49:2480–2485.
96 Tuck KL, Hayball PJ: Major phenolic compounds in olive oil: metabolism and health effects. J Nutr Biochem 2002;13:636–644.
97 Lavelli V: Comparison of the antioxidant activities of extra virgin olive oils. J Agric Food Chem 2002;50:7704–7706.
98 Briante R, Patumi M, Limongelli S, Febbraio F, Vaccaro C, Di Salle A, La Cara F, Nucci R: Changes in phenolic and enzymic activities content during fruit ripening in two Italian cultivars of olea europaea L. Plant Sci 2002;162:791–798.
99 Ninfali P, Aluigi G, Bacchiocca M, Magnani M: Antioxidant capacity of extra-virgin olive oils. J Am Oil Chem Soc 2001;78:243–247.
100 Pellegrini N: Analytical approaches to measure the oxidative stability of olive oils. Food Industry J 2002;5:51–61.
101 Deiana M, Aruoma OI, Bianchi ML, Spencer JP, Kaur H, Halliwell B, Aeschbach R, Banni S, Dessi MA, Corongiu FP: Inhibition of peroxynitrate dependent DNA base modification and tyrosine nitration by the extra olive oil-derived antioxidant hydroxytyrosol. Free Rad Biol Med 1999;26:762–769.
102 De La Puerta R, Martinez-Dominguez ME, Ruiz-Gutierrez V, Flavill A, Hoult JRS: Effects of virgin olive oil phenolics on scavenging of reactive nitrogen species and upon nitrergic neurotransmission. Life Sci 2001;69:1213–1222.
103 Anon: The pursuit of quality: a major quest of the International Olive Oil Council. Grasas Aceites 2004;100:34–38.
104 Rural Industries Research and Development Corporation: Regional Australian Oilve Oil Processing Plants. http:/www.rirdc.gov.au/reports/NPP.01
105 Food and Drug Organization: FAOSTAT data. Food Balance Sheets,1996. http:/www.fao.org.
106 Paraskevopoulou A, Boskou D, Kiosseoglou V: Stabilization of olive oil-lemon juice emulsion with polysaccharides. Food Chem 2005;90:627–634.
107 Nakatami N: Antioxidant and antimicrobial constituents of herbs and spices; in Charalambous G (ed): Spices, Herbs and Edible Fungi. Amsterdam, Elsevier, 1994, pp 251–271.
108 Exarchou V, Nenadis N, Tsimidou M, Gerothanassis IP, Troganis A, Boskou D: Antioxidant activities and phenolic composition of extracts from Greek oregano, Greek sage and summer savory. J Agric Food Chem 2002;50:5294–5299.
109 Antoun N, Timidou M: Gourmet olive oils: stability and consumer acceptability studies. Food Res Intern 1997;30:131–136.
110 Ansorena D, Astiazaran I: Effect of storage and packaging on fatty acid composition and oxidation; in d'Ansorena D, Astiazaran I (eds): Effect of Storage and Packaging on Fatty Acid Composition and Oxidation in Dry Fermented Sausages Made with Added Olive Oil and Antioxidants. Meat Sci 2004, vol 67, pp 337–344.
111 Boskou D: Non-nutrient antioxidants and stability of frying oils; in Boskou D, Elmadfa I (eds): Frying of Food. Lancaster, Technomic Publishing, 1999, pp 183–204.

112 Andrikopoulos NK, Dedoussis GVZ, Falirea A, Kalogeropoulos N, Hatzinikola HS: Deterioration of natural antioxidant species of vegetable edible oils during the domestic deep-frying and pan-frying of potatoes. Int J Food Sci Nutr 2002;53:351–363.
113 Varela G: Some effects of deep frying on dietary fat intake. Nutr Rev 1992;50:256–262.
114 Varela G, Ruiz Roso B: Frying process in the relation fat/degenerative diseases. Grasas Aceites 1998;49:359–365.
115 Cuesta I, Perez M, Ruiz-Roso B, Varela G: Comparative study of the effect on the sardine fatty acid composition during deep frying and canning of olive oil. Grasas Aceites 1998;49:371–374.
116 Bastida S, Sanchez-Muniz FJ, Cava F, Viejo JM, Macros A: Benefits of the consumption of olive oil fried sardines in the prevention of hypercholesterolemia in rats: Effects of some serum lipids and cell-damage marker enzymes. Grasas Aceites 1998;49:375–376.
117 Brenes M, Garcia A, Dobarganes MC: Influence of thermal treatments simulating cooking processes on the polyphenol content in virgin olive oil. J Agric Food Chem 2002;50:5962–5967.
118 Pellegrini N, Visioli F, Buratti S, et al: Direct analysis of total antioxidant activity of olive oil and studies on the influence of heating. J Agric Food Chem 2001;49:2532–2538.
119 Gomez-Alonso S, Fregapane G, Desamparados Salvador M, et al: Changes in phenolic composition and antioxidant activity of virgin olive oil during frying. J Agric Food Chem 2003;51:667–672.
120 Quiles JL, Ramirez-Tortosa MC, Gomezs JA, et al: Role of vitamin E and phenolic compounds in the antioxidant capacity, measured by ESR of virgin olive oil and sunflower oils after frying. Food Chem 2002;76:461–468.
121 Carlos-Espin J, Soler-Rivas C, Wichers HJ: Characterization of the total free radical scavenger capacity of vegetable oils and oil fractions using 2,2-diphenyl-1-picrylhydrazyl radical. J Agric Food Chem 2000;48:648–656.
122 Kalantzakis G, Blekas G, Peglidou K, Boskou D: Stability and radical scavenging activity of heated olive oil and other vegetable oil. Eur J Lipid Sci Technol 2006;in press.

Dimitrios Boskou
Aristotle University of Thessaloniki
School of Chemistry, Laboratory of Food Chemistry and Technology
GR–540 46 Thessaloniki (Greece)
Tel. +30 31 997791, Fax +30 31 997779, E-Mail boskou@chem.auth.gr

Melatonin in Edible Plants (Phytomelatonin): Identification, Concentrations, Bioavailability and Proposed Functions

Russel J. Reiter[a], Dun-xian Tan[a], Lucien C. Manchester[a], Artemis P. Simopoulos[b], Maria D. Maldonado[a], Luis J. Flores[a], M. Pilar Terron[a]

[a]Department of Cellular and Structural Biology, University of Texas Health Science Center, San Antonio, Tex.; [b]Center for Genetics, Nutrition and Health, Washington, D.C., USA

The discovery of melatonin (N-acetyl-5-methoxytryptamine) in plants occurred just over a decade ago [1–3]. For roughly 35 years before that, melatonin was known to be the indole product synthesized in the pineal gland of vertebrates [4]. In the vertebrate classes, however, melatonin is not uniquely produced in the pineal gland but in many tissues including the retinas [5], skin [6], gastrointestinal tract [7], lens [8], Harderian glands [9], and other organs as well. Besides its ubiquitous distribution in vertebrates, melatonin has also been found in every invertebrate that has been examined for its presence [10]. The first investigation reporting the presence of melatonin in a species outside of the vertebrate class was in the dinoflagellate alga *Gonyaulax* (*Lingulodinium polyedrum*) [11]. Subsequently, melatonin was identified in insects, fungi, protists and in prokaryotes [12, 13].

The discovery of melatonin in algae likely prompted investigations into its possible presence in plants. In 1995, two papers [1, 2] and one abstract [3] appeared which claimed the presence of melatonin in tissue of angiosperms. These discoveries stimulated other scientists to consider the possibility that the indole melatonin was common to many, and possibly all, plant tissues. While publications in this research arena are still not numerous, there is a steadily increasing series of reports characterizing melatonin in virtually every plant species investigated, similar to the situation in the animal kingdom [14–17].

The current review summarizes the results of the publications that extracted and identified melatonin in plant tissues. Examination of these reports readily reveals several bits of information: (a) the quantity of melatonin within different plant tissues varies over a very wide range of concentrations, and (b) neither the measurement of melatonin in plant materials nor its extraction is straightforward.

Preparation of Plant Tissues for Melatonin Measurement

The methods of measurement of melatonin in plant tissues have included radioimmunoassay [18], enzyme-linked immunoabsorbent assay (ELISA) [19], high-performance liquid chromatography (HPLC) [20] and, less frequently, gas chromatography-mass spectrometry (GC-MS) [21]. Although these techniques are generally considered reliable, to varying degrees, for animal tissues, their application to plant material is fraught with difficulties. Also, the extraction and purification of the melatonin from tissues is often somewhat more difficult and this is certainly no less true for plant materials. In specific reference to tissues from unicellular eukaryotes and plants, it has been noted that they typically contain molecules including chelated iron and/or redox-active agents that could degrade the inherent melatonin by means of photooxidation or free radical-mediated reactions [11, 22]. In fact, the papers cited made some specific recommendations for the recovery of melatonin from plant tissues. Thus, to limit the potential enzymatic destruction of melatonin they suggest the use of 0.4 M $HClO_4$ for protein precipitation (to prevent the potential enzymatic degradation of melatonin) and the addition of a hydroxyl radical ($^{\bullet}OH$) scavenger. Melatonin rapidly undergoes structural modification in the presence of $^{\bullet}OH$ because it is a highly efficient free radical scavenger [23]. Additionally, the suggestion was made that the extraction procedures should be performed under dim light conditions to curtail photooxidation of melatonin. A number of reports used acetone-, Tris- or tricine-based extraction mixtures which sometimes included antioxidants (e.g. butylated hydroxytoluene), $HClO_4$ or the chelator EDTA [11, 24–28].

When melatonin is directly measured in samples of plant extracts [2, 11, 24, 29], additional sample purification may be important to remove molecules that interfere with melatonin measurement [27]. For example, at least two reports utilized solid-phase extraction on C18 cartridges; in some cases, this also included HPLC fractionation [25, 27]. Some investigators also employed an aqueous extraction solution into an organic solvent, i.e. chloroform or diethyl ether, in order to recover melatonin [1, 30]. Finally, immunoaffinity chromatography may also improve sample purification [31]. This method was included because it has been successfully used in combination with GC-MS to estimate melatonin levels in human serum [32].

The same methods for the measurement of melatonin in animal tissues [18–21] have, as noted above, been used for plant extracts as well. However, the sensitivity and specificity of these techniques differ, so the method employed is determined by the level of melatonin as well as potential interfering molecules in the plant extract being investigated. Although RIA has been occasionally used to measure melatonin in plants [33], plant tissues contain a variety of molecules that may cross-react with the anti-melatonin antibody leading to a potential over-estimation of the actual melatonin values [27]. HPLC with a fluorescence detector proved insufficiently sensitive to identify melatonin in shoots of *Chenopodium rubrum* but was an appropriate method to estimate melatonin values in medicinal herbs [34].

Compared to the fluorescence detector, HPLC with electrochemical detection is more sensitive and has been used to quantify melatonin levels in algae and higher plants [11, 24, 29, 30] even though it is not a highly specific method. This is problematic considering that plants contain a variety of compounds with oxidation potentials and retention times similar to melatonin.

GC-MS or liquid chromatography-mass spectrometry (LC-MS) have high sensitivity and detection specificity and their use in measuring plant melatonin avoids many of the shortcomings of the methods mentioned above. These techniques have been successfully employed to estimate melatonin levels in animal samples as well. With LC-MS, melatonin can be measured directly or after its conversion to a volatile derivative which is analyzed by GC-MS [35]. GC-MS has been used to identify melatonin in plants [1] as well as to estimate its levels [27]. Also, liquid chromatography-tandem mass spectrometry has proven useful in identifying [26, 28, 34] and quantifying melatonin in plant material [25, 31]. This latter method has distinct advantages given that it does not require melatonin derivatization and the double ion selection method provides the greatest melatonin specificity. However, even this method may not be infallible because of what is referred to as the matrix effect [36, 37].

Pape and Lüning [38] used three different extraction methods in combination with ELISA and HPLC to determine the melatonin concentrations in tomato (*Lycopersicon esculentum* Mill.), ginger tuber and the marine macroalga, *Ulva lactura*. The expressed purpose of the study was to define the optimal extraction methods under conditions where the measurement of melatonin is the goal of the investigation. The three extraction methods used were based on Na_2CO_3-ether [1], perchloric acid [22] and acetone-methanol as summarized in figure 1. The latter two methods also included C18 solid-phase extractions (SPE) for the purpose of sample purification and to avoid clogging of the HPLC column. All extractions were standardized to an injection into the preparative HPLC system that was

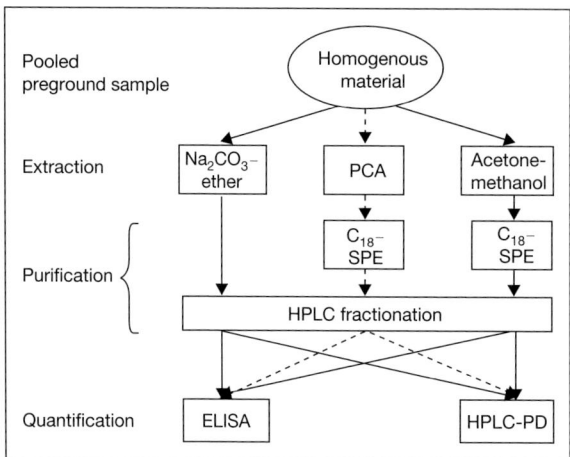

Fig. 1. The methods of extraction, purification and quantification used by Pape and Lüning [38] to identify melatonin in plant tissues. Despite the different methodologies employed, the amounts of melatonin estimated were similar. PCA = Perchloric acid; SPE = solid-phase extraction.

equivalent to 200 mg of fresh plant material. The authors also performed all procedures in dim white light (<0.1 photons/m²/s) and recovery rates were also carried out.

Use of these extraction techniques and the two quantification methods, i.e. ELISA and HPLC, yielded similar melatonin concentrations in each of the three plant products with a very high correlation. The ginger tuber had an average of 5 pg/g fresh weight (f.w.) while tomatoes and green alga contained 1,200 and 12 pg/g f.w., respectively. When considering the recovery rates using synthetic melatonin, no marked differences in the measured melatonin concentration were noted using the different methods of extraction.

In general, to accurately identify and quantify melatonin in plant tissues, precautions beyond those already apparent when animals tissues are used, should be heeded. Additional improvements, refinements and standardizations of currently available techniques will likely be forthcoming and, thereby, improve the reliability of the methods of measurement of plant melatonin levels. Certainly, the recent publication of Pape and Lüning [38] will contribute significantly to the confidence that scientists will have that melatonin in plant material can be accurately measured.

The pitfalls associated with the characterization and quantification of melatonin in plant tissues are not trivial. In the discussion of many of the published reports in this area, the authors introduce precautions for those attempting to conduct similar experiments. In fact, Pape [pers. commun.] recently made the suggestion for an intercalibration study that includes a number of scientists working on characterization of melatonin in plant materials. This idea is highly worthwhile and certainly timely. The completion of this study would help to establish the most reliable extraction and quantification methods and would serve to accelerate research in this highly interesting and important field.

Because of the difficulties experienced by individuals measuring melatonin in plants, in the current report the tabulated material from different publications is not combined. Rather, all the information recorded in a given table is from an individual report since, at this stage, the actual melatonin levels in plant tissues may vary due to different extraction and measurement methodologies.

Melatonin Levels and Proposed Functions in Plant Tissues

To date, only one plant tissue, the potato tuber [1], has been reported to be devoid of detectable levels of melatonin. In all others, melatonin has been identified and the concentrations have an extremely wide range from pg to µg/g tissue. Melatonin has been found in a variety of angiosperms and in both monocotyledons and dicotyledons; however, many higher plants, e.g. mosses, ferns, gymnosperms, have not been examined for the presence of melatonin.

It seems likely that the reason investigators undertook studies of melatonin in plants was that this indoleamine is ubiquitous in the animal kingdom including species on the cusp between the animal and plant kingdoms. It thus seemed possible, if not likely, that melatonin would also exist in plant material.

The two full-length papers that first described the presence of melatonin in plants used slighted different rationales for their investigations. Dubbels et al. [1] noted that serotonin, the precursor of melatonin during its synthesis in the mammalian pineal gland [4], was identified in fruits and vegetables in the late 1950s [39, 40]. Thus, they were curious whether melatonin, a product of serotonin metabolism, would also be present in plant material especially since it had been shown to be a very highly evolutionarily conserved molecule existing in organisms as diverse of humans and algae [4, 11].

In contrast, the report of Hattori et al. [2] noted that most living organisms use annual changes in seasonal environmental variations, i.e. photoperiod, temperature, rainfall or food availability, to regulate circannual fluctuations in physiological events. For example, the changing circadian melatonin rhythm had been shown to mediate seasonal alterations in reproductive physiology of photoperiodic mammals [4]; therefore, they reasoned that similar processes involving melatonin may be operative in plants.

Table 1. Average melatonin levels, measured by radioimmunoassay, in edible foods

Common name	Scientific name	Melatonin pg/g wet tissue
Asparagus	*Asparagus officinalis*	10
Strawberry	*Pragaria magna*	12
Kiwi fruit	*Actinidia chinensis*	24
Cucumber	*Cucumis sativus*	25
Onion	*Allium cepa*	32
Tomato	*Lycopersicon esculentum*	32
Pineapple	*Ananas comosus*	36
Indian spinach	*Basella alba*	39
Apple	*Malus domestica*	48
Japanese butterbur	*Patasites japonicus*	50
Taro	*Colocasis escutenta*	55
Carrot	*Paucus carota*	55
Onion Welsh	*Allium fistulosum*	86
Cabbage	*Brassica oleracea*	107
Chinese cabbage	*Raphamus sativas*	113
Barley	*Hordeum vulagare*	378
Chungitsu	*Chrysanthemum cororarum*	417
Ginger	*Zinigiber officinale*	584
Japanese ashitaba	*Angelica keiskei*	624
Japanese radish	*Bassica campestris*	657
Rice	*Oryza sativa japonica*	1,006
Sweet corn	*Zea mays*	1,366
Oat	*Abena sativa*	1,796
Fall fescue	*Sestvca arundinaces*	5,288

Data from Hattori et al. [2]. These results indicate a wide variation in the concentration of melatonin in plant material.

Hattori and colleagues [2] performed their studies only using plants that were edible with the method of melatonin measurement being RIA. Immunologically identifiable melatonin was found in every plant tested with wide variations in the amounts of melatonin present in various plant species (table 1). In general, the highest levels of melatonin were found in the family *Graminae* (barley, rice, sweet corn, oat and tall fescue). While the melatonin values were estimated using RIA, radish extracts additionally were subjected to high-performance liquid chromatography-fluorescence delection; with this method, authentic melatonin had the same retention time as the major peak in the radish extracts.

Table 2. Average melatonin levels in various plant tissues as measured by HPLC-MS by Dubbels et al. [1]

Common name	Scientific name	Melatonin pg/mg protein
Potato	*Salanum tuberosum* L.	0
Beetroot	*Beta vulgaris*	9
Cucumber	*Cucumis sativus*	93
Tomato	*Lycopersicon pimpinellifolium*	167
Tomato	*Lycopersicon esculentum* (Cultivar 'Rutgers California Supreme')	179
Banana	*Musa sapientum*	236
Tobacco	*Nicotiana tabacum* (BEL-B, young leaves)	350
Tobacco	*Nicotiana tabacum* (BEL-W3, young leaves)	353
Tobacco	*Nicotiana tabacum* (BEL-B, old leaves)	480
Tomato	*Lycopersicon esculentum* (Cultivar 'Sweet 100')	667
Tobacco	*Nicotiana tabacum* (BEL-W3, old leaves)	862

Hattori et al. [2] theorized that if high melatonin-level plants are consumed, ingestion of sufficient quantities of the indoleamine would influence physiological processes. For example, considering that melatonin is a sleep-promoting agent [41], postprandial sleepiness could, theoretically, be a consequence of a meal rich in melatonin. Likewise, considering that melatonin is an antioxidant, the authors note that consumption of foodstuffs rich in melatonin may aid organisms in defeating free radicals and related reactants.

Dubbels et al. [1] primarily used fresh plants grown by the first author of the report; the only exception was banana which was purchased. Melatonin was measured in 11 different plant tissues (table 2) using HPLC-MS. The only plant material in which melatonin was undetectable was the potato. Interestingly, the quantity of serotonin in several plants exhibited a strong parallelism with the amount of melatonin identified; thus, the potato, tomato and banana were previously reported to contain 0, 12 and 28 µg/g tissue of serotonin [40]. The authors point out that there was significant sample-to-sample variability in the amount of melatonin detected in extracts from the same fruit or vegetable. They also note that in the tobacco plants, old leaves contained more melatonin than

Table 3. Mean levels of melatonin in the seeds of edible plants as measured by HPLC [29]

Common name	Scientific name	Melatonin ng/g dry seed
Milk thistle	*Silybum marianum*	2
Poppy	*Popaver somniferum*	6
Anise	*Pimpineal anisum*	7
Coriander	*Coriandrum sativum*	7
Celery	*Apium graveolens*	7
Flax	*Linum usitatissimum*	12
Green cardamom	*Elettaria cardamomum*	15
Alfalfa	*Medicago sativum*	16
Fennel	*Foeniculum vulgare*	28
Sunflower	*Helianthus annuus*	29
Almond	*Prunum amygdalus*	39
Fenugreek	*Trigonella foenum-graecum*	43
Wolfberry	*Lycium barbarum*	103
Black mustard	*Brassica nigra*	129
White mustard	*Brassica hirta*	189

did young leaves from the same plant. Also, in reference to the tobacco leaves in which melatonin was estimated, the BEL-W3 and BEL-W exhibit different susceptibilities to ozone damage [42] consistent with their different levels of melatonin, i.e. high melatonin concentrations in tobacco correlated with the greatest resistance to ozone. Since ozone is an oxidizing agent, this suggests that melatonin may protect tobacco plants from the damaging effects of ozone because of its antioxidant potential.

Given that nuts/seeds contain an abundance of readily oxidizable fats and since melatonin functions as an antioxidant, one might expect that seeds would contain melatonin. Reducing oxidative damage in seeds is important considering they represent the next generation of the plant. Fifteen different edible seeds were purchased from a distributor and, using HPLC, they were investigated as to their levels of melatonin by Manchester et al. [29]. As in other investigations, these workers found widely varying melatonin concentrations in different seeds (table 3). Manchester et al. [29] reasoned that the marked variation in the melatonin levels of seeds may relate to differences in their water content, the abiotic environment in which the plants were grown and intrinsic genetic variability of the plants.

The authors of this report suggested that melatonin may function as a free radical scavenger and antioxidant in seeds [29]. They also introduce the idea that plants rich in melatonin may have a high tolerance for toxic metals taken up from

Table 4. Representative medicinal herbs and their levels of melatonin as measured by high pressure liquid chromatography-fluorescence detector on-line with a mass spectrometer

Common name	Scientific name	Melatonin ng/g dry seed
Zhizi	*Galdenia jasminoides* Ellis	12
Baijing	*Herba Patriniae scabiosaefoliae*	32
Shidagonglao	*Mahonia bealei* (Fort.)	52
Wuwei	*Schisondra chinensis*	86
Shuanhua	*Lonicera japonica* Thunb	140
Juhua	*Dendranthema morifolium*	160
Qinjiu	*Gentiana macrophylla* Pall.	180
Wugong	*Scolopendra subspinipes mutilang*	248
Fupenzi	*Rubus chingli* Hu	387
Luhui	*Aloe vela* L.	516
Danghui	*Angelica sinensis* Oliv.	698
Dahuang	*Rheun palmatum* L.	1,078
Sangye	*Morus alba* L. (leaf)	1,510
Chantui	*Periostracum cicadae*	3,771

This list includes 14 plants of the 64 that were listed in the original table and includes the plant with the lowest level (Zhiji) and the plant with the highest melatonin level (Chantui). Data from Chen et al. [34]. The original publication should be consulted for melatonin levels in other Chinese medicinal herbs. The table illustrates the wide range of melatonin concentrations in these herbs.

the soil in which they are grown. One implication of this statement is that enriching the melatonin concentration of plants may increase their resistance to agents that generate free radicals and, thereby, improve their utility in phytoremediation.

The walnut (*Juglans regia* L.) has also been investigated for its content of melatonin [43]. HPLC measurements indicated an average level of 3.5 ng/g tissue in this widely-used edible nut. Also, the feeding of walnuts to rats also caused a measurable increment in blood melatonin levels and in the total antioxidative status of the blood. Even before melatonin was identified in walnuts, the US Food and Drug Administration allowed the industry to promote their product as a healthful foodstuff since their regular consumption reportedly reduces the risk of heart disease.

A large study was carried out by Chen et al. [34] in which 108 Chinese herbs were analyzed for their melatonin content using HPLC-FD on-line with MS. Of these, 64 herbs contained melatonin in excess of 10 ng/g dry weight. Representative samples of the melatonin concentrations are given in table 4.

According to this report, medicinal herbs have higher melatonin levels, on average, than other plants in which the indole has been measured. Of special interest with regard to this study is that several of the herbs in which melatonin levels are in the µg/g range are used in traditional Chinese medicine to treat diseases associated with free radicals and to slow the processes of aging. The reason these herbal products have reported efficacy against free radical-related conditions has never been satisfactorily explained, and the herbs have not been heretofore known to contain large quantities of antioxidants. Thus, Chen et al. [34] theorized that the high levels of melatonin may provide a potential pharmacological basis for the beneficial effects of the herbs.

The finding reported by Chen et al. [34] are consistent with studies by Murch and co-workers [44–46] who also noted what are considered to be uncommonly high levels of melatonin in select Chinese medicinal plants. Their interest in these herbs was also stimulated by the fact that the ones they investigated, i.e. feverfew, St. John's wort and Huang-qin, have reported beneficial medicinal uses [47, 48]. For the study, feverfew (known synonymously by four botanical names and here referred to as *Tanacetum parthenium* L.) was purchased from a green house while Tanacetum (a commercial preparation of feverfew) was obtained from a health food store. St. John's wort (*Hypericum perforatum*) was harvested from roadside populations. Melatonin was identified by HPLC-eletrochemical detection.

Melatonin was found in all plant preparations. Two varieties of feverfew were compared and the levels of melatonin where significantly higher in the green leaf variety as opposed to the golden leaf variety. Both varieties, however, had melatonin concentrations in the low µg/g range. Similar levels of melatonin were uncovered in St. John's wort and Huang-qin with the highest levels (7.11 µg/g) being detected in Huang-qin [44].

A report by Murch and Saxena [46] provided data to support the supposition that melatonin in St. John's wort may be significant in the regulation of reproductive physiology of this plant. Thus, they report highest concentrations of serotonin in flower buds at the tetrad stage of microspore development while highest concentrations of melatonin were measured during uninucleate microsporogenesis. Furthermore, the regenerative potential of isolated anthers was greatest at the stage of elevated melatonin concentrations. Because of these findings, the authors speculated that melatonin may be involved with flower development and the reproductive capacity of not only St. John's wort, but other higher plants as well [46].

Reports by Tettamanti et al. [49] and Jametti-Tettamanti and Conti [50] also examined melatonin levels in Mediterranean and alphine medicinal plants. In these studies, the applied analytical methodology was HPLC with fluorimetic detection after phase-separation and purification and both official and spontaneous alpine plants were studied. As in other investigations, melatonin was identified in all plant materials tested with values ranging from the pg to the ng/g range. Of interest is that, in general, the reported melatonin levels in wild species of plants were lower than what was observed for the selected officinal species. Iametti-Tettamanti and Conti [50] also emphasize, like other scientists working in this area, that there are inherent difficulties investigating plant material in terms of both extraction and quantification.

The tart cherry (*Prunus cerasus*), a widely used and economically important fruit grown in several countries, was specifically investigated to determine if melatonin is present [30]. Two varieties of cherries, i.e. Montmorency and Balaton, were studied and their melatonin concentrations differed significantly; thus, the Montmorency variety had measurable melatonin levels of 13.5 ng/g while Balaton cherries had an average melatonin concentration of 2.0 ng/g. Interestingly, while Balaton cherries had significantly lower melatonin values, their concentrations of other antioxidants (polyphenols) are considerably higher than in Montmorency cherries [51].

Burkhardt et al. [30] also estimated melatonin levels in tart cherries picked from different trees, e.g., sun-exposed and shaded, and found substantial differences which may be attributable to the amount of direct sunlight that strikes the fruit. Cherries from different orchards had roughly equivalent melatonin levels. This group mentions the possibility that, besides its potential synthesis in the cherry plant, melatonin could be absorbed through the roots and transported to the fruit.

Purslane (*Portulaca oleracea*) is a widely-consumed vegetable especially in the eastern Mediterranean region. The population that consumes this product historically has a reduced incidence of cardiovascular disease and cancer [52]. Purslane is uncommonly rich in highly beneficial omega-3 fatty acids [53] which makes it an important foodstuff in terms of its potential for improving human health. In addition to a high content of omega-3 fatty acids, purslane contains concentrations of melatonin that average 19 ng/g wet weight [52]. The combination of omega-3 fatty acids and melatonin along with many other antioxidants in this plant could make it a nutritionally important food product. Besides melatonin's antioxidant activity, both melatonin and omega-3 fatty acids have similar inhibitory actions on cancer cell growth [54].

Flowering in plants is often dependent upon a specific light:dark environment. Since melatonin had been previously identified in the short-day flowering plant, *Chenopodium rubrum* [25], Kolar et al. [55] used this species to test whether this indole would influence flowering. H-labeled melatonin was applied to the cotyledons and plumules of 5-day-old seedings. Application of either 100 μM or 500 μM melatonin significantly lowered the flowering rate of plants exposed to a single inductive 12-hour period of darkness. To achieve this effect, melatonin had to be applied prior to lights off or during the first half of the dark period. The implications of these findings is that melatonin influences some early steps in the transition to flowering. However, the concentrations of melatonin used to inhibit the flowering response are much higher than those measured in this plant.

In animals, melatonin influences the process of apoptosis, often a result of its free radical scavenging capabilities [56]. In a suspension of carrot cells (*Daucus carota* L.), pretreatment with 43 nM to 86 nM melatonin for 5 days significantly attenuated cold-induced apoptosis as indicated by changes in the number of TUNEL-positive cells, a reduced level of DNA fragmentation and fewer morphological changes associated with programmed cell death [57]. Mechanistically, however, melatonin's antiapoptotic actions seemed not related to its antioxidant effects but, rather, due to its upregulation of polyamine (purtrescine and spermadine) levels.

Evidence of Melatonin Synthesis in Plants

The first study of melatonin synthesis in any plant, St. John's wort, was reported by Murch et al. [26]. Tryptophan, the amino acid precursor of melatonin, has a variety of primary metabolites in plants [58] with the best characterized metabolite being indole acetic acid [59]. This plant hormone exerts strong biological activity at very low concentrations and is necessary for the maintenance of optimal physiological processes in plants. In view of their demonstration of high levels of melatonin in St. John's wort as well as the presence of another tryptophan metabolite (serotonin) in plants [56], Murch et al. [26] reasoned that plants may synthesize melatonin. They did their measurements in in vitro regenerated plantlets of St. John's wort from thidiazuron-induced stem explants. The plantlets were grown in MS basal medium for 2 months. ^{14}C-tryptophan was added to excised plantlets and, among other products, ^{14}C-melatonin was recovered. Chromatographic peak identity was confirmed using HPLC-MS and melatonin was quantified by RIA. Under low light conditions, more radiolabeled serotonin was recovered than was melatonin; as light intensity increased, this ratio was reversed suggesting to the authors that the metabolism of tryptophan to melatonin is influenced by light intensity. This is also the first evidence that the incorporation of the carbon skeleton of tryptophan into serotonin and melatonin in higher plant species.

Previously it had been speculated that melatonin may act as a chemical messenger to the circadian system in plants as it does in animals [60]. The differential synthesis of serotonin and melatonin, depending on the degree of light to which a plant is exposed, suggests that melatonin, in plants, may have functions analogous

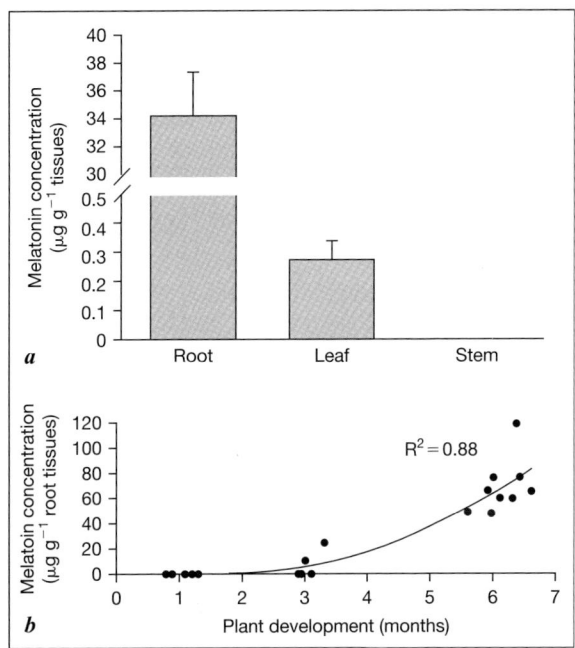

Fig. 2. a Melatonin concentrations in roots, leaves and stems of the medicinal plant *G. uralensis*. *b* Relationship (2nd order polynomial) between plant maturation and the levels of melatonin in the roots. Data from Afreen et al. [61].

to those in animals which provide information about circadian time. This is consistent with the observations of Kolar et al. [25] who reported diurnal fluctuations of melatonin in a short-day plant, *Chenopodium rubrum*, where melatonin levels were highest during the dark phase of the light:dark cycle.

Afreen et al. [61] examined melatonin levels in the seed, root, leaf and stem tissues from the medicinal plant, *Glycyrrhiza uralensis*. This plant is widely used because of its reported antiviral and antitumor effects. In the study, the authors grew the plants, from seeds, under lights of different spectral quality and melatonin levels were quantified. The authors assumed that the changing melatonin concentrations were a consequence of its synthesis by the plant.

After growing the plants for 3 months under red, blue or white fluorescent lamps, the melatonin concentrations in the plants varied according to the spectral quality of the light under which they were maintained as follows: red $\gg$ blue $\geq$ white light. Among the different plant tissues, roots had the highest melatonin levels (fig. 2a). After 6 months of growth, the melatonin levels were much higher in all plant parts compared to their values in younger plants (fig. 2b).

Other plants were exposed to either high-intensity ultraviolet-B (UV-B) radiation (integrated value: 103.20 W/h/m^2) or low-intensity UV-B radiation (integrated value: 54.24 W/h/m^2). Exposure to the former was twice as effective as low-intensity UV-B radiation in stimulating an increase in melatonin concentrations in the roots of G. uralensis. The fact that there were proportional incremental changes in root melatonin levels in plants exposed to high intensity verses low intensity UV-B radiation suggested to the authors that these wavelengths of radiation promote melatonin production as a means of protecting itself from free radicals [15, 17, 23]. This is consistent with the assumptions of Dubbels et al. [1] who also believed that melatonin may protect the tobacco plant from damaging ultraviolet radiation.

Bioavailability of Melatonin from Consumed Plant Material

Melatonin, when consumed in the drinking fluid [33] or taken as a Galenic tablet [62], is readily absorbed into the circulation. Thus, it would be expected that melatonin from foods would also likely be taken up. Only two studies have investigated this. Hattori et al. [2], in their early publication, reported that circulating daytime levels of melatonin were elevated at various times up to 4 hours in chickens that had eaten melatonin-containing foods (corn, milo, beans and rice). The chickens had been fasted for 48 h prior to being fed the melatonin-containing foods. In this study, the daytime melatonin levels were roughly doubled.

In a more recent investigation, 24-hour-fasted rats were given exclusively walnuts (which contain an average 3.5 ng/g) or regular rat chow (melatonin concentration unknown) to eat [43]. Within 4 h, circulating levels of daytime melatonin in the blood of rats that consumed walnuts had more than doubled. Whereas the increase would seem to be larger than expected, the design of the study was such that it maximized the likelihood of a measurable increase in blood melatonin concentrations. Thus, given that the rats had been fasted for 24 h before being fed the walnuts, they consumed large amounts of the food (estimated to be about 3 g) within a short interval and, at least their upper digestive tract, was essentially empty before they did so. While the elevated level of melatonin in the blood after the consumption of a melatonin-containing food is important, the study also examined, in the same blood samples, the total antioxidant capacity of the blood. This showed that the rise in peripheral blood melatonin concentrations was accompanied by increases in the ability of this fluid to resist free radical damage as indicated by the elevated trolox equivalent antioxidant capacity (TEAC) and the ferric reducing ability of plasma (FRAP) levels. It should be noted, as the authors point out, that while the rise in blood melatonin correlated with elevated TEAC/FRAP values, the incremental changes in the latter parameters may not have been exclusively a function of the antioxidant melatonin given that walnuts contain a number of other molecules that function as antioxidants, e.g. γ-tocopherol.

If dietary melatonin is to have general nutritional value, it is obviously essential that it be absorbed. The only two studies to date verify that this occurs and, certainly, pure melatonin when consumed, has beneficial effects. The question remains, however, how important is the dietary intake of melatonin? As a free radical scavenger, even small amounts of melatonin could reduce molecular damage in cells since it, and its metabolites, neutralized several free radicals [63, 64]. Furthermore, melatonin stimulates antioxidative enzymes [65, 66]. It is important to determine whether other components in the diet alter, either augment or diminish, melatonin uptake by the gastrointestinal tract or its metabolism in other organs, e.g. in the liver.

There is one other consideration when melatonin-containing foods are eaten and peripheral blood melatonin levels rise. The gastrointestinal tract itself contains rather high concentrations of melatonin [67], and it may be released in response to eating. Thus, the rise in circulating melatonin values in the walnut-fed rats may have been a consequence of the melatonin consumed and absorbed as well as a result of its release of gastrointestinal melatonin.

Unresolved Issues

There are still many unanswered questions concerning melatonin in terms of its concentrations and functions in plants. Are the reported levels of melatonin in the plants in which it has been measured uniformly accurate? Is melatonin synthesized by plants or is it taken up via the root system from the medium in which the plant is grown? If it is synthesized, in what part of the plant does this occur? If it is taken up via the roots, can the concentration of melatonin in various plant organs be changed by adding melatonin to the growth medium? Is the concentration of melatonin within plant organs influenced by the ambient temperature, the degree of direct sunlight to which they are exposed, or by contaminants in the soil, water or air? What are the most important functions of melatonin in plants? Could melatonin-enriched plants be used in phytoremediation of contaminated soils given that this indole is such a potent free radical scavenger and antioxidant capable of protecting tissues against the toxicity of many soil/water pollutants? How important is the consumption of melatonin-containing plant products for the health of animals including humans? Is the melatonin normally present in plant material conserved when the food is processed? Does the concentration of melatonin in plant organs vary with the age of the plant? Do melatonin levels in plants change on a seasonal basis when they are grown in their natural habitat? Do seasonal variations in day length influence the quantity of melatonin a plant produces/contains? Are their variations in the melatonin concentrations of plants grown at different latitudes? Does consumption of melatonin-containing plants by animals have anything to do with seasonal physiological alterations in these species?

Depending on the particular interests of the research scientist performing the study, answers to the questions posed above will be specifically investigated in the forthcoming years. A major issue for the nutritionist/dietician will be the importance of melatonin in the human diet. Melatonin, as briefly summarized herein and extensively elsewhere, has a wide variety of potential beneficial effects. From preliminary studies under conditions where the animals were fasted before they ate foodstuffs where melatonin is present, the indole is taken up by the gastrointestinal tract and altered circulating levels of the indole. Once in the circulation, melatonin would have access to all cells in the organism where it could have either/both melatonin receptor-mediated and melatonin receptor-independent actions. The diet, as a source of melatonin, will likely become a major area of investigation.

Concluding Remarks and Perspectives

Among a variety of potential functions, melatonin may act as an antioxidant in the plants in which it is found. Additionally, however, the ingestion of melatonin–containing plant tissues by animals including humans may also contribute to the ability of the animals to resist oxidative damage. In this case, the protective actions of melatonin could occur in the gastrointestinal tract before the indole is absorbed as well as in blood and tissues once it is taken up.

It is already known that oxidized lipids contained in the diet are a source of plasma hydroperoxides [68, 69] and also of oxidized lipids in chylomicrons in animal and human serum [70, 71]. Lipid peroxidation is a major mechanism of the deterioration of stored food products, particularly meat. Meat, i.e. muscle tissue, contains a number of endogenous catalysts which participate in the generation of free radicals; these include 'free' iron and methmyoglobin, both of which exaggerate the oxidation of lipids. Lipid hydroperoxides are not only formed in stored food products but also after their ingestion and during digestion. Of particular importance may be the stomach where absorbed oxygen levels are high and the pH is low. It is surmised that chemical interactions in the stomach create an environment where oxidation, especially when high-fat, cholesterol-rich foods are consumed, is enhanced due to the presence of the catalysts mentioned above, i.e. the elevated oxygen concentration and the low pH [72].

This being the case, the presence of melatonin in the diet could work in the stomach to reduce not only oxidative destruction of lipids, but other molecules as well, by the gastric fluid [72]. Additionally, given that melatonin is absorbed when eaten in the diet, it could be effective in limiting oxidative processes in the serum and in tissues. The implication is that, especially when fatty foodstuffs are eaten, including food in a meal that is rich in melatonin, may reduce the generation of toxic oxidation products and limit the total oxidative burden to the organism. In regard to this, other antioxidants contained in the diet have already been shown to be effective [72], so it is likely that melatonin would be as well.

Beyond protecting against oxidation of the consumed food in the stomach cavity, plant-derived melatonin may also assist with preserving the integrity of the gastric and intestinal mucosa. Melatonin is known to protect against ulcer formation that is a consequence of aspirin [73], indomethacin [74], ethanol [75] and stress [76]. Since free radicals are contributory to these conditions, melatonin consumed in the diet may help in preventing pathological damage to the mucosal lining of the gastrointestinal tract. It may be particularly beneficial when contained in food that possesses other antioxidants, e.g. vitamin E and/or C, because of the potential synergy of melatonin with these molecules [77, 78].

The brief investigative history of melatonin in plant tissues, including edible foods, has obviously left many questions unanswered. It seems likely that the next decade will witness a flurry of activity by dieticians and nutritionists in an attempt to identify the importance of melatonin in the food that is consumed.

References

1 Dubbels R, Reiter RJ, Klenke E, Goebgel A, Schnakenberg E, Ehlers C, Schiwara HW, Schloot W: Melatonin in edible plants identified by radioimmunoassay and by high performance liquid chromatography. J Pineal Res 1995;18:28–31.
2 Hattori A, Migitaka H, Iigo M, Itoh M, Yamamoto, Ohtani-Kaneko R, Hara M, Suzuki T, Reiter RJ: Identification of melatonin in plants and its effects on plasma melatonin levels and binding to melatonin receptors in vertebrates. Biochem Molec Biol Int 1995;35:627–634.
3 Van Tassel DL, Roberts NJ, O'Neill SD: Melatonin from higher plants: isolation and identification of N-acetyl-5-methoxytryptamine. Plant Physiol 1995;108(suppl):101.
4 Reiter RJ: Pineal melatonin: cell biology of its synthesis and of its physiological interactions. Endocrine Rev 1991;12:151–180.
5 Tosini C, Chaurasia SS, Ivone MP: Regulation of arylalkylamine N-acetyltransferase (AANAT) in the retina. Chronobiol Int 2006;23:381–391.
6 Slominski A, Fischer TW, Zmijewski MA, Wortsman J, Sernak I, Zbytek B, Slominski RM, Tobin DJ: On the role of melatonin in skin physiology and pathology. Endocrine 2005;27:137–148.
7 Bubenik GA: Gastrointestinal melatonin: localization, function, and clinical relevance. Dig Dis Sci 2002;47:2336–2348.
8 Abe M, Itoh MT, Miyata M, Schinizu K, Sumi Y: Circadian rhythm of serotonin-N-acetyltransferase activity in rats lens. Exp Eye Res 2000;70:805–808.
9 Djeridane Y, Toutiou Y: Effects of diazepam and its metabolites on nocturnal melatonin secretion in rat pineal and Harderian glands. Chronobiol Int 2003;20:285–297.

10   Hardeland R, Poeggeler B: Non-vertebrate melatonin. J Pineal Res 2003;34:233–241.
11   Poeggeler B, Balzer I, Hardeland R, Lerchl A: Pineal hormone melatonin oscillates also in a dinoflagellate *Gonyaulax polyedra*. Naturwissenschaften 1991;78:268–269.
12   Vivien-Roels B, Pevet P: Melatonin: presence and formation in invertebrates. Experientia 1993;49:642–647.
13   Hardeland R, Fuhrberg B: Ubiquitous melatonin – presence and effects in unicells, plants and animals. Trends Comp Biochem Physiol 1996;2:25–45.
14   Reiter RJ, Tan DX, Burkhardt S, Manchester LC: Melatonin in plants. Nutr Rev 2001;59:286–290.
15   Reiter RJ, Tan DX: Melatonin: an antioxidant in edible plants. Ann NY Acad Sci 2002;957:341–344.
16   Caniato R, Filippini R, Piovan A, Puricelli L, Borsarini A, Cappelletti EM: Melatonin in plants. Adv Exp Med Biol 2003;527:593–597.
17   Kolar J, Machackova I: Melatonin in higher plants: occurrence and possible functions. J Pineal Res 2005;39:333–341.
18   Peschke E, Frese T, Chankiewitz F, Peschke D, Preiss U, Schneyer U, Spessert R, Mulbauer F: Diabetic Goto Kakizaki rats as well as type 2 diabetic patients show a decreased serum melatonin level and an increased pancreatic melatonin-receptor status. J Pineal Res 2006;40:135–143.
19   Ackermann K, Bux R, Rub U, Korf HW, Kanert G, Stehle JH: Characterization of human melatonin synthesis using autoptic pineal tissue. Endocrinology 2006;in press.
20   Rowsing S, Bokman F, Bergqvist Y: Determination of melatonin in saliva using automated solid-phase extraction, high performance liquid chromatography and fluorescence detection. Scand J Clin Lab Invest 2006;66:181–190.
21   Nunez-Vergara LJ, Squella JA, Sturm JC, Baez H, Camargo C: Simultaneous determination of melatonin and pyridoxine in tablets by gas chromatography-mass spectrometry. J Pharm Biomed Anal 2001;26:929–938.
22   Poeggeler B, Hardeland R: Detection and quantification of melatonin in a dinoflagellate, *Gonyaulax polyedra*: solutions to the problem of methoxyindole destruction in non-vertebrate material. J Pineal Res 1994;17:1–10.
23   Tan DX, Chen LD, Poeggeler B, Manchester LC, Reiter RJ: Melatonin: a potent, endogenous hydroxyl radical scavenger. Endocrine J 1993;1:57–60.
24   Fuhrberg B, Balzer I, Hardeland R: The vertebrate pineal hormone melatonin is produced by the brown alga *Pterygophora californica* and mimics dark effects on growth rate in light. Planta 1996;200:125–131.
25   Kolar J, Machackova I, Eder J, Prinsen E, van Dongen W, van Onckelen H, Illnerova H: Melatonin: occurrence and daily rhythm in *Chenopodium rubrum*. Phytochemistry 1997;44:1407–1413.
26   Murch SJ, Krishna Raj S, Saxena PK: Tryptophan is a precursor for melatonin and serotonin biosynthesis in in vitro regenerated St. John's wort (*Hypericum perferoration* L. CV. Anthos) plants. Plant Cell Rep 2000;19:698–704.
27   Van Tassel DL, Roberts N, Lewy A, O'Neill SD: Melatonin in plant organs. J Pineal Res 2001;31:8–15.
28   Hernandez-Ruiz J, Cano A, Cernao MB: Melatonin: a growth-stimulating compound present in lupin tissues. Planta 2004;220:140–144.
29   Manchester LC, Tan DX, Reiter RJ, Park W, Mouis K, Qi W: High levels of melatonin in the seeds of edible plants: possible function in germ cell protection. Life Sci 2000;67:3023–3029.
30   Burkhardt S, Tan DX, Manchester LC, Hardeland R, Reiter RJ: Detection and quantification of the antioxidant melatonin in Montmorency and Balaton tart cherries (*Prunus cerasus*). J Agric Food Chem 2001;49:4898–4902.
31   Wolf K, Kolar J, Witters E, von Dongen W, van Onckelen H, Machackova I: Daily profile of melatonin levels in *Chenopodrium rubrum* L. depends on photoperiod. J Plant Physiol 2001;158:1491–1493.
32   Rolcik J, Lenobel R, Siglerova V, Strnad M: Isolation of melatonin by immunoaffinity chromatography. J Chromatogr [B] 2002;775:9–15.
33   Blask DE, Dauchy RT, Sauer LA, Krause JA: Melatonin uptake and growth prevention in rat hepatoma 7288CTC in response to dietary melatonin: melatonin receptor-mediated inhibition of tumor linoleic acid metabolism to the growth signaling molecule 13-hydroxyoctadecadienoic acid and the potential role of phytomelatonin. Carcinogenesis 2004;25:951–960.

34 Chen G, Huo Y, Tan DX, Liang Z, Zhang W, Zhang Y: Melatonin in Chinese medicinal herbs. Life Sci 2003;73:19–26.
35 Lewy AJ, Markey SP: Analysis of melatonin in human plasma by gas chromatography negative ionization mass spectrometry. Science 1978;201:741–743.
36 Matuszewski BK, Constanzer ML, Chavez-Eng CM: Matrix effect in quantitative LC/MS/MS analysis of biological fluids: a method for determination of finasteride in human plasma at picogram per milliliter concentrations. Anal Chem 1998;70:882–889.
37 Smeraglia J, Baldrey SF, Watson D: Matrix effects and selectivity issues in LC-MS-MS. Chromatographia 2002;55:595–599.
38 Pape C, Lüning K: Quantification of melatonin in phototropic organisms. J Pineal Res 2006;41: 157–165.
39 West GB: Tryptamines in edible fruits. J Pharm Pharmacol 1958;10:589–590.
40 Udenfriend S, Lovenberg W, Sjoerdsma A: Physiologically active amines in common fruits and vegetables. Arch Biochem Biophys 1959;85:487–490.
41 Dawson D, Encel N: Melatonin and sleep in humans. J Pineal Res 1993;15:1–12.
42 Haggestad HE: Origin of Bel-W3, Bel-C and Bel-B tobacco varieties and their use as indicators of ozone. Environ Pollut 1998;74:264–291.
43 Reiter RJ, Manchester LC, Tan DX: Melatonin in walnuts: influence on levels of melatonin and total antioxidant capacity of blood. Nutrition 2005;21:920–924.
44 Murch SJ, Summons CB, Saxena PK: Melatonin in feverfew and other medicinal plants. Lancet 1997;350:1598–1599.
45 Murch SJ, Ruposingbe HP, Goodenowe D, Saxena PK: A metabolomic analysis of medicinal diversity in Huang-qin (Scutellaria baicalensis Georgi) genotypes: discovery of novel compounds. Plant Cell Rep 2004;23:419–425.
46 Murch SJ, Saxena PK: Mammalian neurohormones: potential significance in reproductive physiology of St. John's wort (Hypericum perforctum L.). Naturwissenschaften 2002;89:555–560.
47 Murphy JJ, Mitchell JRA, Heptinstall S: Randomized double-blind placebo-controlled trial of feverfew in migraine prevention. Lancet 1988;ii:189–192.
48 DeWeerdt CJ, Bootsma HPK, Hendricks H: Herbal medicines in migraine prevention. Phytomedicine 1996;3:225–230.
49 Tettamanti C, Cerabolini B, Gerola P, Conti A: Melatonin identification in medicinal plants. Acta Phytotherap 2000;3:137–144.
50 Iametti-Tettamanti C, Conti A: Melatonin identification in Mediterranean and alpine medicinal and wild plants. Acta Phytotherap 2002;5:42–45.
51 Wang H, Nair MG, Iezzoni AF, Strasburg GM, Booren AM, Gray JI: Quantification and characterization of anthocyanins in Balaton tart cherries. J Agric Food Chem 1997;45:2556–2560.
52 Simopoulos A, Tan DX, Manchester LC, Reiter RJ: Purslane: a plant source of omega-3 fatty acids and melatonin. J Pineal Res 2005;39:331–332.
53 Simopoulos AP, Salem N Jr: Purslane: a terrestrial source of omega-3 fatty acids. N Engl J Med 1986;315:833.
54 Sauer LA, Dauchy RT, Blask DE: Polyunsaturated fatty acids, melatonin and cancer prevention. Biochem Pharmacol 2001;61:1455–1462.
55 Kolar J, Johnson CH, Machackova I: Exogenously applied melatonin (N-acetyl-5-methoxytryptamine) affects flowering of the short-day plant Chenopodium rubrum. Physiol Plant 2003;118:605–612.
56 Jou MJ, Pang TI, Reiter RJ, Jou SB, Wu HY, Wen ST: Visualization of the antioxidant effects of melatonin at the mitochondrial level during oxidative stress-induced apoptosis of rat brain astrocytes. J Pineal Res 2004;37:55–70.
57 Lei XY, Zhu RY, Zhang GY, Dai YR: Attenuation of cold-induced apoptosis by exogenous melatonin in carrot suspension cells: the possible involvement of polyamines. J Pineal Res 2004;36: 126–131.
58 Radwanski ER, Last RL: Tryptophan biosynthesis and metabolism: biochemical and molecular genetics. Plant Cell 1995;7:921–924.
59 Bartel B: Auxin biosynthesis. Annu Dev Plant Physiol Plant Mol Biol 1997;48:51–66.
60 Balzer I, Hardeland R: Melatonin in algae and higher plants: possible new roles as a phytohormone and antioxidant. Bot Acta 1996;109:180–183.

61 Afreen F, Zobayed SMA, Kozai T: Melatonin in *Glycyrrhiza uralensis*: response to plant roots to spectral quality of light and UV-B radiation. J Pineal Res 2006;in press.
62 Lee BA, Parrott KA, Ayres JW: Development and characterization of an oral controlled-release delivery system for melatonin. Drug Dev Ind Pharm 1996;22:269–274.
63 Allegra M, Reiter RJ, Dan DX, Gentile G, Tesoriere L, Livrea MA: The chemistry of melatonin's interaction with reactive species. J Pineal Res 2003;34:1–10.
64 Hardeland R: Antioxidative protection by melatonin. Endocrine 2005;27:119–130.
65 Rodriquez C, Mayo J, Sainz RM, Antolin I, Herrera F, Martin V, Reiter RJ: Regulation of antioxidant enzymes: a significant role of melatonin. J Pineal Res 2004;36:1–9.
66 Tomas-Zapico C, Coto-Montes A: A proposed mechanism to explain the stimulatory effect of melatonin on antioxidative enzymes. J Pineal Res 2005;39:99–104.
67 Bubenik G: Gastrointestinal melatonin: localization, function and clinical relevance. Dig Dis Sci 2002;47:2336–2348.
68 Ursini F, Zamburlini A, Cazzolato G, Maiorino M, Bon GB, Sevanion A: Postprandial plasma lipid hydroperoxides: a possible link between diet and arthrosclerosis. Free Radic Biol Med 1998;25:250–252.
69 Williams MJ, Sutherland WH, McCormick MP, de Jong SA, Walker RJ, Wilkins GT: Impaired endothelial function following a meal rich is used cooking fat. J Am Coll Cardiol 1999;33:1050–1055.
70 Staprans L, Rapp JH, Pan XM, Kim KY, Feingold KR: Oxidized lipids in the diet are a source of oxidized lipid in chylomicrons of human serum. Anterioscler Thromb 1994;14:1900–1904.
71 Strapans I, Hardman DA, Pam XM, Feingold KR: Effect of oxidized lipids in the diet on oxidized lipid levels in postprandial serum chylomicrons of diabetic patients. Diabetes Care 1999;22:300–306.
72 Kanner J, Lapilot T: The stomach as a bioreactor: dietary lipid peroxidation in the gastric fluid and the effects of plant-derived antioxidants. Free Radic Bio Med 2001;31:1388–1395.
73 Sener-Muratogul G, Porskaloglu K, Arbak S, Hurdag C, Ayanogul-Dulger G: Protective effect of farmotidine, omerprazole and melatonin against acetylsalicylic acid-induced gastric damage in rats. Dig Dis Sci 2001;46:318–310.
74 Ganguly K, Maity P, Reiter RJ, Swarnakar S: Effect of melatonin on secreted and induced matrix metalloproteinase-9 and -2 activity during prevention of indomethacin-induced gastric ulcer. J Pineal Res 2005;39:307–315.
75 Bendyopadhyay D, Chattopadhyay A: Reactive oxygen species-induced gastric ulceration: protection by melatonin. Curr Med Chem 2006;13:1187–1202.
76 Brzozowski T, Konturek PL, Zwirska-Karczala K, Konturek SJ, Brzozowski I, Drozdowicz D, Sliwowska Z, Pawlik M, Pawlik WW, Hahn EG: Importance of the pineal gland, endogenous prostaglandins and sensory nerves in the gastroprotective actions of central and peripheral melatonin against stress-induced damage. J Pineal Res 2005;39:375–385.
77 Gitto E, Tan DX, Reiter RJ, Karbownik M, Manchester LC, Cuzzocrea S, Fulia F, Barberi I: Individual and synergistic antioxidative actions of melatonin: studies with vitamin E, vitamin C, glutathione and desferrioxamine (desferoxamine) in rat liver homogenates. J Pharm Pharmacol 2001;53:1393–1401.
78 Lopez-Burrillo S, Tan DX, Mayo JC, Sainz RM, Manchester LC, Reiter RJ: Melatonin, xanthurenic acid, resveratrol, EGCG, vitamin C and alpha-lipoic acid differentially reduce oxidative DNA damage induced by Fenton reagents: a study of their individual and synergistic actions. J Pineal Res 2003;34:269–277.

Russel J. Reiter
Department of Cellular and Structural Biology
The University of Texas Health Science Center, 7703 Floyd Curl Drive
San Antonio, TX 78229–3900 (USA)
Tel. +1 210 567 3859, Fax +1 210 567 6948, E-Mail Reiter@uthscsa.edu

Author Index

Bogani, P. 162
Boskou, D. 180

Castillo-Garzón, M.J. 114

de Lorgeril, M. 1

Flores, L.J. 211
Friberg, P. 52

Galli, C. 67
Gentile, M. 85
Gutierrez-Sainz, A. 114

Johansson, M. 52

Kallithraka, S. 139

Leighton, F. 33

Maldonado, M.D. 211
Manchester, L.C. 211
Mancini, F.P. 85
Mancini, M. 85
Marangoni, F. 67
Martiello, A. 67

Ortega, F.B. 114

Reiter, R.J. 211
Rubba, P. 85
Ruiz, J.R. 114

Salen, P. 1
Simopoulos, A.P. XI, 211

Tan, D. 211
Terron, M.P. 211

Urquiaga, I. 33

Visioli, F. 162

Zeghichi-Hamri, S. 139

Subject Index

Algeria, *see* Maghreb diet
Antioxidants, *see also* specific antioxidants
  cancer studies 163, 164
  coronary heart disease prevention studies 10
  Cretan diet composition 6, 7
  endothelial function 170
  olive oil studies
    free radical scavenging 195, 196
    isoprostane formation 195
    low-density lipoprotein oxidation 193, 195
    reactive nitrogen species scavenging 196
  oxidative stress 162, 163
Apoptosis, melatonin inhibition 222
Arachidonic acid (AA), metabolism 14
Ascorbic acid
  cancer protection 100
  Cretan diet composition 6

Body composition
  Mediterranean adolescent cardiovascular risk factor studies
    fat distribution 130–133
    total body fat 129, 130
  Mediterranean diet effects 61, 62

Cancer
  Cretan diet selenium and protection 16–18
  Italian diet studies 98–104
  Maghreb diet protection studies 155–158

oxidative stress and diet protection 163, 164
Cereals, Maghreb diet 144, 158
Cholesterol, intake recommendations 5
Coronary heart disease
  epidemiology studies of Mediterranean diet
    HALE Study 54
    Italian diet macronutrient studies 90–94
    Lyon Diet Heart Study
      modified Cretan diet features 4–8
      summary of findings 3, 4
    metabolic syndrome study 40, 41
    overview 1–3
    tea protection 21, 22
  inflammation role
    markers 8, 9
    plaque rupture and progression 9, 10
  Mediterranean adolescent cardiovascular risk factor studies
    body composition
      fat distribution 130–133
      total body fat 129, 130
    cardiorespiratory fitness 120, 121, 124–127
    muscle strength 127–129
  risk factors 114

Docosahexaenoic acid (DHA)
  anti-arrhythmic activity 34
  anti-platelet activity 36
  cancer protection 103
  Cretan diet composition 53

Eicosapentaenoic acid (EPA)
  anti-arrhythmic activity 34
  anti-platelet activity 36
  cancer protection 103
  Cretan diet composition 53
  metabolism 14
Enzyme-linked immunosorbent assay
  (ELISA), melatonin 213, 214
Estrogen, cardioprotective effects 35
Exercise
  diet interaction studies
    maximum oxygen consumption 119, 120
    physical fitness 118, 119
    plasma lipids 116–118
  health benefits 115
  Mediterranean adolescent cardiovascular risk factors
    body composition
      fat distribution 130–133
      total body fat 129, 130
    cardiorespiratory fitness 120, 121, 124–127
    muscle strength 127–129
  metabolic syndrome protection 42
  Spanish-Mediterranean lifestyle 115, 116

Fat intake, Mediterranean diets
  animal fats 71–74
  comparison of diets 69, 70
  fatty acid profile and content 74, 77, 78
  Italian diet and coronary heart disease 90–92
  Maghreb diet
    consumption of animal fat and vegetable oil 151–153
    nutritional aspects 153–155
  plant foods 72
  vegetable visible fats 70, 71
Fatty acids, see also specific fatty acids
  diabetes and elevation in plasma 38
  Mediterranean diet
    composition and coronary heart disease 12–15
    Cretan diet composition 12–15, 53
    metabolism effects 13, 33–35

Fiber, Italian diet and coronary heart disease 93
Fish oil, see Docosahexaenoic acid; Eicosapentaenoic acid
Folate
  cardioprotection mechanisms 15, 16
  Cretan diet composition 15
  Italian diet 96
Fruits and vegetables
  cancer protection 99–102
  Maghreb diet
    consumption patterns 146, 147
    nutritional aspects 147–149

Healthy Diet Indicator (HDI), diet scoring 89
Heart rate, Mediterranean diet effects 62
High-density lipoprotein (HDL)
  transport 35
  wine response 34, 35
High-performance liquid chromatography (HPLC), melatonin assay 212–214
Hydroxytyrosol, neuroprotection 168
Hypertension
  Italian diet studies 94
  Mediterranean diet effects 60, 61

Inflammation
  markers 8, 9
  plaque rupture and progression role 9, 10
  wine anti-inflammatory effects 43, 44
Insulin, alcohol and sensitivity 39, 40
Isoprostanes, olive oil inhibition of formation 195
Italian diet
  cancer studies 98–104
  changes over time 86, 87
  elderly studies 104–106
  hypertension and stroke studies 94
  macronutrients and coronary artery disease 90–94
  obesity studies 97, 98
  scores 88–90
  vitamin intake 95, 96

Leukocyte count, Mediterranean diet effects 58

Libya, *see* Maghreb diet
Lignans, dietary sources 22, 23
Linoleic acid (LA), Cretan diet composition 5
α-Linolenic acid (ALA)
  Cretan diet composition 5, 12, 53
  desaturase competition 13
  health benefits 80
  Mediterranean food content and intake optimization 81, 82
Low-density lipoprotein (LDL) oxidation
  coronary heart disease 9–11
  diet effects 10, 11
  olive oil studies 193, 195
Lycopene
  biological activity 165
  health benefits 166
  tissue distribution 165
Lyon Diet Heart Study
  modified Cretan diet features 4–8
  summary of findings 3, 4

Maghreb diet
  animal products 144, 149–151
  cancer protection studies 155–158
  cereals 144, 158
  changes over time
    1968–1970 144, 145
    1990–1992 144, 145
    recent trends 140–144
  countries 140
  fats
    consumption of animal fat and vegetable oil 151–153
    nutritional aspects 153–155
  fruits and vegetables
    consumption patterns 146, 147
    nutritional aspects 147–149
Mass spectrometry (MS), melatonin assays 213
Maximum oxygen consumption, physical fitness 119, 120
Mediterranean Adequacy Index (MAI), diet scoring 88, 89
Mediterranean diet
  changes over time 69, 85, 86
  common features 67, 68
  definition 52, 67, 139, 140
  historical perspective 85
Mediterranean Diet Score (MDS), diet scoring 89
Melatonin
  antioxidant activity 218, 227
  apoptosis inhibition 222
  plants
    bioavailability 224, 225
    edible plant levels 215–222
    functions 218, 220
    prospects for study 225–227
    synthesis 211, 222–224
    tissue preparation and assay 212–216
  species distribution 211
  synthesis in vertebrate 211
Metabolic syndrome
  alcohol and insulin sensitivity 39, 40
  Cretan diet effects 18, 19
  definition 39
  exercise protection 42
  Mediterranean diet
    nitric oxide synthase induction and metabolic syndrome protection 42–44
    studies of coronary risk 40, 41
  nitric oxide synthase in pathogenesis 41, 42
  risk factors 39
Morocco, *see* Maghreb diet
Muscle strength, Mediterranean adolescent cardiovascular risk factor studies 127–129

Nitric oxide (NO)
  Cretan diet effects 15, 16
  endothelial function 37, 38, 170
Nitric oxide synthase (NOS), endothelial
  antioxidant interactions 38, 39
  fish oil induction 36, 38
  insulin activation 36
  Mediterranean diet induction and metabolic syndrome protection 42–44
  metabolic syndrome pathogenesis role 41, 42
  phenolic antioxidant effects 170
  thrombosis role 36

Obesity
    Italian diet studies 97, 98
    Mediterranean diet effects 61, 62
Oleic acid
    health benefits 78, 79
    omega-6 fatty acid inverse relationship 79, 80
Olive oil
    antioxidant studies
        free radical scavenging 195, 196
        isoprostane formation 195
        low-density lipoprotein oxidation 193, 195
        reactive nitrogen species scavenging 196
    biological activity 167, 168
    cognitive benefits 168
    composition
        diterpene alcohols 186
        fatty acid profile and content 78, 79, 181, 182
        fatty alcohols 185, 186
        phenols
            heating effects 203, 204
            polar phenols 189, 190
            polyphenols 79, 166, 190–192
        phospholipids 187–189
        squalene 182, 183
        sterols 183–185
        tocopherols 186, 187
        triacylglycerols 181, 182
        triterpene acids 187
        triterpene alcohols 185
        volatile compounds 187
    consumption trends 201
    extraction processes 199, 200
    market 20, 201
    prospects for study 205
    quality assessment 197–199
    shelf life 190, 191
    types 196, 197
    unfiltered oil 204
    uses 201–203

Peroxisome-proliferator-activated receptor (PPAR), metabolic syndrome pathogenesis 42

Phytomelatonin, see Melatonin
Polyphenols
    antioxidant activity 38, 39
    cancer protection 101
    classification 19, 20
    flavonoids 20, 21
    metabolic syndrome protection 44
    olive oil 79, 166, 190–192
    phenolic acids 20
    stilbenes 21
    tea 21, 22
    wine 22, 44

Radioimmunoassay, melatonin 213, 216
Reference Mediterranean Diet (RMD), diet scoring 88, 89
Resveratrol, biological activity 169

Selenium
    cancer protection 18
    Cretan diet composition 16
Stroke, Italian diet studies 94
Swedish diet
    composition 55
    Mediterranean diet switching effects
        body composition 61, 62
        endothelial function 58, 59
        heart rate 62
        hypertension 60, 61
        leukocyte count 58
        plasma lipids 55–57
        vascular endothelial growth factor 56

Tea, polyphenols 21, 22
    Tissue plasminogen activator (t-PA), alcohol induction of expression 35
Total antioxidant capacity (TAC), Mediterranean diet effects 15
Tunisia, see Maghreb diet

Urokinase plasminogen activator (u-PA), alcohol induction of expression 35

Vascular endothelial growth factor (VEGF), Mediterranean diet effects 56
Vitamin B6, Italian diet 96
Vitamin C, see Ascorbic acid

Vitamin E
    cancer protection 100
    Cretan diet composition 6
    olive oil 186, 187

Wine
    anti-inflammatory effects 43, 44
    French paradox 169
    hemostasis effects 35
    high-density lipoprotein response 34, 35
    metabolic syndrome protection 44
    polyphenols 22
    resveratrol actions 169